Prozac on the Couch

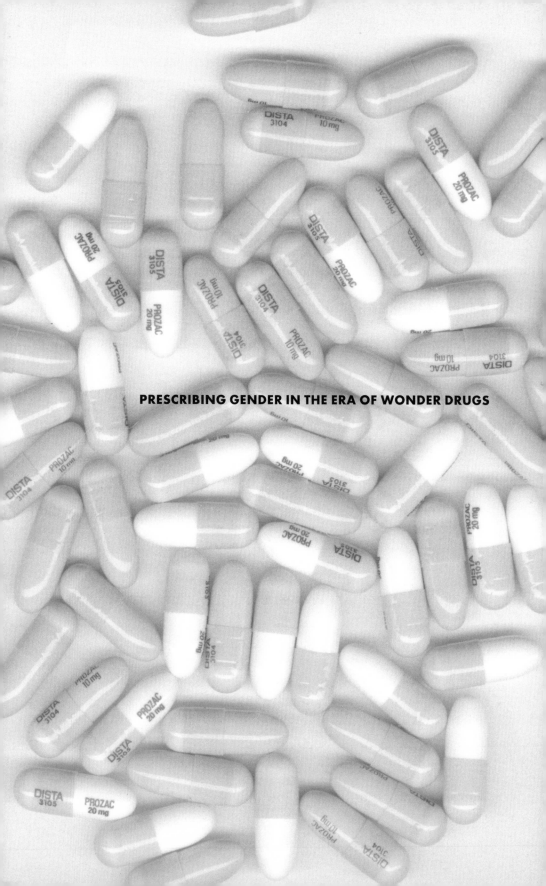

PRESCRIBING GENDER IN THE ERA OF WONDER DRUGS

JONATHAN MICHEL METZL

Prozac on the Couch

DUKE UNIVERSITY PRESS *Durham and London* 2003

© 2003 Duke University Press

All rights reserved. Printed in the United States of America
on acid-free paper ⊗ Designed by Amy Ruth Buchanan. Typeset
in Carter & Cone Galliard by Tseng Information Systems, Inc.
Library of Congress Cataloging-in-Publication Data appear
on the last printed page of this book.

This publication is made possible in part by awards from the
Office of the Vice President for Research, the Department of
Psychiatry and Rachel Upjohn Scholars Program, the Robert
Wood Johnson Clinical Scholars Program, and the Women's
Studies Program, all at the University of Michigan.

Contents

List of Figures

Acknowledgments

Individual authorship is a false front, inasmuch as this project represents my place in a network of relationships. Simply, this book would not have been possible without the unqualified love of my family, the support of my friends, and the guidance of my teachers. Kurt, Marilyn, Jordan, Jamie, and Joshua Metzl have been unwavering in their enthusiasm from the instant I decided to pass on my former life and came to Michigan to pursue a Ph.D. My father sent me a stupid joke a day, my mother learned to email, my brothers delivered flowers to celebrate when I succeeded and encouragement when I was unsure. In the process of a potentially isolating undertaking, they taught me, yet again, about the importance of belonging. My great friends Elise Frasier, John Carson, Elizabeth Wingrove, and Gina Bloom were always *there,* never tired of hearing me, and helped me find my voice. Amanda Lewis and Tom G. Gugleilmo have been thoughtful readers and excellent critics. I also wish to thank John Greden, Pamela Trotman Reid, Earl Lewis, and Tim Johnson for their support of my career and for their unique abilities to think outside the box. On an institutional level, support from the Robert Wood Johnson Clinical Scholars Program, the Rachel Upjohn Clinical Scholars Program, the University of Michigan's Institute for the Humanities and Institute for Research on Women and Gender, and the Stanford University Master's of Liberal Arts Program have enabled my research.

Sidonie Smith, Abigail Stewart, Tobin Seibers, and Walter Ricci have been giving with their time and insightful with their comments and have provided an important sense of overview. Tricia Mcelroy, Meredith Martin, Bill Hirsch, and Clair James generously lent me their left brains. I would also like to thank my editors at Duke University Press, Ken Wissoker, Christine Dahlin, and Pam Morrison, for piloting this project as well as Joseph Brown for his meticulous copyediting. I cannot begin to express my gratitude to Domna Stanton and Joel Howell, under whose tireless advocacy, careful mentorship, and acute vision I have learned to become a scholar. Finally, Parna Sengupta, my companion and closest confidant, surely knows the text that follows by heart, a text that bears her love and friendship on every page. Thank you, all.

*   *   *

Some of the material presented in this book has previously appeared elsewhere: an early version of chapter 3 in *Gender and History* (vol. 15, no. 3 [2003]); excerpts from chapter 4 in the *Journal of Medical Humanities* (vol. 24, no. 1 [2003]); and an early version of chapter 5 in *Signs: Journal of Women in Culture and Society* (vol. 27, no. 2 [2001]).

List of Abbreviations

DSM-I	*Diagnostic and Statistical Manual of Mental Disorders.* 1st ed. Washington, D.C.: APA Press, 1952.
DSM-II	*Diagnostic and Statistical Manual of Mental Disorders.* 2d ed. Washington, D.C.: APA Press, 1967.
DSM-III	*Diagnostic and Statistical Manual of Mental Disorders.* 3d ed. Washington, D.C.: APA Press, 1980.
DSM-III-R	*Diagnostic and Statistical Manual of Mental Disorders.* 3d ed., rev. Washington, D.C.: APA Press, 1987.
DSM-IV	*Diagnostic and Statistical Manual of Mental Disorders.* 4th ed. Washington, D.C.: APA Press, 1995.

The factor of the repetition of the same thing will perhaps not appeal to everyone as a source of uncanny feeling. From what I have observed, the phenomenon does undoubtedly, subject to certain conditions and combined with certain circumstances, arouse an uncanny feeling, which, furthermore, recalls the sense of helplessness experienced in some dream states.

SIGMUND FREUD, "The Uncanny"

About "and/or of psychoanalysis" . . . it seems to me that this elaboration is surely not possible so long as psychoanalysis remains within its own field.

LUCE IRIGARAY, *The Sex Which Is Not One*

We conducted an open pilot study of repetitive transcranial magnetic stimulation in a group of seven outpatients who had been free of antidepressant medication for at least 2 weeks. All patients were female and ranged in age from 41 to 66 years. Their initial scores on the 17-item Hamilton rating scale ranged from 20 to 29 points. We used a Cadwell rapid-rate stimulator and a Cadwell water-cooled figure-8 coil. Motor threshold was determined, as usual, by use of an electromyogram. We stimulated patients 10 times within a 2-week period, over the left prefrontal cortex. If after four treatments there was no effect, intensity was raised to 100% of motor threshold. Results were assessed on the Hamilton rating scale on Mondays after the first and second weeks. After 2 weeks, we conclude that repetitive transcranial magnetic stimulation was unsuccessful in these patients. Only one patient (F) improved more than 50% on the Hamilton rating scale, with a reduction from 22 to 10 points. Of the seven patients, one restarted antidepressants after 1 week, and two started antidepressants the day after the last treatment. Our preliminary conclusion is that a clinically relevant effect of repetitive transcranial magnetic stimulation over the left prefrontal area on depression remains questionable.

A. M. EUGENE, A. ALFREDO, W. NOLEN, et al., "Mood Improvement from Transcranial Magnetic Stimulation"

Chapter One

INTRODUCTION: THE FREUD OF PROZAC

he history of contemporary American psychiatry is often written with the presupposition of a paradigm shift. Psychoanalysis was the power structure of the profession through the 1950s and into the 1960s. Analysts chaired the country's leading academic psychiatry departments and headed important grant-making institutions.[1] A psychoanalyst served as a brigadier general in the army.[2] And psychoanalysts dominated the American Psychiatric Association's 1951 Committee on Nomenclature and Statistics. Their presence helped shape the first postwar national classification of psychopathology, the *DSM-I*, published in 1952. The manual was filled with psychoanalytically inflected disorders such as *psychoneurosis, conversion, displacement,* and other terms that assumed presenting symptoms, and, indeed, personality itself, to be the result of early-life conflicts that were mapped onto the unconscious psychical apparatus for the remainder of life. As a result, analytic concepts affected the ways in which all psychiatrists, analysts and nonanalysts alike, conceptualized mental disease.[3]

Somewhere in the 1970s, according to this narrative, American psychiatry began to change when a series of randomized, often placebo-controlled clinical research studies reported the success of biological psychiatry and psychopharmacology. Scientific findings laid bare neural pathways that exposed the inner workings of the mind. Psychogenetics, evoked potentials, and the discovery of key neurotransmitters ushered in the creation of an "objectifiable, biological" psychiatry that eschewed the role of early-life experience to identity formation and instead looked beneath these constructs to the level of the anatomic substrate.[4] Split-brain research found that each hemisphere of the brain specialized in mediating certain functions, thereby demonstrating that what Freud (himself a neurologist) had mistaken as the "unconscious" was in fact the domain of a new neuroscience. "Music appreciation and the comprehension of puns and jokes" were, thereby, discovered to come, not from a repressed unconscious, but rather from the governance of a nondominant, wholly observable cerebral hemisphere.[5] And, most important, biological mental illnesses were treated, not only with psychotherapy or psychoanalysis, but primarily with tranquilizers, benzodiazepines, antidepressants, and other forms of psychotropic medication.[6]

It then follows that, as a direct result of these events, present-day academic psychiatry often rejects its psychoanalytic origins.[7] To be sure, psychoanalysis and psychotherapy are still widely practiced by clinicians who also prescribe medications, and many voices within psychiatry now tout the importance of "combination" therapy—an arrangement in which psychiatrists prescribe medications while non-M.D. therapists provide therapy.[8] Yet evidence points to the fact that biological psychiatry has replaced psychoanalysis as the dominant paradigm in the field. Psychoanalysts rarely hold leadership positions in academic psychiatry departments or major funding organizations.[9] The *DSM-IV* emphasizes immediately observable criteria of illness.[10] Leading journals such as the *American Journal of Psychiatry* (*AJP*), *Archives of General Psychiatry,* and *Biological Psychiatry* employ genetics, structural and functional neuroimaging, neurochemistry, and other methods in order to demonstrate the commonly held belief that mental illness has a constitutional, "biological substrate."[11] These conditions are then treated with psychotropic medications—antidepressants, anxiolytics, antipsychotics, and mood stabilizers—that correct imbalanced levels of neurotransmitters within the central nervous system and inhibit or stimulate mood, affect, or behavior accordingly. Finally, the notion that personality and identity result primarily from early-life experiences is often called into question by contemporary psychiatric researchers. Gender identity, for example, is frequently defined in structural rather than developmental terms. As the academic psychiatrists Peg Nopoulos and Nancy Andreasen write, "Modern day advances in brain imaging technology minimize if not eliminate social and environmental con-

founders [of sex difference] and suggest the existence of a substrate of biological sex differences in brain-behavior relationships."[12] In other words, the
social environment is no longer considered a primary source of information
when brain-imaging technology can determine sex differences.

The notion that these events represent a paradigm shift from psychoanalytic to biological sensibilities suffuses the ways in which the recent history
of psychiatry is understood in contemporary academic writing and in many
histories of psychopharmacology. True to Thomas Kuhn's analysis in *The
Structure of Scientific Revolutions,* the success of pharmacological treatments
for mental illness, modern-day advances in brain-imaging technology, and
discoveries in psychogenetics are widely assumed to have catalyzed "a community's rejection of one time-honored scientific theory in favor of another
incompatible with it," causing "a subsequent shift in the problems available
for scientific scrutiny."[13] For example, Loyd Rogler describes the events of
the 1970s as causing a "paradigm shift in psychiatry," in which new diagnostic
presuppositions and treatment options "became largely discontinuous with
previous formulations."[14] Similarly, the psychiatrist Michael Stone describes
a "biological revolution in psychiatry" between 1970 and 1997, leading to
an environment in which mental illness, personality, and even object choice
are "now realized to be primarily constitutional rather than psychodynamic
in nature."[15] The former Johns Hopkins psychiatry chair Paul R. McHugh
writes in "The Death of Freud and the Rebirth of Psychiatry" that "as psychiatry becomes more coherent . . . psychiatrists can present themselves to
the public just as physicians and surgeons do, and no longer as practitioners
of a mystery cult, condescendingly proposing crude, sexualized ideas about
human nature."[16] Likewise, the neuropsychologist Eliot Valenstein's critique
of contemporary psychiatry is constructed on the assumption that psychiatry has undergone a "shift from blaming the mother to blaming the brain":
"The value of this [psychoanalytic] approach and the theory underlying it is
now widely questioned, if not totally rejected, by most mental health professionals. Today, the disturbed thoughts and behavior of mental patients
are believed to be caused by a biochemically defective brain, and symptoms
are not 'analyzed' but used mainly as the means of arriving at the diagnosis
that will determine the appropriate medication to prescribe."[17] Finally, the
historian Edward Shorter prefaces his argument that psychiatry has moved
"from Freud to Prozac" in the latter half of the twentieth century with the
contention that "a revolution took place in psychiatry," in which,

old verities about unconscious conflicts as the cause of mental illness were pitched out and the spotlight of research turned on the brain itself. Psychoanalysis became, like Marxism, one of the dinosaur ideologies of the nineteenth century. Today it is clear that when people experience a major mental illness, genetics and brain biology have as much to do with their problems as do stress and their early childhood experiences. And even in the quotidian anxieties and mild depressions that are the lot of humankind, medications can now lift the symptoms, replacing hours of aimless chat. If there is one central, intellectual reality at the end of the twentieth century, it is that the biological approach to psychiatry—treating mental illness as a genetically influenced disorder of brain chemistry—has been a smashing success. Freud's ideas, which have dominated the history of psychiatry for the past half century, are now vanishing like the last snows of winter.[18]

In this book, however, I challenge the notion that biological psychiatry replaced psychoanalysis. I question the binary that Shorter, Valenstein, Nopoulos and Andreasen, McHugh, and other academic psychiatrists, anthropologists, and historians of psychopharmacology assume exists between these two modes of treatment and explore the stakes in their rejection of Freud. No doubt, many important and beneficial changes have taken place in the profession of psychiatry over the past half century, leading to very real changes in the diagnosis and treatment of mental illness. Moreover, even the American Psychiatric Association has come to realize clinical interactions to be more complicated than an often-artificial division between biological substrates and environmental confounders.[19] Yet arguments such as Shorter's serve a purpose: asserting that a biological approach to a person's problems has replaced "aimless chat" about early-life experiences, or dismissing social and environmental factors as "confounders," effaces the ways in which socially, environmentally, and culturally produced tensions and anxieties play a part in even the briefest or most prescriptive clinical encounters. Psychoanalysis knew this very well. Concepts such as *transference* and *countertransference,* for example, are contingent on the notion that the expectations that doctors and patients bring into an examination room shape the content of their interaction. To claim that such considerations have vanished, or are replaced by pharmaceuticals, often works to the contrary, reinforcing preexisting hierarchies surrounding the positions *doctor* and *patient* while making it more difficult for psychiatrists and other health-care workers to think critically about the implications of the treatments they prescribe.

I should state at the outset that I am not a structuralist, an essentialist, or even a psychoanalyst. Rather, I am a psychiatrist who trained in a residency program that put a great deal of emphasis on chemical and neurophysiological definitions of mental illness. I now work in a university-run outpatient psychiatry clinic and, thus, spend much of my life writing prescriptions for medications similar to those described above. I believe in, and have seen firsthand, the many ways in which psychotropic medications ease pain and suffering and often help people lead happier, more productive lives. I also believe that the success of these medications has vastly improved the reliability, efficiency, and even the quality of the treatments that psychiatrists can offer their patients.

Yet I am made constantly aware of the inaccuracy of the belief that biology has replaced psychoanalysis, or that medications and talking cures work on entirely different axes, whenever a woman comes to my office requesting a prescription for Zoloft after seeing an advertisement in *Marie Claire* magazine; or whenever a male patient tells me that he believes that, owing to her strange behavior, which has ruined their intimate relations, his wife requires Valium, lithium, or Haldol; or whenever I find myself thinking that Effexor might help a woman patient cope with the depression that she experiences as a result of marital stress even though I know that her husband's attitude is largely to blame for her emotional state; or even at times when a woman requests medication to help her cope with intense feelings of sadness during her menstrual periods, a condition defined in the *DSM-IV* as *premenstrual dysphoric disorder,* for which fluoxitine is now a known indication. At issue in these moments is not the question whether medications may or may not be helpful in this particular case—they may be, or they may not be. Rather, there is the clear possibility that the patient and I may not be talking about medications at all, at least not about those medications prescribed, bought, sold, or ingested. These interactions suggest that psychotropic medications are imbued with expectation, desire, gender, race, sexuality, power, time, reputation, countertransference, metaphor, and a host of important factors that a putative paradigm shift from interaction to prescription tacitly eliminates from psychiatry's purview. At these moments, I and other practitioners of psychiatry have much to learn from the "social environment" because social and environmental "confounders" accompany patients into the examination room. More important, these confounders also help shape psychiatry itself, and psychiatry is revealed to be a part of the same social environment when it looks back at patients or thinks about itself and its place in the world. In these instances, medications convey a host of multiple meanings often occluded by an emphasis on the replacement of talking cures with prescribing cures. And the notion of a paradigm shift works to efface the ways in which biological psychiatry generally, and psychopharmacology specifically, often functions in many of the same ways as psychoanalysis. Assuming a move from Freud to Prozac, in other words, precludes the awareness of Freud as Prozac.

I argue that the biological revolution in psychiatry needs to be read socially, environmentally, historically, and, indeed, psychoanalytically if we are to understand how a narrative claiming change—and specifically a changed notion of the relevance of gender—also risks reinventing and rearticulating the same gender hierarchies for which psychoanalysis was widely critiqued. To understand how this process has taken place, however, is to consider the possibility that psychotropic medications accrue meanings in both medical and popular cultures, meanings that then come back to inform clinical practice. My project shifts the origins of the "biological revolution" to American popular culture in the 1950s and then explores the interrelation between popular and medical, or psychoanalytic and biological, sensibilities as they appear in representations of psychotropic medications in American print culture between 1955 and 2002. My specific focus is, in fact, the castrating mothers, shrunken fathers, and other psychoanalytically inflected representations that appear and reappear in pharmaceutical discourse, contrary to all explicit claims.

Over the course of this fifty-two-year period, as electrophysiology gave way to lactate infusion and neuroreceptor binding (which were in turn replaced by positron-enhanced neuroimaging), the terminology of psychiatry claimed to minimize, if not eliminate, social and environmental confounders while suggesting the existence of biological substrates in brain-behavior relations. Yet the sharp divide between the biological and the social/environmental explanations seems an inadequate means of understanding, for example, how in 1956 a *Cosmopolitan* article reported the research of Dr. Frank Ayd in "curing" frigid women with tranquilizers ("after treatment, frigid women who abhorred marital relations responded more readily to their husbands' advances"), or how a 1970 advertisement in the *Archives*

of General Psychiatry introduced Jan, the unmarried "psychoneurotic" lesbian who "needs" Valium in order to find a man, or how Peter Kramer describes the process whereby his patient "Mrs. Prozac" meets her husband
after beginning treatment.[20] These and other sources bring to the fore how
psychoanalytic assumptions helped shape the construction of biology and
how, as a result, psychoanalytic and biological models were often similarly
employed in maintaining traditional gender roles, even as the language for
defining symptoms underwent drastic revision. I ultimately argue that these
sources reveal the ways in which psychotropic medications often redeploy all
the cultural and social baggage of the psychoanalytic paradigms, but without the awareness of gender, and its socially constructed dimensions, that
those Freudian paradigms reveal and, in my view, render problematic.

My use of the term *psychoanalysis*—as in the psychoanalytic function
of psychopharmaceuticals—implies a specific definition: psychoanalysis is
Freudian psychoanalysis, a historical object of study, a heuristic tool, and a
set of concepts that ironically reappear in and help explain the gender implications of psychotropic medications. Like psychoanalysis, this "Freudian"
function of psychopharmaceuticals is both connotative and discursive. I return to this point more fully below, but for now it will suffice to examine the psychoanalytically inflected condition of Prozac through a reading
of Carolyn Stack's "Psychoanalysis Meets Queer Theory." A psychoanalyst
who, like Shorter, argues for a rejection of Freud, Stack critiques "traditional
(Freudian) psychoanalytic categories" of gender, sexuality, and desire for the
same reason that appears in the work of Peg Nopoulos, Nancy Andreasen,
and Eliot Valenstein: for turning sample bias and observer bias into a master
narrative. Stack contends that Freudian psychoanalysis assumed normalizing, universalizing, heterosexist notions of gender identity and gender development that still influence contemporary thought. For example, "As long
as psychoanalysis promulgates the concept of 'penis envy,' and as long as we
use this image no matter how we understand its symbolic meaning, we reify
the phallocentric narrative that men have/are the desired object that women
lack. This heterosexist trope of desire rambles through our personal lives,
our work with patients, and our professional relations, reinforcing and reenacting its belief in itself every time it shows up."

Stack attempts to retheorize psychoanalytic models in response to what
she describes as "heterosexist tropes of desire." While many Freudian theorists assume "an underlying commitment to heterosexist norms," Stack

and other "nontraditional" thinkers express a primary commitment to "an emerging postmodern queer sensibility" in which a consideration of "fluid categories" allows for "new narrative strategies," new considerations of "gender," and new notions of "what constitutes a family." Stack explains that many contemporary psychoanalytic thinkers reject traditional, modern, master-narrative definitions of the Oedipus complex, castration anxiety, the superego, civilization, and other concepts that presuppose requisite, developmental binaries of culture versus nature, conscious versus unconscious, and even man versus woman. These theorists instead suggest that an "understanding of sexed bodies and of gender is always a complexly determined, contextually driven, individual process."[21]

Stack's analysis complicates the notion that biological models replaced psychoanalytic models at the end of the twentieth century. For example, she suggests that psychoanalytic ideas have not vanished but are, rather, involved in a continued process of adaptation and negotiation—even if this process takes place in a small journal (*Gender and Psychoanalysis*) that is not funded by pharmaceutical companies and in an essay written by a psychoanalyst without *M.D.* at the end of her name. Further, Stack's analysis implies the existence of subtle similarities between contemporary psychoanalytic and biological projects, each of which works to rethink long-held assumptions concerning developmental differences between "women" and "men." Both Stack's notion of psychoanalysis and Nopoulos and Andreasen's functional magnetic resonance imaging (fMRI) reject "traditional stereotypes" while attempting to define individualized notions of identity and pathology on the basis of the evidence at hand.[22]

Most important, however, the notion that biological psychiatry depends on the rejection of psychoanalysis breaks down in a small, first-person vignette at the beginning of "Psychoanalysis Meets Queer Theory," which Stack presents and then almost entirely ignores in the remainder of the text. The vignette describes the author's conversation with "John," her "gay male friend." Stack presents John as an embodied example of someone attempting to negotiate the performativities of desire in an era when Freud's outdated notions of gender are no longer relevant: "We were discussing the assumed identification in sadomasochistic sex—how it gets decided who's bottom, who's top, and what each of those designations means at any specific time to each partner." Instead of functioning within fixed, Freudian, and often self-evident categories of mothers and fathers or the expectations of husbands and wives, John and his male lovers are involved in a constant negotiation of roles and role-playing in which the designation of "gender" depends almost entirely on the context of their interaction. Maybe John meets a sadist, thereby requiring him to play the passive role; or perhaps John feels the dominatrix on a particular day. All is negotiable in this postmodern canvas. Yet, "In the same spirit of discussing getting to know a new sexual partner, John said that his new boyfriend was on Prozac, which made it difficult for him to sustain erection. 'Anyway,' he said, 'that whole business about hardness is so overrated. There's so much one can do sexually, and besides, there are far worse sexual dysfunctions than impotence.'"[23]

Impotence is a major clinical side effect of Prozac, suffered by up to 40 percent of patients. In the case of John and his new boyfriend, however, the impotence caused by Prozac leads to another untoward effect: it creates a "traditional" binary between the two men and determines identification in sadomasochistic sex—how it gets decided who's bottom, who's top, who's hard, and who's not. In John's case, the division of roles—masculine and feminine—is not contingent on negotiation. Rather, these categories are predetermined, metabolized, and protein bound and appear on the suddenly corporeal body of John's lover: biologically, John's lover cannot become erect and is, thereby, relegated to the role of submissive; John, always already the man, is, therefore, hard by comparison.

Prozac's brief cameo appearance at the beginning of Stack's article thereby works to enact the very binary against which Stack protests. The possibility of reworking traditional terminology, or reinscribing traditional categories, is undermined by Prozac. And the notion that biology might bring liberation from these outdated norms, or freedom from the biases of social and environmental confounders, is called into question by Prozac as well. Instead, in Stack's analysis at least, Prozac ascribes gender in a traditionally Freudian sense, forging a division between having and wanting as an established fact: Prozac both castrates the man and maintains the structure whereby *masculine* is defined as the opposite of *feminine*.[24] In the process, the threat of undermining a notion of gender contingent on the division of passive and active, top and bottom, father and mother, is effectively contained.

In the pages that follow, I present case studies that illustrate how the medications assumed to replace hours of chat can at the same time work to restore those gender roles defined and popularized by Freudian psychoanalysis. My deployment of Freud is not meant to revive his theories or to prove them universally correct. At best, Freudian psychoanalysis proved during its heyday in the 1940s and 1950s to be an inegalitarian mode of treatment; at worst, it was often guilty of institutionalizing cultural biases as pathologies. Yet Freud's theories provide insight into the role and function of psychopharmaceuticals in contemporary American academic psychiatry and, thus, illuminate those aspects of academic psychiatry that reflect specific gender biases. Examining the Freud of Prozac allows me to consider those historical aspects of Freudian psychoanalysis still imbricated in biological discourse, as if they were repetitively expressed components of its pharmaceutical DNA. Moreover, a consideration of how such late-Freudian concepts as *the Oedipus complex, the superego, anxiety,* and *neurosis* inherently assumed a developmental binary of conscious/paternal placed above unconscious/maternal realms lets me think about the ways in which biological concepts often function in a similar manner, restoring traditional notions of civilization while oppressing (in the name of repressing) homosexuality, feminism, and other "symptoms." Ultimately, I employ Freud as an object of study and as an analytic tool in the process of thinking about how tensions disavowed by contemporary psychiatry, and rejected through the rhetoric of a paradigm shift, are still very much a part of its conversation. Again, I do not argue for an overthrow of a guild of which I am a practitioner. I believe that a great majority of clinical interventions, research trials, and pharmaceutical innovations are well intentioned. Yet biological psychiatry needs to become more self-aware of the form of its content, the assumptions and acts of disavowal contained within its diagnoses, treatments, and core beliefs, lest it manifest its own compulsive acts of repetition.

Pharmaceutical Mothers and Pills for the Mind

The psychiatrist Joseph Glenmullen's *Prozac Backlash* is an often-poignant critique of psychopharmacology. Glenmullen analyzes an overwhelming range of data—including laboratory notes, articles from the *AJP* and other leading medical and psychiatric journals, published research reports from scientific laboratories, published interviews with scientists, outcome studies of drug effectiveness, and other sources—in the project of rethinking the effective implications of selective serotonin reuptake inhibitor (SSRI) antidepressants. "The highly touted 'selectivity' of the Prozac group is an illusion," Glenmullen explains. "In fact the extreme emphasis these drugs place on serotonin may be a liability, because changes in serotonin levels can trigger secondary, or indirect changes in dopamine." Yet the precision of these criticisms is undermined by Glenmullen's descriptions of clinical interactions with his patients. Anne began an SSRI—Zoloft—in her first month at the Harvard Graduate School of Design after becoming "upset" over her boyfriend breaking up with her. The result: "We got back together a few months later. We've been married for two years now, quite happily." Similarly, Maura, "lying back in a chair in my office, . . . leaning her head back into the soft headrest, closing her eyes and relaxing her body," is a "thirty-nine-year-old native of Ireland" with "milk-white skin and soft, delicate features, framed by ringlets of auburn hair."[25]

The psychologist Lauren Slater often writes against the notion, so painfully apparent in Glenmullen's narrative, that white, middle-class, middle-aged women are the texts on which psychopharmacology is enacted. In her first published essay about Prozac, "Black Swans," Slater describes herself as a young, single, graduate student whose main focus is her academic career. Prozac helps her win a research grant and leave her male roommate. She then leaves Prozac, through the discovery of her true self. Yet, through the corpus of her work, Slater ultimately finds maternity through chemistry in much the same way as does Stack's friend John and Glenmullen's patient Anne. By the end of "Black Swans," Slater admits that she longs for "a superego . . . the angel in the self who rises above an ego under siege."[26] Her subsequent book, *Prozac Diary,* is dedicated to Ben, the man whom she met and married after taking Prozac. Finally, in December 1999, Slater completes the trilogy when she holds her newborn son in a picture on the cover of the issue of the *New York Times Magazine* containing her essay "Prozac Mother and Child."

Like Stack, Glenmullen and Slater are clinicians whose keen sensibilities provide insight into the theory and practice of clinical interactions. Yet, in all three cases, the authors' critiques also serve to reproduce preconceived categories of having and wanting. Glenmullen's blind spot, the unanalyzed "fact" that Zoloft leads to a happy marriage, is the same point reenacted by Slater over time. Prozac is exposed in all three works as the product of questionable science or of an often-impersonal system of care. But Prozac also works to restore traditional pairings between *women* and *men,* defined differently in three different texts.

The connection between Prozac and ringlets of auburn hair, mothers and sons, or tops and bottoms is a historical, developmental connection that can be traced through time. The process whereby—unlike most other types of medications—psychotropic medications become connected with both curing disease and maintaining certain specific notions of gender roles is a mechanism of action that evolved over the latter half of the twentieth century. Yet Glenmullen, Stack, and even Slater reveal that this effect cannot be wholly explained by the narratives of clinicians—perhaps because diagnostic knowledge often privileges the immediately observable, at the expense of the cultural or the contextual.[27] Neither can the Prozac that divides John from his lover be wholly conceptualized by the work of academic psychiatrists, many of whom argue against the notion that culture determines psychiatric definitions of gender, its constitutional pathologies, or its largely chemical cures. For example, Ellen Leibenluft, the chief of the Affective Disorders Unit at the National Institute of Mental Health, writes that "gender differences" in depression and anxiety are "no longer conceptualized as the result of social supports, life events, and life course" but are, instead, "observed by functional neuroimaging": "Clinical psychiatric research is being revolutionized by insights derived from basic neuroscience (including but not limited to those related to genetic mechanisms) as well as by relatively new structural and functional neuroimaging techniques."[28] Finally, the psychoanalytic function of Prozac cannot be entirely understood through outcome studies of prescription patterns, anthropological analyses of medical communication, or other studies that focus on the medical interaction at the expense of contextualizing it.[29]

Instead, the process whereby psychotropic medications work ironically to reinscribe Freudian beliefs is forged in the very cultures and contexts with which the profession of psychiatry claims no longer to be concerned. I come to this conclusion by closely reading representations of psychotropic medications in sources from American print culture over the latter half of the twentieth century, including articles from popular news and fashion magazines from the mid-1950s through the early 1960s (*Newsweek, Time, Cosmopolitan, Look*) describing the "new fad" in medical treatment, pills for emotional worries; long-running psychopharmaceutical advertisements from professional journals (the *AJP, Archives of General Psychiatry*) from 1964 to 1997, promoting new pharmaceutical "innovations"; and selected works of American literature produced between 1990 and 2002 in which SSRI antidepressants appear as characters. These three time periods roughly correspond to the life spans of psychiatry's three American "wonder drugs": psychotropic medications that became the objects of American popular frenzies in the latter half of the twentieth century. Miltown—a muscle relaxant with sedative properties—introduced the notion of a chemical treatment for outpatient neurosis in the 1950s and provided a wildly popular cure for neurosis, hysteria, and other conditions once treated exclusively by psychoanalysis. Valium—and the other benzodiazepines, medications that calmed "the activity of serotonin neurons" and "reduced the activity of norepinephrine neurons"—resulted, on its release in the 1970s, in "Valiumania," at least until widespread concerns about habit formation led to a decrease in use.[30] Finally, Prozac, the first and surely best named of the SSRIs, became the most prescribed and most profitable psychopharmaceutical in history, before suffering its own recent backlash.

The types of sources that I include under the rubric *print culture* are also meant to suggest the new relations between doctors, patients, and medications catalyzed by psychotropic medications at different points in time. *AJP* research reports and articles from popular news magazines in the 1950s, for example, often focus on the new relationships between doctors and patients brought about by tranquilizers. Both describe clinical encounters in which emotional ills are treated without the work of a prolonged interpersonal interaction. *Newsweek* articles thus describe wonder drugs that offer peace of mind without the necessity of spending years on the couch, leading to quick office visits for the harried well.[31] Not surprisingly, pharmaceutical advertisements in professional journals in the 1970s and 1980s promote new relations between doctors and medications. During this era, psychiatry's shift from being psychotherapy focused to drug-management focused forced many psychiatrists to rethink the theoretical foundations of their profession. Finally, literary works from the 1990s suggest new relations between patients and medications. Characters analyze decisions whether to take Prozac in a manner reminiscent of the ways in which psychoanalysts once analyzed their patients. These characters are concomitantly empowered by their autonomy as consumers and wary of the threat of pharmaceutical hegemony.

Over and beyond their obvious differences are the similarities among these sources, points of connection where the discourse of wonder drugs works to break down established divides between high and low, medical and popular, and the many other axes separating professional journals, news magazines, and literary texts. In all these sources, white men are assumed to be doctors, and doctors are almost always assumed to represent white men.

Meanwhile, women, and specifically white, middle-class women, are consistently scripted into the role of patient. Finally, notions of *mental illness* are often expressed through representational strategies that are clearly influenced by Freudian concepts of gender development—enlarged, threatening mothers, for example, who pathologize their cowering sons. These elements have, of course, been well documented in scholarship examining the interactions of American psychiatry and American popular culture in the latter half of the twentieth century.[32] What have not been examined, however, are the ways psychotropic medications became imbricated in this process and how this imbrication serves to destabilize the separateness of biological and psychoanalytic schools of thought from a historical perspective as well as a functional one. Far from rejecting psychoanalysis, pharmaceutical discourse (in popular culture as well as in the writings of clinicians such as Glenmullen, Slater, and Kramer) works to prove the ongoing relevance of psychoanalytic categories—as cultural scripts and as social and narrative resources—in ways that attest to the ongoing salience of the gender identities to which those categories give shape.

A key component of my intervention in this work is to argue that the biological revolution in psychiatry took on many of its gender characteristics not, as many have claimed, in the 1970s but in popular culture in the 1950s, a time when many scholars rightly argue that Freudian concepts were even more influential in popular culture than they were in academic psychiatry. Movies, Broadway plays, and the popular press were so dominated by depictions of analysts and analysis that the historian Nathan Hale cites the mid-1950s as the beginning of the "Golden Age of psychoanalytic representation" in the United States.[33] More important for my purposes, the conflation by psychoanalysis of individual and communal psychology gave voice to an often-ambiguous set of anxieties about mothers during an era when a host of social, political, and economic issues combined to create what the historian Mari Jo Buhle and other scholars describe as a "crisis in patriarchal authority" in postwar America.[34]

Within this milieu, the first public products of biological psychiatry appeared: pharmaceutical cures for chemically defined mental illnesses. Released in 1955, Miltown and the tranquilizers were posited as replacements for psychoanalysis—and specifically the assumption that mental illness resulted from early-life mother-child interactions—in both medical and popular literatures. Neuroscientists claimed that advances in psychopharmacology in the 1950s "liberated psychiatry from its primitive and outdated ways" —an argument that grew in influence with the reported success of psychopharmacology.[35] However, popular definitions of the new treatments owed a great deal to primitive ways of speaking, inasmuch as psychotropic medications became known as cures for a neurosis explicitly caused by mothers. Between 1955 and 1960, articles about pharmaceutical miracle cures for psychoanalytically inflected "mental illnesses" ranging from a woman's frigidity, to a bride's uncertainty, to a wife's infidelity filled leading mass-circulation periodicals. *Newsweek* described biological cures for women's neuroses, *Cosmopolitan* showed castrating mothers suddenly tranquilized, and *Time* introduced "pills for the mind" that restored a mother's maternity, fidelity, and sexuality all at once.[36]

Themes emerging from the 1950s then played out in the 1960s and 1970s, when the women's movement questioned "patriarchal institutions" such as marriage and the "male-female role system" that they represented. Kate Millett's argument that women's oppression originated in men's "sexual power over women" and Jill Johnson's claim that "a true political revolution would not occur" until "all women are lesbians" were aimed directly at Freudian psychoanalysis.[37] Yet appropriating this same Freudian psychoanalysis proved a remarkably successful strategy in numerous Valium advertisements depicting visually threatening, "feminist" women who were tamed by the new miracle cures for anxiety (see fig. 1).

In the 1990s and the early years of the twenty-first century, Paxil, Prozac, and Peter Kramer all suggested that work, not home, was the domain where gender lines were contested and redrawn. Kramer describes Prozac as a medication that allowed women such as "Mrs. Prozac" to achieve a state of being "optimistic, decisive, quick of thought, charismatic, energetic, and confident."[38] Prozac advertisements, Kramer's own case studies, and Slater's essays all present women who become productive and successful after taking Prozac—in "Black Swans," for example, the medicated Slater returns to her studies and works feverishly on her research.[39] Yet each text's claim of liberation is called into question by the ways in which psychotropic drugs reinscribe traditional categories of maternity, sensitivity, and other forms of femininity that exist in requisite opposition to masculine reason.

At the end of the line (although at the beginning of my narrative) is the June 1999 *AJP* special issue on gender. "Gender, What's the Difference?" asks Nada Stotland in a lead editorial meant to explore the viability of tradi-

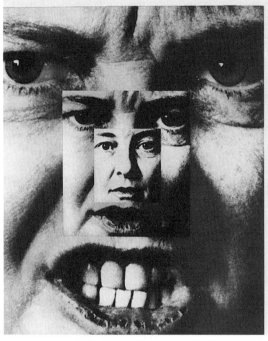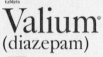

1. A threatening, "feminist" woman was tamed by the new miracle cure for anxiety in a Valium advertisement (*American Journal of Psychiatry* 121 [1965]: xii–xiii).

tional gender categories in an era when difference is determined by deeper levels of exploration. "Men and women are more alike than they are different," Stotland claims, a point then reinforced by key articles that openly discount "gender roles and life experiences" on the grounds that these can be attributed to molecules, receptors, pharmaceuticals, and other substrates that function beneath the level of social expectations. Yet binaried notions of gender work their way back into the narrative nonetheless, uncovered at the moments when the journal's insistence on a gender that functions free of social expectation reads against the social expectations of contemporary psychiatry: "Why is it that the same gene can have different effects depending on whether it comes from the male or the female parent? How do differences in hormones interact with differences in rearing and circumstances to cause differences in behavior both simple and complex (parenting being behavior that is fundamental to survival of the species but very complex)?"[40]

It is not my intention to flatten out the many, often intentionally conflicting notions of gender and gender roles at play within and between these sources. Kramer's case studies are anything but Valium's strung-out heroes, such as Neely in Jacqueline Susann's *Valley of the Dolls.* The notions of "male or female parenthood" expressed in the *AJP* in 1999 are often poised in rejection of a 1950s notion of fatherhood (one that Kramer and Glenmullen oddly recuperate). Slater writes, speaks, works, and in the process recuperates many other forms of agency denied women in *Time* magazine and Valium advertisements. Books such as Meri Nana-Ama Danquah's *Willow Weep for Me* then serve to complicate Slater's assumptions about motherhood by writing from a perspective of a single mother, caring for an "intelligent daughter," with the support of Paxil, therapy, and "black women whom I call colleagues and friends [who] battled or were battling depression." Finally, Danquah's experience of combining medication with therapy in order to find the "beauty on the other side" surely would not describe the experience of characters such as Jam, the narrator of Persimmon Blackbridge's *Prozac Highway,* who employs Prozac in the project of lesbian cybersex seduction.[41]

Yet, once again, these differences are always in tension with the many similarities among texts, the works at once poised in rejection and in reification of the normal and the normalizing across time, space, and genre. Housewives in the 1950s, angry feminists in the 1970s, and writers in the 1990s all become mothers when they take medication. Jam returns to feminine "nature" when Prozac fails her during her attempts at love. Danquah paraphra-

ses research from the *AJP* that assumes a maternal transfer of mental illness.[42] At these moments and others that I examine throughout this study,
psychotropic medications can be seen to participate in traditionally psychoanalytic projects. And the notion that psychiatry has moved from blaming
the mother to blaming the brain is complicated by the confounding fact that
the mother keeps showing up in places where psychopharmacology is introduced, negotiated, and familiarly redefined.

Science, Popular Culture, and the Use of Freud

To think that psychopharmacology can be read through *Newsweek,* advertisements, essays, and other sources, however, is to consider the possibility that housewives in need of meprobamate, feminists on benzodiazepines, or other stereotypical cultural images of medicated masses who go
running for a "mother's little helper" are not simply products of science pol-
luted by popular culture or distortions of the true concepts of psychopharmacology. Rather, they also represent psychopharmacology as the product
of multiple, interrelated discourses, each of which comes to inform the other.
Genetics, neurochemistry, and pharmacology might claim to uncover universal facts. But these facts are interpreted only through the cultural moments in which they are given meaning, mediated through the particulars of
specific time periods, philosophies, aesthetics, genres, and other broad contexts into which pharmaceuticals come to circulate. Such statements may
seem self-evident for medications such as Valium, Prozac, and other wonder
drugs constructed both by science and by desire, by the media and by the
medical establishments. Yet to believe that popular culture creates the context for psychopharmacology or produces a form of pharmaceutical knowledge independent of psychiatry is to read against the prevailing narratives
that shape how psychopharmacology is written about and is understood.

For instance, assumptions that psychiatric knowledge is constructed free
of social supports, life events, and other qualitative variables are also at play
in contemporary histories of psychiatry and psychopharmacology written
by men who are often clinicians, scientists, or academic psychiatrists turned
historians. Included among such works are high-profile attempts to docu-
ment the clinical impact of psychopharmacology as well as works that take
a more critical stance. Examples of the former are Ayd, "The Early History
of Modern Psychopharmacology"; Shorter, *A History of Psychiatry;* Healy,

The Antidepressant Era; Stone, *Healing the Mind.* Examples of the latter are Valenstein, *Blaming the Brain;* Glenmullen, *Prozac Backlash;* and Breggin and Breggin, *Talking Back to Prozac.* Each of these histories narrates a trajectory that begins in the laboratory, moves to the clinic, and then concludes with often cursory references to popular culture.[43] Each author also assumes that pharmaceutical companies and marketing firms are involved in producing discourses of pharmacology. Healy compellingly argues that drugs and drug companies, and then doctors and patients, "create their own markets" by defining everyday ailments as pathology and then supplying the treatment for this newly realized disease state.[44] Similarly, Shorter presents depression as a condition "familiar for many centuries" whose "boundaries have been expanded relentlessly outward" by the collusion between the marketing and development of antidepressants such as Prozac and the "American Psychiatric Association's continual hammering of the depression theme." Citing utilization and prescription data to support his version of the argument that drugs create their own markets, Shorter contends that the availability of drugs such as Prozac has "doubtless contributed to the diagnosis of depression: Physicians prefer to diagnose conditions they can treat rather than those they can't."[45]

Finally, each author presupposes that, as the products of biological science and adept marketing, wonder drugs then filter into popular consciousness. Each uniformly employs evidence from popular magazines, advertisements, works of fiction, and other "nonscientific" sources to illustrate the ways in which an initially specialized knowledge informs, misinforms, and, ultimately, explains popular actions and beliefs. Taking cues from many related works in science and technology studies, each author thus assumes that the societal metabolism of wonder drugs shifts from the scientific narrative to the popular narrative and, by extension, from scientific practice to the practice of everyday life.[46] Ayd, for example, begins his history of Miltown in medical journals, traces it through marketing campaigns, and concludes by citing references from popular magazines. Shorter similarly casts popular culture as the end point of the psychopharmacology phenomenon, in which laboratory discoveries are ultimately "reported" in unexamined citations from *Newsweek* and *Time.* Finally, Healy claims to examine the ways in which "a new biological language in psychiatry" has "come to be part of popular culture."[47]

To be sure, pharmaceutical companies certainly do play a major role in researching, treating, and ultimately shaping mental illness—a point well illustrated by a brief examination of the acknowledgments section of published studies of drug effectiveness or a quick walk through the exhibition hall at the annual meeting of the American Psychiatric Association.[48] The nonmedical public often eagerly awaits and then warmly embraces new forms of therapy. As the now-realized SSRI phenomenon reveals, market forces, consumer demand, and the thermodynamics of trial and error can often combine to expand the indications for new medications well beyond what the historian of pharmacology Mickey Smith calls "rational use."[49] Prozac, Paxil, and Zoloft were all initially approved as treatments for one illness but have subsequently been used for an ever-widening spectrum of conditions and disorders.[50]

Yet, when read together, a clear problematic emerges from the established conventions of writing about psychotropic drugs that provides a point of entry for my intervention: the a priori assumption of a trickle-down economy of psychopharmacology works to organize the telling of the history of psychopharmaceuticals in accordance with the same, predetermined hierarchy often insisted on by psychiatry itself. Here, hermetic knowledge originates in a laboratory or a pharmaceutical company and ends only with popular consumption. For instance, books such as the Breggins' *Prozac Backlash* often read like scientific reports whose purpose is to counter research with research. In the process, however, these works reinforce a traditionally gendered model of dissemination in which science is the phallic signifier, the source and origin of knowledge, and culture is, thereby, defined as its female receptacle, the place where such information "goes." Like Prozac in Stack's "Psychoanalysis Meets Queer Theory," the very notion of a top and a bottom, with the science of mankind on top and the instability of gender below, perpetuates and stabilizes the selfsame gender binary that Edward Shorter, Frank Ayd, and Eliot Valenstein all claim no longer exists.[51]

What then falls out of the established conventions of writing about the impact of psychotropic drugs is the very point that a study of popular culture helps explain: the possibility that psychiatry itself is gendered by, or prescribes information shaped by, the cultures that it deems to be artifact. Left unexamined are the questions raised by the realization that, in the process of enabling and mediating interactions between doctor and patient on the page, the "case studies" in *Time, Cosmopolitan, Prozac Backlash,* the *AJP,* and the other materials that I examine present women whose marital status is threatened by "mental illness," doctors whose powers of observation allow them to recognize ringlets of auburn hair, and medications that divide hard from soft.

As feminist literature has shown, knowledge flows in directions other than from the top down. I am indebted to feminist scholars in the social sciences who connect stereotyped representations of women in magazines, advertisements, and works of fiction to the white, middle-class, middle-aged women who have been historically overprescribed these same medications in real life.[52] Meanwhile, historians and cultural critics such as Mari Jo Buhle, Nathan Hale, Jacqueline Zita, Elizabeth Lunbeck, and Tamar Garb provide evidence to support the contention that, like all revolutions, the biological revolution is a product of history.[53] Finally, feminist critics of science have shown how clinical interactions reveal the gendered nature of scientific discourse. Over the past three decades, these scholars have written against the notion of essential differences between women and men that biological psychiatry ironically claims to recuperate. Psychopharmacology, neuroimaging, and, of course, Freud might posit structural notions of mothers, fathers, and sons. Yet Donna Haraway, Evelyn Fox Keller, Sandra Harding, and others argue that these differences are interpreted only through what Keller calls the "symbolic work of gender," in which "norms associated with masculine culture are taken as universal."[54] In other words, both popular and psychiatric representations of psychopharmaceuticals function within a notion of gender that normalizes married women, men doctors, and other requisite components of a heterosexual symbolic order while pathologizing the lesbian, the ambitious woman, the homosexual man, and other threats as diseases in need of a cure.

Ultimately, however, the conceptual apparatus that I employ for understanding the Freud of psychopharmacology comes from Freud himself—despite the fact that Freud's theories are overlooked or overtly rejected by many feminist, Foucaultian, and cultural-studies scholars as well as by most academic psychiatrists. By *Freud,* I mean the Freud who insists on the identification and inscription of requisite, relational binaries, and surely biological binaries, of man/woman, mother/father, culture/nature, or phallus/absence. This is the later-era Freud of *Inhibitions, Symptoms, and Anxiety* (1925) and *Civilization and Its Discontents* (1930), who reappears in the work of Theodore Reik, Irving Beiber, and the *DSM-I* definition of *psychoneurosis* in 1952, among many other sources.[55] In these works, Freud assumes that the castration crisis is a requisite step in the development of individual and communal man, an event "of the profoundest importance in the formation alike of character and of neuroses."[56] During the Oedipal crisis, the male child is overcome with the fear of the loss of his penis. In response, the child undergoes a painful act of compromise, resulting in the formation of what Freud calls a "moral superego"—a structure that (for structural reasons) is more developed in a man than in a woman. As a result, the child internalizes the father's moral authority and specifically the prohibition of desire for the mother.[57] The male superego's authority provides, not only the "rules" by which the child may live in "culture," but also the rules that organize culture itself. The child, Freud argues in *Civilization and Its Discontents,* becomes civilized and takes "his" place in a like-structured civilization.[58] The desire for the mother, meanwhile, is repressed—placing the emotions and memories that constitute the very notion of mother below the radar of consciousness—and, in the act of repression, the unconscious is formed. Thus, Freud argues that civilization is built on the renunciation of "instinct."[59]

The notion that Freudian psychoanalysis is important as an object of study and as a heuristic model for understanding the function of psychopharmacology in scientific research reports, theoretical essays, advertisements, works of fiction, and other sources is admittedly a somewhat tenuous position. As someone writing at the beginning of the twenty-first century, I have been influenced by the many coexisting and competing interpretations and revisions of Freudian concepts. Karen Horney, Alfred Adler, Jacques Lacan, Julia Kristeva, Jessica Benjamin, Deanna Holtzman, Nancy Kulish, Peter Blos, Slavoj Žižek, and Heinz Kohut are but a few of the theorists whose work has reshaped concepts once attributed to Freud. These revisions, on top of Freud's often competing topographies of development, make the very notion of a unified "Freudian" narrative all but impossible. Finally, as I hope the following chapters reveal, I am not arguing that a Freudian ur-narrative "correctly" provides universal truths about gender formation and gender identity. Indeed, I share the Foucaultian assumption that psychoanalysis incites the production of knowledge that is cultural rather than natural and that contributes to maintaining specific power relations in the guise of liberation—a concept that surely holds true for biological psychiatry as well.[60]

Following Judith Butler, however, I mean to say that psychoanalysis allows for a critical engagement with questions of gender that helps explain why pharmaceutical discourse behaves the way it does. Psychoanalysis also helps expose the inherent limitations of a strict reliance on Foucault present throughout contemporary work in the cultural studies of psychiatry.[61] This is because the history of Freud is specifically the history of Prozac, and, thus a consideration of certain key Freudian concepts is necessary to address the question of why psychoanalytic themes, and psychoanalytic notions of gender keep showing up in representations of biological psychiatry at times when "nontraditional" claims are undermined by the traditional effects of psychotropic medications. This lineage—or this "social temporality," to use Butler's term—differentiates the history of psychopharmacology from the history of American culture, or family culture, or popular culture, or antibiotic culture, or any of the other cultures intimately concerned with neurotic housewives who may or may not be sleeping around.[62] As an object of study, a historical understanding of Freud's concepts helps explain those aspects of the representation of wonder drugs shaped by the influence of psychoanalysis on American popular culture, circa 1955, which then played out in the scientific press in the 1970s. A historical understanding of psychoanalysis also helps explain those shards of seemingly vanished Freudian concepts that still shape the ways in which pharmaceuticals are defined, discussed, and understood.[63]

Scholars of the history of science might counter that the psychoanalytic function of psychopharmacology simply illustrates how a paradigm shift is always incomplete. The new paradigm is defined through the terminology of the paradigm that it claims to replace. The postmodern, for example, always depends on awareness of the modern. However, close inspection of the behavior of these "remnants," a term that I appropriate from Žižek to imply those pieces of the prior regime that remain imbricated after the shift, shows that they can govern the form and the function of the regime that takes its place. These remnants are often expressed in moments of anxiety, as when John's homosexuality, Kate Millett's feminism, or other destabilizations of traditional gender roles are experienced as deviations from a norm.[64] Not only does the modern appear within the postmodern, but it also helps it recognize, cast off, and disavow the modern in its own design. The modern, in other words, works against the possibility of difference by the compulsive recognition of its own, abject similarity.

Here is where Freud as a heuristic model then comes in—or, more to the point, a heuristic understanding of the gender assumptions inherent in Freud's model. The notion that *civilization* is the realm of reason, superego, and morality is surely one of the more widely criticized aspects of Freudian theory. Scholars as far afield as Luce Irigaray, Catherine Bates, Frederic Crews, Carolyn Stack, and, most important, Nancy Andreasen and Ellen Liebenuft are joined in the supposition that the Oedipal model posits a troubling binary of having and wanting when it comes to discussions of the gendering of the world. Boys, in individual and in communally essential evolution, have. Girls, meanwhile, lack. This division leads to marked differences in development. Since the fear of castration, or of being turned into a girl, is one of the most powerful forces in male psychical development, according to Freud, it serves as a "forceful . . . motive towards forming the superego." Girls, meanwhile, have less to lose and accept castration as "an established fact": since girls see themselves as already castrated, they thus have relatively less impetus to form a strong superego. This key difference then leads to differences in moral character between the sexes. As Freud wrote, "I cannot escape the notion that for women the level of what is ethically normal is different from what it is in men. Their super-ego is never so inexorable, so impersonal, so independent of its emotional origins as we require in men. . . . [Women] show less sense of justice than men, that they are less ready to submit to the greater necessities of life, that they are more often influenced in their judgments by feelings of affection or hostility."[65]

Biology works to ablate this divide by constructing a world of all-consciousness. By replacing the "social," the "environmental," and the unknown with the all-seeing eye of the fMRI, biological theories and practices often claim to denature the unconscious entirely. Freud's ideas are "pitched out," and biological markers, visualized by neuroimaging technologies, determine sex differences. Yet the point that I make throughout this work is the same point that Freud ironically illuminates: the notion that biology replaced psychoanalysis is undone in the moments when biology is expressed as psychoanalysis, or performs the cultural work of psychoanalysis, or assumes the same definition of *civilization* as psychoanalysis, or looks at a patient with ringlets of auburn hair and soft, delicate features as psychoanalysis does. What Freud successfully realized was, I believe, not that the organization of the world into civilization and unreason, conscious and unconscious, is a universal truth, but, rather, that there seems to be a universal truth in the need to restore order against a threat long after the threat itself has disappeared. The model answers questions of obsession, repetition, disavowal, the uncomfortable state between desire and discomfort, and other instances where the response does not seem entirely commensurate with the stimulus. At these times, psychoanalysis promises to maintain a certain structure, even when the drive seems confoundingly irrational or unprofessional. The notion of civilization justifies the irrationality of these moments and then maintains order, reason, and rationality in the face of seen and unseen threats—maintains family values, one might say, in the face of the erosion of the nuclear unit. Psychoanalysis maintains the familiar when the familiar is in peril. Civilization justifies the irrationality of these emotions and then maintains order, reason, and rationality in comfortable and uncomfortably problematic ways.

In spite of its protestations to the contrary, biology works the same way every time frigid housewives, Mrs. Prozacs, homosexuals, or other non-normative subjects are constructed as symptoms, points of rupture in the otherwise coherent facade of civilized reason. But, more to my concerns, these popular representations also help illuminate the ways in which practitioners and historians of psychiatry make the same assumption whenever they tacitly assume that pharmaceutical knowledge disseminates downward from the realm of reason to the confounders of culture or that environmental biases alter the practice of objectifiable medicine. The persistence of this form of reason, this ideological work, might be called *the ahistorical kernel of psychiatry*.[66] At these moments, biological psychiatry works to reify gender, in the Freudian sense, as a cultural, developmental, division that justifies imbalances between the self-defined categories *woman* and *man*. The symptom remains the same, even if its treatment differs. Psychoanalysis then forms the unconscious of biological psychiatry: like all things from the repressed, Freud's return both ruptures the flow of biology's argument and restores an uncanny sense of familiarity in the system.

Traced over the latter half of the twentieth century, the Freudian components of Prozac then open a space in which to retheorize the meaning of psychotropic medications in the texts that I examine—a problematic that I set as my project in the chapters that follow.[67] To be sure, medications are those denotative entities bought, sold, and ingested. But, unlike penicillin, insulin, the polio vaccine, or other nonpsychiatric miracle cures, psychotropic medications also come to represent the illusive promise of potency and social restoration that is the result of their specific, psychoanalytic history. Here, sex, gender, and civilization do not mean that psychotropic medications enhance corporeal enjoyment, prolong physical stamina, or provide means for liberation—although many late-twentieth-century popular sources might suggest otherwise.[68] Rather, I mean that medications perform the work of phallic symbols, in much the same way phallic symbols are "traditionally" defined by Stack, as characters in a "phallocentric narrative that men have/are the desired object that women lack": "This heterosexist trope of desire rambles through our personal lives, our work with patients, and our professional relations, reinforcing and reenacting its belief in itself every time it shows up."[69] Psychotropic medications serve this same purpose, even as Freud falls out of fashion. Rambling through personal lives, professional relations, even articles trying to deconstruct heterosexist assumptions, these medications signify a narrative in which men have and are the desired object that women lack. Developed in the interdisciplinarities of time, space, and genre, Prozac promulgates, helps define, and works to maintain seemingly outdated gender norms, reenacting its belief in itself every time it shows up, often listening and always talking back in the project of normalization.

Prozac on the Couch

The following chapters are organized as case studies, meant to rethink the interrelation between scientific innovation and popular perception. My analysis is organized into four genre-specific sections, each of which explores the various genders that are shaped by, and then in turn shape, the notion of chemical treatments for emotional problems. Chapter 2 is a rewriting of scientific narratives that implicitly assume that the history of psychiatry represents the conquest of feminine nature by masculine science. Reading *AJP* research reports against a backdrop of Freud's case studies and theories (the "Wolf Man," the negative Oedipus complex), I take at face value the notion that the biological revolution in psychiatry occurred in the 1970s while at the same time pointing out the inconsistencies in that narrative with regard to masculine character and its vicissitudes. To do so, I trace the alleged demise of psychoanalysis and the ascent of biological psychiatry through the formation of a new "doctorhood" in which the talking skills of psychotherapy are replaced by writing skills involved in prescription. The role of medication expands significantly over the fifty-two-year period of my study, while at the same time physicians literally disappear from view. This dynamic forces a reconceptualization of the power of the psychiatrist in relation to the power of pharmaceuticals. On the one hand, psychotropic medications enhance the psychiatrist's position as guardian and perpetuator of a mental health whose parameters are circumscribed by the mutually exclusive interactions of "men" and "women." But, on the other, the notion that these categories are maintained by psychotropic medications, not psychiatrists themselves, threatens to upend the "gender" of psychiatry itself.

Having opened a space in the standard narrative, I then return to popular culture in the 1950s in order to explore the larger historical and cultural contexts that shape that narrative's form and content. My rereading of the *AJP* begins in chapter 3, which examines the implicit assumptions of scientific progress and innovation defined in "information" articles in American newsmagazines announcing the discovery of Miltown in 1954–60. My analysis is shaped by Freudian notions of anxiety, by feminist critiques of Freud, and by feminist histories of psychoanalysis. Over the course of the chapter, I reexamine psychoanalysis' fall from grace through a series of articles from the mainstream popular press, culminating with a discussion of the ways in which psychoanalysis is shown to be unable to treat the anxiety caused by women's discontent and how, as a result, women threaten to rupture civilization's progress narrative. I also read scientific and popular articles announcing the success of Miltown and other tranquilizers for the ways in which they respond to this failure of psychoanalysis: untreated by psychoanalysis, women were assumed to be the source of an epidemic of "cultural anxiety." In Miltown, however, culture found its restorative cure.

This mechanism of action then becomes my point of entry into chapter 4, where I look more closely at the gender of the patients constructed in advertisements for psychotropic medications in professional journals. I approach these ads as sites where cultural representations commingled with medical "information" to produce a system of representation directed at physicians who were overtly assumed to be men, in spite of the fact that women were entering the profession in increasing numbers. I show how problematic connections between mothers and pharmaceuticals from popular culture in the 1950s are repackaged as successful marketing techniques in the 1970s, 1980s, and 1990s. Each of the images that I examine overtly links marital status and mental illness, whether by depicting a wedding ring or by identifying woman as "single." However, marriage is represented differently at different points in time—a progression that allows me to connect changes in advertisements to the threats to normalcy specifically presented by the waves of the women's movement.

If advertisements reveal the construction of a new doctorhood brought about by psychopharmacology, then the American fictional and autobiographical accounts of women suffering from mental illness in the 1990s—the subject of chapter 5—speak to a new patienthood. I focus on one essay and three works of fiction narrated in the first person by women in various forms of relation to Prozac. In each narrative, Prozac represents the possibility of a new selfhood, described as a chemical liberation from past expectations and outdated gender norms. Prozac also allows for a new sense of connectedness and new possibilities of being. In many ways, these four works successfully conceptualize new categories of being. Each effectively co-opts the language of "Prozac science" in the name of specific feminist critiques of past structures of oppression (psychoanalysis, literary genre) and, ultimately, of Prozac itself. At the same time, each illustrates how resistance is often expressed within existing narrative frameworks, developed over time and in direct relation to the "gender" of medication. As in Stack's "Psychoanalysis Meets Queer Theory," the Freudian assumptions that Prozac is engineered to replace work their way into the narratives, as if returning from the psychopharmacologically repressed.

My goal throughout this project is to work as much as possible within the stereotypes presented in the texts of mainstream popular sources. By *stereotypes,* I mean the ways in which the discourse of wonder drugs seems to insist on transparent and self-limited definitions of race and gender over time, embodied in the persistence of white, male doctors and middle-aged, white, women patients despite overwhelming evidence of the outdated nature of these characterizations. This consistency is in one sense largely a result of the sources that I examine—newsmagazines directed at a mainstream, white readership; advertisements in leading professional journals; essays and works of fiction by white, women writers. I am aware that mine would be a different narrative were I to spend more time looking at sources that bring other voices to the fore. These might range from the few published first-person mental-illness narratives written by persons of color (e.g., Danquah's *Willow Weep for Me*) to the narratives of persons denied access to health care.

By working within raced and gendered stereotypes, I risk perpetuating the existence of, and the divide between, the categories *inside* and *outside, control group* and *deviant, gender* and *sex.* Yet part of the point that I am trying to make in this study is that the persistence of certain forms of representation is important in and of itself because it serves to create stealthily a two-tier system, a binary on top of a binary, dividing the seen from the unseen. In the realm of the normal are the circumscribed categories *illness* and *health, man* and *woman, biology* and *psychoanalysis,* and other modes of expression that presuppose the stability of unstable categories (*race* as "whiteness," e.g., or *gender* as "woman"). I believe that there is much to be learned from close examination of these stereotypes and from the ways in which they reappear through time, as if regenerating neurons. In the heterosexuality of Prozac advertisements, the whiteness of Valium, or the unstated markings of a petite, blonde housewife, we see an unabated (if differently construed) path of resistance to social change. Here, not only wellness and power are defined but disease as well. Illnesses threaten straight, white print culture and are treated by straight, white, middle-class medications, always already within the domain of the neurotic.

Yet such artifacts must always be read with the awareness that certain sensibilities are diagnosed as outside this particular pharmaceutical discourse.[70] Appearing as outside (by taboo, foreclosure, or some other mechanism) is everything placed within the abject category *psychosis.*[71] Here lies the unspoken and the unacknowledged, deemed so as a result of race, or social class, or resistance to treatment, or object choice. It took thirty years, for example, for persons of color to appear in pharmaceutical advertisements in the *AJP,* and, when they did appear in the mid-1970s, they did so only as patients in antipsychotic medication advertisements—either as medicated inpatients on psychiatric wards or as assaultive and belligerent, threats to society during an era when the journal pathologized the "Black Power class of reactions."[72] Neurosis is a problem that we can understand; it is, as Lacan argued, of us. Psychosis is of the exogenes, and thus do we create neuroleptics (fig. 2).

I conclude this introduction on a personal note, writing from the often-conflicted position of someone who both prescribes and criticizes psychotropic medications. This position forces a concomitant awareness of the therapeutic and the hegemonic, of treatments for conditions that are more prevalent in women and of treatments that reinscribe the category *woman.* I struggle with the tension of this position on a daily basis, and this book is in part meant to be a search for often-elusive answers. My authorial position as a doctor, a white male, and a graduate of a biological psychiatric training program surely structures many of my observations, if not my belief that I can speak about this issue in the first place. In my clinical practice, I would be entirely wrong to refuse treatment to any persons who may call on stereotypes, or employ discursive tropes, or make assumptions that I describe in

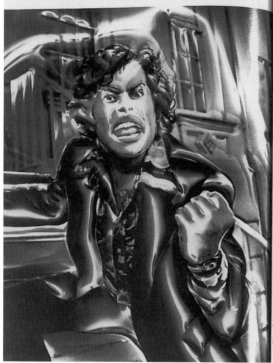

2. Drugs for the assaultive and the belligerent appeared during an era when psychiatry pathologized the "Black Power" class of reactions: Haldol advertisement (*Archives of General Psychiatry* 131 [1974]: 732–33).

this study as problematic. Women longing for maternal, auburn hair or men requesting Paxil because they feel stuck in their jobs often come to the psychiatric clinic in which I work because they are in pain, or unhappy, or desiring a change that they cannot seem to bring about on their own. "I have a chemical imbalance that keeps me from getting married," a person might say, or, "I saw the Prozac advertisement in *Self* magazine and realized, 'This is *me*.'" When these persons express themselves and give voice to deep emotions, they often do so in ways that utilize cultural stereotypes, assumptions, and tropes. These ways of speaking surround us—this is in part my point— and affect how patients and doctors talk about disease. And, to be sure, such ready availability is in many ways necessary for human interaction. Tropes, for example, imply a common language that facilitates talking about a person's emotional state, making such communication more nuanced and often more meaningful.

Yet, as a psychiatrist, I am also made constantly aware of the dangers of accepting these specific medications, stereotypes, and tropes as ends rather than as points of entry into larger questions and concerns. The astonishing biological language that David Healy contends has "come to" popular culture is in many ways a language that insists upon such shorthand.[73] As I argue throughout this book, biological language often constructs an eternal present tense, a science that claims to see with the technical neutrality of the SPECT scan, diagnose at the moment of the office visit, and treat with the objectivity of medications that work largely the same in men and women, white and brown, gay and straight.

Mine is not an appeal for a return to mass psychoanalysis. As I mention above, during its golden age in the 1940s and 1950s, psychoanalysis was often guilty of normalizing and institutionalizing misogyny and racism, surely paving the way for the biological revolution that would follow. Yet psychoanalysis also forced awareness of the very tensions to which the culture of biology seems, in its demand for technical, scientific language, to want to block access. Psychoanalysis understood how the anxieties of the patient are defined only in relation to the anxieties of the doctor and how even the most unconfounded discoveries come to be defined in a process of mutual negotiation when they enter into conversation. My insistence on the authority of magazine articles, works of fiction, and strategies of representation is meant to show that biology has a great deal to learn from the popular cultures within which it is given meaning. These sources reveal the ways in which objective knowledge is itself contextual and is often contextually problematic. And they reveal how this project is ultimately as much about myself, and about my own biases, fears, and assumptions, as it is about the biases, fears, and assumptions of the persons who become my patients. This awareness, I believe, can only heighten the relevance of the interaction, be it in a fifty-minute hour or a seven-minute medication evaluation, a talking cure or a cure that requires no talking, a 1950s culture enamored of psycho-analysis or an early-twenty-first-century culture that listens and speaks back only to Prozac. In each case, the strength of progress is more fully under-stood, not as a continuum of transparent and self-evident facts, but as a con-versation of important knowledges that are at the same time deeply shaped by cultural perceptions, if not interpreted through individual structures of expectation and desire.

Chapter Two

THE NAME OF THE FATHER, THE PLACE OF THE MEDICATION:

A BRIEF HISTORY OF PSYCHIATRY, 1955–2002

On the cover of the June 1999 *American Journal of Psychiatry (AJP)* special issue on gender is reproduced a detail from a retro, black-and-white photograph of twin young women from the 1950s, so identified by their matching sorority pins, tight, clinging sweaters, and Doris Day hairdos. The women's visages reappear, enlarged and in shades of green and white, behind the detail, ghostlike and blurred, contrasting sharply with the pair of phrases—"stressful life events," "major depression"—superimposed on them, phrases reduced to acronyms and repeated in a scientific flowchart. Read temporally, the women serve as foils for the science, their dated black-and-whiteness obviously out of place among the late-twentieth-century psychiatric terminology ("temperament—SLE—MD"). Superimposition of the science onto the women then suggests a progress narrative in which the "gender" of mental illness, once read through body parts and their adornments, is now understood through twin studies, genetic analysis, and other disembodied levels of exploration.

At the same time, this progress narrative is complicated by a glaring absence: there are no psychiatrists pictured on the cover. The two women are unaccompanied by a physician, even though physicians always appeared with patients in 1950s medical iconography in general and in images reproduced in the *AJP* in particular. During that era, not only did representations of psy-

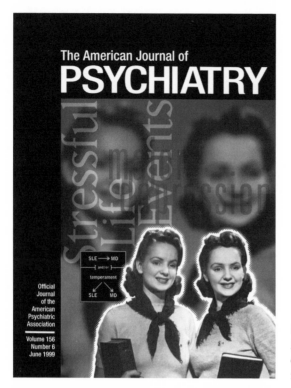

The American Journal of

PSYCHIATRY

Stressful Life Events

Official
Journal
of the
American
Psychiatric
Association

Volume 156
Number 6
June 1999

3. A special issue on
gender (*American Journal
of Psychiatry* 156 [1999]:
front cover).

chiatrists and psychoanalysts appear throughout the journal, but they were
configured in a manner that shored up the position of the male clinician,
placing him in a superior vantage point vis-à-vis the female patient. These
women patients were, thus, defined in opposition to, and in deference to,
the clearly marked gender of the psychiatrist. What we see, however, on this
special-issue cover is an important act of replacement: neuroscience holds
the place of authority; and an image claiming to be of the 1950s is recast from
an entirely 1990s point of view.

The June 1999 *AJP* special-issue cover serves as the jumping-off point for
my interventions in this chapter, in which I trace the gendered assumptions
of psychiatry though the pages of the *AJP*—the official organ of the American Psychiatric Association (APA) and the most widely circulated American
psychiatric journal of the past half century. Open any copy of the journal
from the end of the twentieth century or the beginning of the twenty-first,
and it will be immediately apparent that hardly a psychiatrist appears within

its pages. Instead, the psychiatrists have been replaced, the gender positions that they once held occupied by neuroscience—and, more specifically, by the psychotropic medications that bring advances in neuroscience into the bodies of women and men. For instance, the lead editorial of the June 1999 special issue asks the question, "Gender, What's the Difference?" and proceeds to call for assurance that psychotropic medications "work as well for our female patients as for the male patients on whom they were tested."[1] Throughout the editorial, gender is similarly presented as a binary in which "differences" between women and men are reified by individuals' responses to medications—a binary that is later explained to be requisite for the "fundamental survival" of the species.[2] However, while the gender of patients taking medications is described in minute detail, no mention is made of the gender of the psychiatrist, who is notably absent from the relations in which the categories *women* and *men* are defined.[3]

Clinicians are also missing from the issue's many research articles, which, although they once foregrounded the perspectives of individual practitioners, now attend solely to the interactions of patients and pharmaceuticals. "Placebos, Drug Effects, and Study Design," "Suggested Minimal Effective Dose of Risperidone based on PET Measured D2 and 5HT2A Receptor Occupancy," "Rapid Release of Drugs from Dopamine D2 Receptors," and "Persistence of Haloperidol in Human Brain Tissue" all stake their claims to efficacy on the actions of psychotropic medications while revealing nothing about the psychiatrists who provided them. Finally, not a single prescriber appears in the very pharmaceutical advertisements that once promoted the paternal physician as a component of the therapeusis. Instead, the over sixty pages of ads present an uninterrupted flow of images of medicated women— smiling, walking hand in hand with their young children, proudly displaying wedding rings—images in which gender is marked by interactions between patients and psychotropic medications.[4]

In what follows, I argue that a gender that is both devoid of psychiatrists and enforced by medications represents the end point of the replacement of men with medications in psychiatric journals over the past half century. *Men* are, in this case, the male psychoanalysts who dominated the profession of psychiatry through the 1950s and whose influence is my initial focus, in an examination of the ways in which psychoanalysis and psychoanalysts inscribed a binaried, paternalistic notion of gender on the profession's diagnostic purview. Even the most cursory tour through the pages of the *AJP* at midcentury reveals the dominating presence of psychoanalysts, who were shown in portrait and described in articles and who authored first-person editorials and research studies. So, too, Oedipal notions of gender development served as the foundations of a psychiatry that regarded interactions between mothers, fathers, and sons as the templates for neurosis, hysteria, neurasthenia, homosexuality, and countless other conditions in need of talking cures. At the same time, close inspection of the role of psychotropic medications in several key research articles subtly suggests that psychoanalysis was unable to uphold the Oedipal structure that it had defined and, thus, required pharmaceutical support.

In the 1970s, however, a self-described "revolution" claimed to overturn privileged psychoanalytic assumptions about early-life experiences—which were, it was argued, alienating psychiatry from the rest of the civilized world —in place of "organic" explanations of identity based in neurochemistry, genetics, and, most important, psychopharmacology.[5] Specifically, biological psychiatry claimed to replace the Oedipal model, and its assumptions of binaries such as conscious/unconscious and father/mother, with a less-"gendered" model of care. *AJP* articles decried that psychiatry had come to rely on "diagnostic biases" instead of empirical observations. At the same time, leading practitioners such as Bertram Brown asserted that psychiatry was primarily a medical specialty that was "overstepping its boundaries in attempting to treat problems of living, and was too involved with social questions," claims that found resonance among an increasingly biologically oriented academy.[6] Such arguments were enhanced by the fact that medications came to play an increasingly important role in the *AJP*, both because scientific reports attested to their vastly expanded clinical use and because the growing advertising sections spoke to psychiatry's close connections with the pharmaceutical industry.

Finally, I explore the complexity of a current situation in which medications defend the sanctity of relationships between men and women against the forces of depression, obsessive-compulsive disorder, and even the effects of the medications themselves ("Significantly less orgasm dysfunction with Wellbutrin SR than with Zoloft"), while male psychoanalysts are nowhere to be seen.[7]

Many political, economic, and social factors help explain the process whereby psychotropic medication became imbued with what I describe as *gender tensions,* relatively few of which I attempt to examine here. Instead, I call on prominent articles, editorials, and advertisements to focus on a shift over a fifty-two-year period in which medication came to occupy a space in the *AJP* that is often described, in intended and unintended ways, as replacing practitioners of psychotherapy and psychoanalysis. Thus, the rise of medication takes place against the backdrop of the evanescence of men. In subsequent chapters, I argue that this chiasmus is a space in which to explore the gender of the "patient" and that of the "medication," as they played out in a biological revolution taking place in popular magazines, advertisements, and literary works at least two decades before the alleged revolution in psychiatry. These popular sources ultimately support my contention that the representations of women patients in the *AJP* in the 1950s and in the early years of the twenty-first century are more similar than they are different. Here, however, my concerns are specifically with the gender of the psychiatrist, as it has been historically negotiated with the support of, and at times under the threat of, psychotropic medication. The complexities of this lineage ultimately yield two possible readings of psychiatry as it comes to terms with the role of medication in an age when gender may or make not make a difference: the emergence of psychotropic medication may have enhanced a psychiatrist's power by offering new forms of disciplinary regulation; or, in the light of the emergence of HMOs and conglomerated pharmaceutical companies and encroachment from other medical specialties, medication may have forced psychiatrists to consider the tenuous nature of their own professional identities.

The Gender of Psychoanalysis and the Neurosis of Imprisonment

Psychotropic medications for outpatient conditions were not treatments unto themselves in the *AJP* in the late 1950s and early 1960s. Rather, medications were clearly presented as the helpers of men. "Men," in this case, were the white, male psychotherapists and psychoanalysts whose presence, and the Freudian model that they imposed on psychiatric diagnoses and treatments, dominated the pages of the journal in the decades following the war. White male psychiatrists authored first-person articles and delivered prestigious lectures whose content was reproduced verbatim in "special articles" at the front of the journal. White male psychiatrists also appeared in images throughout the journal, from full-page photographs of leading psychoanalysts, to images representing the psychotherapeutic and psychoanalytic treatments that they administered, to advertisements for psychotropic medication that always put the psychotherapist front and center.

This was not surprising, of course, given the demographics of psychiatry in the 1950s and 1960s. In 1958, for example, John Maciver and Fredrick Redlick's "Patterns of Psychiatric Practice" found that all university psychiatrists and most private-practice psychiatrists demonstrated an "analytic and psychological (A-P) orientation." These "psychodynamic" practitioners were all men, graduates of "approved" medical schools, residency programs, and, often, psychoanalytic institutes whose clinical interactions with patients averaged forty-five to fifty minutes per session. A-P sessions were "almost entirely psychological and non-directive," with an emphasis on "the gaining and application of insight" through modifications of the prevailing "Freudian techniques" of free association, dream analysis, and other means by which the unconscious was made conscious. A-P practitioners reported high rates of satisfaction with their incomes and with the practice of "learning how people think." By contrast, "directive and organic (D-O) psychiatrists" worked largely in state hospitals, where they practiced a psychiatry whose goal was to "change patient attitudes and behavior by means of directive methods (such as suggestion, reassurance, advice, and reproof) and organic methods such as medical and neurological examination, the prescribing of drugs, and shock treatments." D-O psychiatrists spent far less time with their patients by meeting with them in groups or in "short" sessions of fifteen minutes or less and earned lower incomes than did A-P psychiatrists. Over 50 percent of these D-O psychiatrists—who were, it was pointed out, often "Republicans and Protestants"—had "incomplete psychiatric residencies" or had no psychiatric training at all.[8]

The *AJP* was an A-P journal in the mid- to late 1950s, as was the American psychiatry it claimed to represent. To be sure, large segments of the profession practiced in D-O settings, and many D-O psychiatrists published research reports. But psychodynamically oriented psychiatrists dominated leading academic departments, residency training programs, research and funding agencies, and editorial boards.[9] And, most important, the presence of Freudian psychoanalysts on the APA's 1951 Committee on Nomenclature and Statistics helped shape the first edition of the *Diagnostic and Statistical Manual of Mental Disorders (DSM-I)*, the first postwar national classification of psychopathology and a resource used by psychiatrists, A-P and D-O alike. Many *DSM-I* diagnoses, and especially outpatient diagnoses such as neuroses and psychophysiological disorders, thus carried the Freudian assumption that mental disorders were the result of early-life experiences with fathers and mothers that became internalized in adulthood through the explicit binary of conscious and unconscious.[10] The diagnosis of a "neurotic disorder," as the most commonly used example, depended on a mix of those symptoms observed by the clinician at the time of evaluation—feelings of inferiority, anxiety, or incompleteness—and on his trained, psychodynamic understanding of the ways in which these presenting symptoms were but extensions of a "neurotic process" begun during the Oedipal crisis, when a child was forced to make a life-altering decision between the desire for mother and the desire for (male) potency throughout the remainder of life.

In the context of the late-Freudian model that lay beneath the *DSM-I, Oedipal* implied both the specifically gendered castration crisis of childhood and the "structural" psychical apparatus that evolved as a result.[11] Before the Oedipal crisis, the male child was believed to exist in a blissful, if wholly narcissistic, union with his mother. The castration crisis began, however, when the child became aware of "parental threats" that, as the mother in the case study of Little Hans put it, "I shall send for Doctor A. to cut off your widdler."[12] The child, suddenly consumed by castration anxiety, recognized his sexual difference from his mother, who appeared to him as castrated, as well as his guilt and murderous feelings toward his father–turned–rival for his mother's emotions. In the Oedipal crisis, the child was overcome with the fear of the loss of his penis and, with it, his primary source of both pleasure and power. A painful act of compromise was then the result: in what Freud called a "symbolic castration," the post-Oedipal child acknowledged and then identified with the superior power of the father, gave up his primary identification with the mother (who was lost to the father), and proceeded, wounded but intact, to develop.

Reading temporally, the psychical events thought to take place in the process of resolving the crisis allowed for the formation of the male psychological apparatus. The identification with (and fear of) the father, first of all, created the policing conscience of the unconscious, the superego, representing the child's acceptance and internalization of the father's moral authority and specifically the prohibition of desire for the mother. Since the fear of castration, or of being turned into a girl, was, according to Freud, one of the most powerful forces in male psychical development, it served as a "forceful motive" toward the creation of a "moral" superego.[13] However, the child did not entirely give up the desire for the mother—instead, he placed the emotions and memories that constitute the notion of mother below the radar of consciousness, and, in this act of repression, the unconscious was formed. Thus, the child not only entered the adult world but, in most cases, became "neurotic" as a result, inasmuch as the disavowal of intimacy was never as complete as the imagined castration—a point demonstrated by sensations of low self-esteem, feelings of incompleteness, drives for control, and other remnants of a path not taken.[14]

The ultimate result of these developments was an uneasy equilibrium between the superego and its repressed components (and, by extension, between the remnants of father and mother) that became the core of many disorders defined in the *DSM-I,* a diagnostic system that in many instances inscribed a fragile paternal order as the essentialized template for mental illness and mental health. Hysteria, homosexuality, conversion reaction, and psychoneurosis were but a few of the diagnoses that took as their foundational point the naturalness of the father-mother dyad, whose psychical remnants needed to be exposed, analyzed, and understood if they were to be effectively treated. Meanwhile, psychiatry institutionalized a system that held the "phallus" as the site of a power that divided men and women, in unequal proportion, if for no other reason than that accepting the rules of the father became the condition for entering the neurosis of adult life.[15]

Given this constitution, it is far from surprising that much of the psychiatric establishment voiced skepticism about the use of the major and minor tranquilizers that were becoming increasingly popular in the practice of psychiatry in general, and psychotherapy in particular, in the mid- to late 1950s. These medications were thought to be the tools of D-O psychiatrists who worked in state institutions and, thus, carried class and status implications for patients and physicians alike.[16] Moreover, the very notion of a chemical quick fix or a treatment that ablated tension and anxiety manifestations of deep, psychological processes read against the concept of illnesses that developed over lifetimes and treatments guided by specially trained clinicians over years of fifty-minute hours. Throughout the decade and into the 1960s, the *AJP* published numerous articles and editorials by leading psychiatrists who were critical of, or hostile to, the use of psychotropics and who openly questioned the qualifications of those who prescribed them. R. Finley Gayle's "Presidential Address," published in July 1956, warned against undue enthusiasm about medication, while Lothar Kalinowsky's "Appraisal of the 'Tranquilizers'" attacked "misconceptions, discrepancies, confusion, and sketchy contradictions" surrounding the use of the tranquilizers and the "lack of psychopathological observations in individual cases"—a clear reference to D-O experience and training.[17] And Percival Bailey's erudite "The Great Psychiatric Revolution" argued for closer readings of Freud while employing Freud's binary of masculine reason and feminine nature to mock the use of drugs that "may calm the patient long enough to make him more accessible to other forms of therapy, or long enough to let nature take her course, and so make him easier to care for . . . but that have also deleterious effects and cannot be given indefinitely. They are not replacement therapies."[18]

Bailey's insistence that medications were not "replacement therapies" illustrates an important theme: from the earliest descriptions of their clinical effects, prescription psychotropic medications were defined in the *AJP* by their capacity to assist in, but not to replace, the embodied psychotherapeutic and psychoanalytic interactions between therapists and patients. Medications and other "organic" therapies may have decreased patients' resistance and bolstered their self-image. But such effects were, it was often pointed out, performed wholly in the service of the psychotherapist or psychoanalyst and the theoretical system that he served. For instance, as the prolific academic psychiatrist Paul Hoch wrote in an October 1955 "special article" entitled "Progress in Psychiatric Therapies," "There has recently been a great deal of activity in the biochemical and pharmacological approach in psychiatry. . . . An increasing number of chemical compounds are offered which influence mental symptomatology to varying degrees." And, while Hoch acknowledged that "their value in psychiatry is still not properly assessed because they have been used for a comparatively short time," he criticized research showing that "new compounds such as Rauwolfia serpentia and chlorpromazine are very effective in certain psychiatric conditions, for example, in controlling excitement states, reducing or eliminating confusional states, and in many instances clamping down on tension and anxiety manifestations." Hoch made clear that, while such effects had the potential to alter "the psychotherapeutic procedure" by providing exogenous means of reducing an individual's anxiety and increasing "his" ego strength, "the underlying (neurotic) disorder still remains" until it is "psychodynamically" extracted.[19]

Similar sentiments were expressed in "regular articles" as well. For example, in his June 1956 "The Uses of Drugs in Psychiatric Research," the

National Institute of Mental Health psychiatrist Abraham Wikler explained that "drugs have interested psychiatrists mainly because of their possible uses in therapy" and that the bulk of clinical research on psychotropic agents "consisted of therapy-oriented studies, the results of which are expressed in terms of percent 'cured' [of neurotic conditions] or 'improved.'"[20] Meanwhile, "research reports" and "clinical notes," such as the State University of New York College of Medicine professor Jerome Schenk's "Anxiety-Depression and Pharmacotherapy" and Joseph Barsa's "Use of Chlorpromazine Combined with Meprobamate," both published in June 1958, described the "alteration, through anxiety reduction, of the patient's psychodynamic equilibrium" via talk therapies enhanced by tranquilizers.[21]

Even drug advertisements, surely aware that they were playing to a skeptical audience, presented their products as helpers of, rather than replacements for, the male psychotherapist's ability to analyze and expose the neurotic remnants at play in interpersonal interactions. *Augmentation* and *adjunct* thus became common terms: "Sandril facilitates psychiatric treatment," a 1956 advertisement for the tranquilizer claimed above a picture of a psychotherapy interaction; "Miltown moderates tension and anxiety, affording better accessibility and rapport in psychotherapy," added a 1960 promotion for the tranquilizer meprobamate, under the heading "Miltown: An Effective Adjunct to Psychotherapy."[22] As Janet Walker rightly argues in her analysis of pharmaceutical advertisements from the late 1950s and early 1960s, these advertisements were almost always configured to demonstrate the superior vantage point of the psychotherapist, whose position allowed him to look down on the patient; medications, moreover, were simply never pictured in the images. Walker discusses Sandril advertisements in which "a beam of light projects from behind the white-haired doctor, onto the anxious woman . . . a bright light that isolates her fundamental details or supposed essence as it isolates her figure, presenting her for psychotherapy and the rehabilitation with which it is coupled."[23] Supporting this point are also advertisements for the sedative Deprol promoting the notion that medications "help" the psychotherapist by improving the neurotic depressive patient's "ability to work with you toward emotional and social readjustments."[24] The assumption in each case was that medications had clinical validity only within a system where psychotherapy remained the economy of interaction (see figs. 4 and 5). Psychotropic drugs may have helped patients reach a neurotic "equilibrium," thereby rendering them more amenable to therapeutic intervention. But such actions took place only in the service of A-P psychia-trists and the Oedipally gendered, psychodynamically maintained system that they represented. Therapist remained divided from patient, father from mother, conscious from unconscious, thereby enabling (with the assistance of pharmaceutical adjuncts) the transference-countertransference interaction to take place.

Despite the rigid insistence on the primacy of psychodynamics, however, the 1950s were also a time when the A-P treatments promoted by the *AJP* came increasingly under attack for their lack of scientific rigor and proof of outcome. Discontent with the scientific validity of psychoanalytic theory and practice grew ever louder through the decade, exemplified in its most extreme form in the British psychologist Hans J. Eysenck's notorious 1957 study "The Effects of Psychotherapy." Eysenck evaluated nineteen studies of psychoanalytic and psychotherapeutic treatment reported in leading journals including the *AJP* and noted "little agreement among psychiatrists relating even to the most fundamental concepts and definitions." "In the absence of agreement between fact and belief," he wrote, "there is urgent need for a de-crease in the strength of belief, and for an increase in the number of facts available. Until such facts as may be discovered in a process of rigorous analy-sis support the prevalent belief in therapeutic effectiveness of psychological treatment, it seems premature to insist on the inclusion of training in such treatment."[25]

Although Eysenck's review concluded with a radical damnation of the psychotherapies ("there thus appears to be an inverse correlation between recovery and psychotherapy; the more psychotherapy, the smaller the re-covery rate"), his call for scientific analysis, evidence, and uniformity were mirrored in the *AJP*.[26] As but one of many examples, Hoch's "Progress in Psychiatric Therapies" argued that "there is great need for better scientific evaluation of psychiatric therapies. . . . [W]e lack a comprehensive method-ology of evaluating improvement in a patient. Criteria of improvement are judged by different psychiatrists in different ways, because there is no agree-ment as to criteria."[27]

In articles that did, in fact, present outcomes research for psychodynamic methods, however, the paucity of externally validated efficacy was not the only arena in which psychoanalytically influenced treatments were found to be lacking: A-P formulations also failed to maintain the internal structure of psychoanalysis itself and specifically the Oedipal structure whereby the

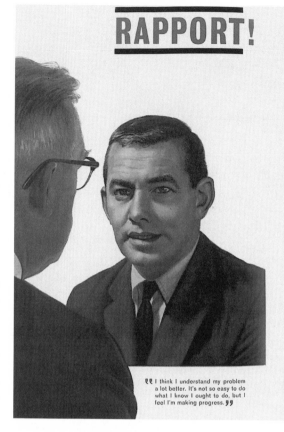

4. As promoted, Deprol helps the patient work with you: Deprol advertisement (*American Journal of Psychiatry* 120 [1964]: xxx–xxxi).

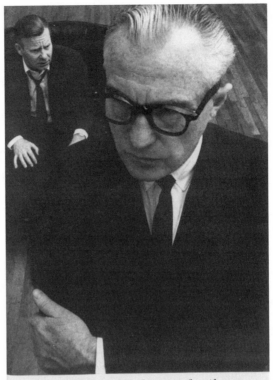

5. Augmenting a man's authority: Taractan advertisement (*American Journal of Psychiatry* 123 [1966]: xlxi–xlxii).

A particularly useful therapy for the anxious patient with coexisting depression

rejection of the "mother" and identification with the "father" provided the point of entry into functional adult life. Studies that were otherwise supportive of psychodynamic treatments reinforced a less-hegemonic reading of the ways in which psychotropic medications acted as the helpers of men. As a key example of this point, Bernard C. Glueck wrote in the February 1956 *AJP* that "the clinical material which forms the basis for the discussion and conclusions presented in this paper has been gathered during the past 3 years by the members of the Sex Delinquency Research Project of the New York State Department of Mental Hygiene." The paper to which Glueck referred, "Psychodynamic Patterns in the Homosexual Sex Offender," described a study comparing thirty "homosexual pedophiles" imprisoned at Sing Sing Prison to thirty "rapists" and fifty "burglars, forgers, and other nonsexual offender controls" with regard to "etiology, prognosis, and ther-

apy of these antisocial acts."²⁸ As the article title implied, the orientation of
the study was entirely psychoanalytic. Each prisoner underwent three "extensive" psychiatric interviews complete with Rorschach tests and dream
analysis. Rapists and controls were most often diagnosed with "character disorders," while homosexual pedophiles overwhelmingly suffered from
pseudoneurotic, pseudopsychopathic, and overt schizophrenia.

Like many psychoanalytic studies of the *DSM-I* era, "Psychodynamic
Patterns in the Homosexual Sex Offender" pathologized "homosexuals" by
their "marked fear of sexual contact with the adult female," accompanied by
"genital diminution fears." "Homosexual" men reported diminished heterosexual interests, marked impairment of heterosexual activity and functioning, and overwhelming "post-intercourse anxiety," characteristics that were
in sharp contrast to those seen in "the rapists and the controls." In response
to a Thematic Apperception Test image of a "seminude female lying in a bed
with a man in the foreground," 93 percent of these men rejected "the usual
heterosexual theme" and exhibited "marked hostility toward the mature
female sex object," who was often described as "sick, dying, or dead." Too,
in evaluating their adult sexual performance, the study found that "60% of
the homosexual offenders have never married, even though they are all older
than 21 years old." The men expressed various "rationalized and distorted"
reasons for their lack of marriage, ranging from sexual and personal difficulties to economic hardships.²⁹

"Psychoanalytic" exploration uncovered deeper and more long-standing
explanations for the men's failure to marry, and, indeed, for their homosexuality, explanations having to do with past history and self-image. Seventy-
eight percent of the "homosexuals" demonstrated some level of "femini-
zation," compared to only 26 percent of the rapists and 20 percent of the
controls. The former category of men also showed a complete inability to
produce a "compensatory 'tough guy' attitude," the direct result of "restric-
tive, punitive, and threatening" parental attitudes toward the child's early
sexual interests and activities. "In the present study, less than 10% of the
men were given any kind of structured sexual information," the text explains, while "only one was given adequate information." Not surprisingly,
these findings pointed to a "serious impairment of *conscious* formation, and
resultant impairment of restraining effects of *conscience* on overt behavior,"
with the terms *conscious* and *conscience* implying the domains of selfhood
formed through a specific interpretation of Oedipal resolution. Over 50 per-

cent of homosexual sex offenders described an "absent father," whose lack of presence caused incomplete separation from the mother, poor conscious/unconscious division, and, ultimately, an impaired ability to enter and adhere to the mores of civilized, heterosexual society. These characteristics defined the "homosexuals" as such—all the more since their "pedophilia" was simply never mentioned in the article and the other groups of men were continually described as "heterosexuals."[30]

Freud had at various points described homosexuality in more liberal terms. He argued in his early writings that male homosexuality was potentially more complicated than a mere gender switch since "a large proportion of male inverts retain the mental quality of masculinity." Pushing beyond the notion that humans were constitutionally bisexual, his case study of the Wolf Man described a so-called negative Oedipus complex, a "pre-Oedipal narcissistic masculinity" construed through a boy's desire for his powerful father and jealousy toward his mother.[31] *Narcissistic* in this context implied a fixation with similarity that, in the case of certain "homosexuals," undermined their need for attraction to "difference" in the castration complex. The Wolf Man was simply not attracted to women because he was already attracted to men—a point that, although it threatened to read against the notion of a gender binary, fell out of Freud's later work.[32] So, too, this notion of homosexuality was explicitly negated in "Psychodynamic Patterns in the Homosexual Sex Offender," which makes it clear that homosexuality was an entirely post-Oedipal condition. Following *Civilization and Its Discontents* and, to be sure, the *DSM-I,* "homosexual" men were not wholly men in the neurotic sense, having never fully identified with their absent fathers, and were, thereby, differentiated from the rapists, burglars, and other neurotic "controls" who were so defined, not by the severity of their crimes, but by the strength of their superegos.[33]

The study's explicit goal (as determined by its funding source, the legislature of the state of New York) was to develop treatments that would allow the homosexuals to reenter society successfully. Yet, while psychoanalysis was shown to be excellent at diagnosis, in effect interpreting homosexuality as supporting evidence for psychoanalytically defined heterosexuality, the study was despite its best efforts confoundingly unsuccessful at providing a cure. Therapist teams composed of psychiatrists, psychologists, and psychiatric social workers, "all with considerable professional experience and skill," provided individual and group therapies in accordance with "psychoanalytic dynamics" for periods of up to three years per prisoner. These interventions yielded a complete "lack of significant improvement," and permission was then obtained to use "organic therapies of various types on the inmates." The article's final paragraph explained that electroshock therapies then brought about improvement in 53 percent of the men, as measured by a decrease in "symptoms," a lessening of "anxiety," and greater control of "impulses." Moreover, "a number of the men have been started on some of the newer drugs that have been introduced in the field of psychiatry in the past year," including major and minor tranquilizers. The "promising results" of these organic therapies led the author to conclude by calling, not for expanding psychoanalysis, but for increasing the availability of the D-O treatments that were, according to Maciver and Redlick, widely held to be psychoanalysis' antithesis.[34]

In "Psychodynamic Patterns in the Homosexual Sex Offender," medications were helpers of men because they helped homosexuals become the men that psychoanalysis wanted them, but could not help them, to be. Psychoanalysis effectively identified and articulated the threat posed by homosexuals to a specific, Oedipally derived notion of gender, manifest through a rejection of the "usual" heterosexual response. Yet, in three years of therapy, psychoanalysis brilliantly diagnosed the problem—and failed to posit a cure. Even so, medications and other organic treatments reduced impulsivity, anxiety, and other symptoms of a malformed superego, now strengthened by chemical reinforcement. Homosexuals were then rendered more amenable to individual and group therapy and dream analysis and were, ultimately, better able to function as "men." In other words, organic therapies helped psychoanalysts provide psychoanalytic answers to entirely psychoanalytic problems, and medications helped men because these psychiatrists were not up to the task in and of themselves.

In summary, psychotropic medications were complex entities in the *AJP* in the late 1950s and early 1960s. Psychotropic medications cast A-P psychiatrists as men who embodied knowledge, authority, and an institution that was overtly resistant to organic, directive, or other nonspecialized forms of treatment. Articles, research reports, and public lectures, often written in first person by single authors, voiced wariness about psychopharmaceuticals, except when used within the strict parameters of psychoanalysis. In this sense, psychoanalysis supplied the interpretive grid whereby the problems of the patient were conceptualized in a manner that stabilized the gender of the psychiatrist, who was often in a position of guarding the integrity of the hetero-sexual binary by employing the paternalistic terminology of the *DSM-I* or by treating homosexuals to ensure their successful reintegration into civili-zation. At the same time, medications also illuminated a lack of the potency that they claimed to enhance. The very need for a product that helped the doctor treat the patient carried with it the a priori assumption that the doctor had not been able to treat the patient before. Psychiatrists could not, in other words, maintain order well enough on their own. Rather, once within the prison walls, they required medication to help them control their patients and to differentiate their patients from themselves.

Crisis, and the Biology of Change

In the November 1973 *AJP,* Manheimer, Davidson, Balter, et al. pub-lished "Popular Attitudes and Beliefs about Tranquilizers," reporting on the results of a nationwide survey. Their study, conducted between 1970 and 1971 in collaboration with the Psychopharmacology Research Branch of the Na-tional Institute of Mental Health, reported evidence from interviews with 2,552 Americans between the ages of eighteen and seventy-four concern-ing the rise in popularity of tranquilizers over the past decade. Interview techniques included word association ("What comes to mind when I say tranquilizer?"), agree/disagree/don't know questions reflecting general atti-tudes and beliefs about efficacy ("Tranquilizers work very well to make a person more calm and relaxed"), and a series of open-ended scenarios meant to test participant willingness to condone tranquilizer use ("Let's assume that someone has a supply of pills on hand that a doctor prescribed and said take as needed. These pills calm you down or make you feel more relaxed [*or* These pills make you feel more energetic or alert, or lift your spirits]"). In prefacing the scenarios, the authors asked readers to "notice that the em-phasis was on the effects the drugs produce rather than on names of drug classes."[35]

After extensive analysis, the authors found "considerable evidence that Americans believe in the efficacy of psychotherapeutic drugs," although con-siderable divergence with regard to the implications of such efficacy. "Gen-eral information" was also statistically significant, for almost 70 percent of respondents had "adequate knowledge about the tranquilizers' desired effect —to calm, relax, or relieve anxiety." Much more significant, however, was the glaring omission in the article's text: through eight journal pages, six tables, and numerous clinical vignettes, no mention was made of psychotherapy or psychoanalysis. Indeed, psychotherapy and psychoanalysis were notable for their absence from the places that they had occupied in earlier decades. The article mentioned no A-P psychiatrists in its references, for example, instead citing the work of such academics as the prominent psychiatrist Gerald Klerman, who would lead a call for a biological revolution against psychoanalysis and psychotherapy in the years immediately following the article's publication. Even more glaring, the questions asked of participants, and, indeed, the article's text, uniformly assumed that the medications—not the men who had prescribed them—were the agents of psychological change. Tranquilizers "worked" to render patients more relaxed, "calmed" anxious nerves, "made" them more energetic or alert, and ultimately "produced" clinical effects. Medications were, thus, imbued with the same powers once attributed to psychotherapy, only, in "Popular Attitudes and Beliefs about Tranquilizers" at least, the psychotherapist was nowhere to be found.[36]

Given the prevalence of this approach, it is easy to understand why the 1970s are commonly thought to be the point of origin of the biological revolution in psychiatry: if in the *AJP* medications were helpers of men in the 1950s, then medications *became* men two decades later. Throughout the 1970s and 1980s, clinical reports, research articles, and topical papers, often authored by teams of neuroscientists, described the ways in which psychotropic medications performed the actions once carried out by psychotherapists. Tranquilizers, sedatives, antidepressants, and, most of all, benzodiazepines, calmed anxious nerves, made people feel relaxed, allowed for insight, and lifted mood and affect all at once. At the same time, the pages of the *AJP* filled with images of medications and medical technologies, from pharmaceutical advertisements that showed oversized capsules and tablets to fluoroscopic depictions of the actions of the benzodiazepines at benzodiazepine-gammaaminobutyric receptor complexes in the hypothalamic-pituitary-adrenal axis. All the while, representations of A-P men faded away like neurotransmitter molecules at a synapse. First-person descriptions of clinical interventions and transcripts of presidential addresses and keynote lectures no longer highlighted the thoughts, actions, or expertise of A-P men, and, beginning in the late 1970s, A-P men never appeared in images, in advertisements, or in the "Images in Neuroscience"—formerly "Clinical Images"—section.

The timing of such a transformation was, of course, far from happenstance. Psychiatry experienced a serious crisis in the mid-1970s, when its operational methods no longer met professional norms. "Psychiatry today faces sociopolitical, economic, and philosophical pressures that threaten its existence as a valued medical specialty," Eaton and Goldstein wrote in "Psychiatry in Crisis," which appeared in the April 1977 *AJP*. "Forthcoming legislation and federal health policies will be related to the ability of the profession to demonstrate its unique role in the provision of mental health and health services."[37] The sociopolitical and economic pressures to which the authors referred were, indeed, many and were often expressed as external forces that were imposed on, and thereby threatened, psychiatry's everyday practices and provisions. For example, numerous articles in the journal in the mid-1970s decried the decision by private insurance programs and "federal health policies" to withdraw fiscal support for long-term psychotherapy, in part because of a perceived resistance by the psychotherapy community to providing proof of efficacy, and in part because psychotherapy was increasingly perceived as ineffective. Sharfstein and Magnas's "Insuring Intensive Psychotherapy" described the trend to eliminate psychoanalysis and other "intensive psychotherapies" from the range of covered treatment options as well as the practice of limiting payments to a decreasing number of office visits. This then led to difficulties maintaining the economic structure, not only of private practice, but of academic institutions as well—a point highlighted in Daniels's "The Crisis of Financing Residency Training in Psychiatry." Such changes took place within a climate in which psychiatry in general, and psychotherapy in particular, was also under attack from social movements and political theorists, such as the "antipsychiatry" movement led by R. D. Laing, Thomas Szasz, and others who sought to expose the "myth" of mental illness and the "repressive" institutions constructed for its perpetuation. "The so-called neuroses are but illness-imitative behavior," Szasz wrote in *The Myth of Psychotherapy*, "and psychotherapy the habituation of faking."[38] Even patients joined the fray: reports throughout the 1970s described physical attacks against the ineffective psychotherapist, whose methods rendered him defenseless against the unleashed anger of those under his care. Whitman, Armao, and Dent's "Assault on the Therapist" concluded that such attacks were "almost inevitable" and urged the development of "techniques for coping with assaultive patients that therapists can use in crisis situations."[39]

Meanwhile, the internal critiques of psychotherapy and psychoanalysis that were subtexts in the 1950s became master narratives two decades later. Once the foundation of psychiatric classification systems, psychoanalytic formulations of mental illness (and, indeed, of character itself) were widely condemned as "debatable etiological theories" whose validity was impossible to ascertain. Psychodynamic "uncongenial viewpoints," argued Spitzer, Endicott, and Robins, among many other critics within the emerging biological faction of academic psychiatry, led to porous categories, with little agreement regarding "clinical criteria" for diagnosis or standards for assessing improvement.[40] In "The Evolution of a Scientific Nosology," Klerman added that the interposing of "unverified [psychoanalytic] assumptions of causality into diagnostic function" resulted in nonconformity with standard "medical principles of causation in the classification of disease."[41] This point was rearticulated in many articles of the mid- to late 1970s that posited what became the widely held belief that psychoanalysis had led psychiatry on a path away from the standards and the economics of medical practice. Koran's "Controversy in Medicine and Psychiatry" attributed medical students' "disinterest" in psychiatry to the perceived disconnect between medical and psychiatric modes of sense making.[42] Sharfstein and Clark's "Why Is Psychiatry a Low-Paid Medical Specialty?" cited the extended periods that psychiatrists spent with patients as the reason why, "since 1970, the income of psychiatrists has been losing ground compared with that of other medical specialists."[43] At the same time, articles such as McCarley's "The Psychotherapist's Search for Self-Renewal" and Russell, Pasnau, and Taintor's "Emotional Problems of Residents in Psychiatry" spoke to a growing belief that the practice of psychotherapy was dangerous for a psychiatrist's well-being. "The role of psychotherapist carries with it special stresses to which many professionals react with depressive feelings, particularly in mid-life," McCarley wrote. "Psychotherapists who participated in small group sessions at two annual institutes of the American Group Psychotherapy Association revealed their depressive feelings in a striking way." The article concludes with a previously unimaginable call for the "continuing necessity for the caretaker to acknowledge and seek care for his emotional needs."[44]

Psychiatry's response to this external, internal, and, ultimately, existential crisis was to force the disappearance of men. At the most denotative level, *men* were the A-P psychotherapists and psychoanalysts who were deposed as chairs of many American academic programs and the editorial boards of leading journals such the *AJP,* to be replaced over the coming decades by psychiatrists who were, according to Bertram Brown, "concerned with biological issues and not with social problems."[45] Yet, much more important, *men* also stood for the discredited, psychoanalytically biased diagnostic system that assumed binaries of father/mother and conscious/unconscious as requisite components of normativity. Changes negotiated over the 1970s and culminating in the *DSM-III* (1980), for example, led to a radical removal of the psychodynamic underpinnings of psychiatric diagnosis. Voicing concerns symptomatic of the era, Klerman successfully argued that, as a branch of medicine, psychiatry should become "scientifically oriented, should focus on the biological aspects of mental illness, and should attend explicitly to the codification, reliability, and validity of psychiatric classifications."[46] These concerns led to the *DSM-III,* in which the developmental analytic "theories" that lay beneath psychiatric diagnostic categories were replaced by "sound empirical principles" and by a focus on discrete, "atheoretical" observational disorders.[47]

Such changes were enacted by eliminating psychiatry's most common, most notorious, and surely its most psychoanalytic diagnosis, that of one of the neurotic disorders. In the *DSM-I* (and again in the *DSM-II*), neurotic disorders were assumed to be conduits to an Oedipal past, present-day manifestations of an earlier crisis in which unconscious desire was created and subjugated beneath the evenly hovering level of consciousness, only to reemerge in dreams, slips of the tongue, or psychodynamic extraction. In the *DSM-III,* however, not only were the neurotic disorders eliminated, but their symptoms were atomized into affective, somatiform, dissociative, and anxiety disorders, diagnosed by direct observation in the examination room and "with the lowest order of inference necessary."[48] In so doing, neurosis was translated from a set of symptoms that revealed an unconscious and a past into a set of immediate observations that disavowed the very existence of, and, indeed, the notion of, the unconscious, thereby negating the theoretical bias of the observer and the gendered structure from which he observed.

Men and their biases were made to disappear from scientific reports as well. Emerging research in psychogenetics, evoked potentials, and neural pathways and neurotransmitters ushered in the creation of an "objectifiable, biological" psychiatry that eschewed the role of gender in identity formation—and, instead, looked beneath these constructs to the level of the anatomic substrate.[49] Split-brain research found that each hemisphere of the brain specialized in mediating certain functions, thereby demonstrating that what Freud (himself a neurologist) had mistaken as the "unconscious" was in fact the domain of a new neuroscience. "Music appreciation, the comprehension of puns and jokes," came, not from a repressed unconscious, but rather from the governance of a "non-dominant" but wholly, consciously observable cerebral hemisphere.[50] Hobson and McCarley's "The Brain as a Dream State Generator" discounted the role of the unconscious in the dreams that were once the royal roads to its existence, arguing that "recent research in the neurobiology of dreaming sleep provides new evidence for possible structural and functional substrates of formal aspects of the dream process. The data suggest that dreaming sleep is physiologically determined and shaped by a brain stem neuronal mechanism that can be modeled physiologically and mathematically."[51]

Even gender was removed from its psychoanalytic point of capitation. Guze's "The Validity and Significance of the Clinical Diagnosis of Hysteria" found that the condition long thought the hallmark of repression was, instead, just a disease: "A valid diagnostic classification based on the medical model is a sine qua non for progress in psychiatric research and treatment. To illustrate this point, this research reports on studies showing that hysteria, or Briquet's syndrome, is a valid clinical entity that follows a predictable course."[52] Similarly, articles published in the years after the APA claimed to have "depathologized" homosexuality, such as Tourney, Petrilli, and Hatfield's "Hormonal Relationships in Homosexual Men" and Newmark et al.'s "Gonadotropin, Estradiol, and Testosterone Profiles in Homosexual Men," assumed that homosexuality was not the result of early-life experiences and conflicts with absent fathers and castrating mothers but was instead caused by imbalanced levels of "sex hormones" and other immediately quantifiable, physiological and endocrinological absolutes. In each case, the implicit assumption was, not merely that biology had rescued psychiatry from its own biases, but that it had done so by denaturing the previously essential divide between unconscious and conscious. Split brains, neurobiological dreams, and chemical homosexuals made a larger point about the invalidity of the unconscious as a category and as an entity. The unconscious had, in other words, been rendered conscious when it was exposed as directly observable, medically predictable, and, it then followed, chemically treatable.

Psychotropic medications were the ultimate replacements for men because they carried the promise of delivering the objective, biological, and truly medicalized advances of psychiatry into the realm of treatment while eliminating theoretical gender bias once and for all. Created in neuroscience laboratories beginning in the 1950s (see chapter 3), these drugs were then tested with the "double-blind," randomized-control research methods that came into vogue in clinical trials. When psychoanalysts ran psychiatry in the 1950s, the testing of drugs had been rendered inaccurate by the frictions at play in an interpersonal interaction. Patients altered their responses on the basis of the expectation of a cure, and clinicians stepped more vigorously into the role of healer when they knew their treatments to be potent. Beginning in the late 1960s and early 1970s, however, patients and clinicians were kept "blind" as to whether the drug or the inert compound, called a *placebo,* was being administered. This setup allowed researchers to control for, and thus eliminate, the tensions that were previously the foundations of psychiatric treatment. Psychoanalysis had based its interventions on the recognition of transference and countertransference, processes that were implicitly connected to the parent/child, conscious/unconscious dialectic, later transposed onto the expectations of doctors and patients (see chapter 4).[53] Yet such erotics were rendered artifactual by an approach that meant to eliminate the unconscious through a process of randomization, thereby allowing for an unbiased, wholly conscious interaction between patient and medication. And, again, if there was no unconscious, there was no binary—a realization that freed psychiatry from the shame of its past and allowed it to join the rest of the civilized world.

Once the clinical success of the drugs was demonstrated, albeit from within a system suddenly structured to highlight their efficacy, medications were held up as sole methods of treatment, thereby replacing the need for psychotherapy.[54] Articles such as Ludwig and Othmer's "The Medical Basis of Psychiatry" cited psychotropic drugs as providing a means for altering the delivery of psychiatric treatments along the lines of the standards of other medical specialties ("the medical model represents the most useful and appropriate model available for the practice of psychiatry"), while Greden and Casariego's "Controversies in Psychiatric Education" described advances in pharmaceutical science as forcing a change in resident education in order to fulfill the prediction that "tomorrow's psychiatrist will be a complete psychobiologist."[55] And, in "The Psychiatrist," Hackett wrote that "psychiatry's historical estrangement from general medicine" and alienation from standard medical practice could potentially give way to the "hope for reconciliation, due to the recent progress of psychopharmacology" and the subsequent expansion of "liaison psychiatry within the general hospital."[56]

Similar changes took place in pharmaceutical advertisements, where the psychiatrist—who had been lauded and glorified in prior generations—was replaced by medication. While in the 1950s the interaction between doctor and patient was promoted as the therapeutic relationship, in the 1970s this interaction became secondary to the doctor's interaction with medication. Corporeal representations of psychotherapists and psychiatrists quite literally disappeared from the images of psychotropic advertisements.[57] In their stead appeared representations of patients and, ever more frequently, of capsules and tablets that grew ever larger throughout the era, assuming an agency once the sovereign domain of men. Medications drove "action," "treating," "providing," and "effecting change," and men were relegated to the passive role of prescribers. No longer adjuncts or helpers, these medications were, instead, constructed as primary visual agents.[58]

The replacement of men with medications in the 1970s and early 1980s was often interpreted in the *AJP* as the first step in the transformation of the profession from an imprecise, secretive guild to a valid, objectifiable science. To be sure, many A-P psychiatrists remained overtly hostile to the use of medications. For instance, the 1976 Survey of Psychoanalytic Practice cited an alarming reduction in the profitability of psychoanalytic practice owing to "the proliferation of other forms of treatment," most notably "the increasing use of psychotropic drugs in the management of patients who previously would have been referred for psychotherapy and psychoanalysis."[59] Yet such protests were largely superseded by the articles and research reports of an increasingly biological academy that touted the unqualified successes of these medications. True to Klerman's vision, articles by biological psychiatrists in the *Annals of Internal Medicine, JAMA,* and other standard publications of the medical establishment even came to describe "effective" psychopharmaceutical treatments, validated by double-blind, placebo-controlled trials.[60]

Together, these sources conveyed the prevailing notion that the unconscious had been defeated and that the progress of biological psychiatry and psychopharmacology in the 1970s and 1980s represented a "victory for medical science."[61] Both Spitzer, Endicott, and Robins (in 1975) and Klerman (in 1984) argued that, in the 1970s, psychiatry was transformed into an investigative science concerned with "proof claims" and that the *DSM-III* (which ap-

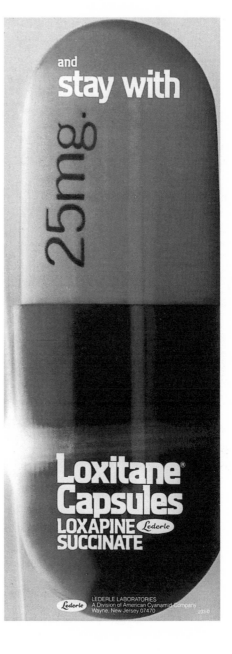

6. Capsules that command respect:
Loxitane advertisement (*Archives of
General Psychiatry* 37 [1980]: 921).
Note: For further illustration of this
point, see *Archives of General
Psychiatry* 36 (1979): 1108–9.

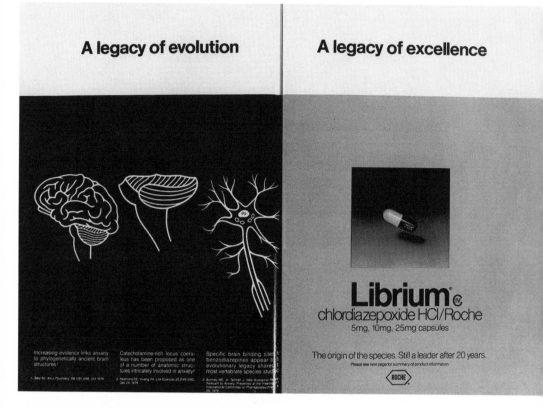

7. Evolution encapsulated: Librium
advertisement (*Archives of General
Psychiatry* 38 [1981]: 68–69).

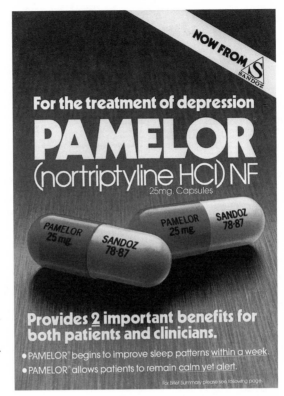

8. The benefits of
Pamelor: Pamelor
advertisement (*Archives of
General Psychiatry* 66
[1979]: 826–27).

peared in 1980) represented, according to Klerman, psychiatry's realization of "the importance of getting the diagnosis right."[62] This line of argument is taken up in Mitchell Wilson's claims that the events of the 1970s and early 1980s served to "narrow the psychiatric gaze" from a system that regarded symptoms as conduits to earlier, traumatic events to one that represented the precision of science, "laying the groundwork" for the changes that would take place over the remainder of the twentieth century and beyond.[63] And T. M. Luhrman's careful study *Of Two Minds* states that, after 1970, the "peak of public confidence in the psychoanalytic method," a decline took place with the advent of psychotropic medication.[64] In each case, the 1970s are identified—wrongly, as I argue below—as the time when psychiatry "pitched out" the notion of the unconscious in a manner that altered psychiatric practices and the profession split into "two minds," one that spoke in talking cures and another that prescribed medication.

Conclusion: The Psychodynamics of Psychopharmacology

At first glance, the end of the twentieth century and the beginning of the twenty-first represent a time when psychiatry has become medicalized beyond even Klerman's wildest dreams. Research in neurogenetics and neuroimaging, the products of a successful "decade of the brain" in the 1990s, put psychiatric research front and center, relegating gender to an object of study. While the profession enjoys a relatively secure place in many of the nation's clinics, hospitals, and academic centers, psychiatrists themselves have become harder to find in the midst of the many others who can use their diagnoses and prescribe their treatments. The *DSM* has grown larger with each successive volume, at the same time requiring less necessary inference, to the point where seemingly anybody armed with a copy of the *DSM-IV* can diagnose a psychiatric illness—and seemingly everybody has one. Depression, social phobia, premenstrual dysphoric disorder, and other shards of an exclusively skilled, religiously guarded psychoanalytic past have, thus, become the common fare of psychologists, social workers, and other practitioners of the psychotherapy that psychiatry has given up in its rush to medication.[65]

Similarly, psychotropic medications require ever less training to prescribe, in direct proportion to their ease of dosing, relatively uncomplicated side-effect profiles, and safety in the event of overdose. Treatments once argued to represent the precision of neuropsychiatry have turned into medications that are used by internists, nurse-practitioners, psychologists, pediatricians, and veterinarians.[66] For instance, in 1998, Kathleen Fairman, Wayne Drevets, et al. studied 3,101 adults who were started on either selective serotonin reuptake inhibitors (ssRIs) or tricyclic antidepressants by a psychiatrist or by a "nonpsychiatrist" internist, family practitioner, or obstetrician/gynecologist. They reported that, "among tricyclic-treated patients, psychiatrists' patients were significantly more likely than nonpsychiatrists' patients to continue in treatment for more than one month (72 percent versus 62 percent)" but that, "for ssRI-treated patients, rates of termination and therapeutic dosing did not differ significantly by prescriber type" (a somewhat uninspiring discovery for psychiatrists since the overwhelming number of prescriptions were, in fact, for ssRIs).[67]

Any victories from the revolutions of the 1970s are complicated, however, by the possibility that, at the end of the twentieth century and the beginning of the twenty-first, certain binaries are reemerging but have changed in important ways: medications, and not men, now hold the position of authority. This mechanism of action is often difficult to see among the mu-receptors, PET scans, and 5HT2 assays—a central problematic of the remainder of this project that explores the "gender" of medications and patients. For now, suffice it to say that evidence suggests that medications hold the power to ascribe new gender divisions between women and men or mothers and sons. Pharmaceutical advertisements are the most obvious example of this mechanism of action. Such advertisements occupy the first sixty printed pages of the June 1999 *AJP,* for instance, while the articles and research reports begin somewhere in the middle of the journal. As a matter of course, these advertisements leave little to the imagination with respect to gender relations or the treatments that enable them. "Power that Speaks Softly: Proven efficacy in major depression, OCD, and panic disorder," reads the Zoloft advertisement that occupies the inside-front-cover spread, above an image in which a woman wearing a centrally placed wedding ring walks hand in hand with her two male children. "Power to Relieve Depression and GAD: Effexor means effective," claims an Effexor XR ad, above a similarly contented woman who smiles as she holds her young son. In each case, the power of ordering lies, not in the hands of men, but in medications whose proven efficacy and enacted agency—to "mean," to "speak," and to provide extended release—enable these women to perform their duties as mothers to their sons. In each, the parameters of interaction are *DSM-IV* disorders—panic disorder, generalized anxiety disorder, obsessive-compulsive disorder—that represent the final remnants of neuroses, now disarticulated from their common, psychoanalytic past. And, in each advertisement, as with all others in the journal, the women are marked as married, but doctors, fathers, and other A-P psychiatrists are nowhere to be found.[68]

Drugs act as guardians of a newly created gender divide in research articles as well. Numerous late-twentieth- and early-twenty-first-century research reports, often funded by pharmaceutical companies, describe the ways in which interactions with medications differentiate women from men in a manner that attests to the newness of the treatment and the persistence of the binary in which it functions. As but one example, the prominent biological psychiatrists Susan Kornstein, Alan Schatzberg, et al.'s "Gender Differences in Treatment Response to Sertraline versus Imipramine in Chronic Depression" finds a distinction between "women" and "men" based, not on the strength of their superegos, but entirely on their responses to psycho-

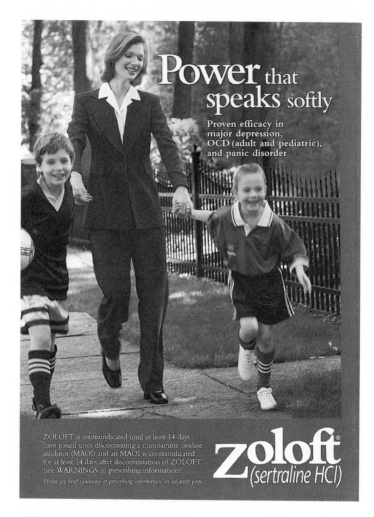

9. The power of drugs (a woman walks
hand in hand with her two children):
Zoloft advertisement (*American Journal
of Psychiatry* 156 [1999]: back cover).

tropic medications: "Women were significantly more likely to show a favorable response to sertraline than to imipramine, and men were significantly more likely to show a favorable response to imipramine than to sertraline. Gender and type of medication were also significantly related to dropout rates; women who were taking imipramine and men who were taking sertraline were more likely to withdraw from the study." Unknowingly connecting the psychoanalysis of the 1950s with the biology of the 1970s, the study then creates a structure whereby women are separated from other women on the basis of their "sex hormones" while providing clinicians an appropriate framework for their interactions with their "patients" by concluding that "the differing response rate between the drug classes in women was observed primarily in premenopausal women. Thus, female sex hormones may enhance response to SSRIs or inhibit response to tricyclics. Both gender and menopausal status should be considered when choosing an appropriate antidepressant for a depressed patient."[69] Like psychoanalysis of years past, medications both treat the symptoms and teleologically maintain the categories in which the symptoms operate.

The most compelling evidence that medications have become the new authority in psychiatry, however, comes from the position of psychiatrists themselves. In the 1950s, psychiatrists were the makers of rules and the drivers of diction. By the end of the century, however, the "treatment" relationship is assumed to be between patient and medication, continued or terminated on the basis of the nature of their interaction, while psychiatrists and other prescriber types are often discursively relegated to the role of conduit. Meanwhile, psychiatric journals that had argued that psychotropic medications were requisite for the survival of the profession now subtly suggest that the profession is in danger of falling into irrelevance owing to the success of psychotropic medications. "In the decade between 1985 and 1995," Mark Olfson, Steven Marcus, and Harold Pincus lament in a study entitled "Trends in Office-Based Psychiatric Practice," "visits in office-based psychiatry became shorter, less often included psychotherapy, and more often included a medication prescription. The proportion of visits that were 10 minutes or less in length increased." Perhaps overlooking psychiatry's own essential role in bringing about this change, the authors conclude that the situation resulted from external forces that had acted "on" a suddenly passive psychiatry: "Changing financial arrangements and new pharmacologic treatments may have contributed to these changes in practice style."[70]

Books such as *The Doctor-Patient Relationship in Pharmacotherapy*, by the psychoanalyst and APA president Alan Tasman, Michelle Riba, and Ken Silk, paint this change in a positive light by arguing that medications carry the potential to enhance the interaction between prescriber and ingestor. "It's the relationship that matters!" boasts the back cover. "Even when medication are the primary modality of treatment and the sessions are brief, the psychiatrist-patient relationship is the hinge on which the efficacy of treatment depends." However, the book jacket's insistence on the primacy of the doctor-patient relationship is undone by the text inside, which explains that the ultimate goal of the interaction is to ensure that the medications are taken, thereby allowing the "real" treatment to begin: "Ensuring compliance with medications can be accomplished more smoothly, effectively, and safely when a clinician attends to and conveys to a patient an interest in who she is, her daily life, and how the medication affects different aspects of her life. Compliance with the medication regimen is essential to a reasonable outcome in many psychiatric cases, and a mutually respectful doctor-patient relationship can only enhance compliance."[71]

In the cruelest twist of all, A-P psychiatrists finally work their way back into the *AJP* in a January 2001 special issue devoted to the topic "Empirical Evidence and Psychotherapy." The issue's lead articles highlight the advances of psychotherapy in meeting the criteria of the scientific community, linking "mind" and "brain" as it were, while "new research" reports by leading psychoanalysts tout the renewed relevance of that approach. Yet, far from celebrating a return to glory, the content of the two lead articles makes it clear how deeply and permanently the psychodynamics of the profession have shifted: both Ciechanowski et al.'s "The Patient-Provider Relationship" and Bateman and Fonagy's "Treatment of Borderline Personality Disorder" conclude that psychoanalytic methods help patients become more compliant with treatment—with psychotropic medications. To be sure, Glen Gabbard's lead editorial, "Empirical Evidence and Psychotherapy," touts the importance of psychoanalytic theories and techniques in addressing "the nemesis of both medical and psychiatric practice—noncompliance."[72] Yet, when taken as a whole and read in historical context, the issue makes exactly the opposite point: the interpersonal relationship is given meaning only in the context of the more important relationship with pharmaceuticals; and A-P men are validated, ultimately, by their ability to work in the service of medications.

It thus seems fair to say that, at the beginning of the twenty-first century, in an era when gender may or may not make a "difference," the relation between psychiatry and psychotropic medication is complex. This is because the very medications that embody the promise of psychiatry's transition "from Freud to Prozac," to recall Edward Shorter's phrase, between the years 1950 and 2002 at the same time enact conflicting implications for the profession.[73] Moreover, the profession's devaluation of the developmental theories in which binaries exist makes it more difficult for psychiatry to comprehend its own process of development, one in which standards, practices, and philosophies of care have changed with time and against time, like psychotherapy the result of real external forces and of external forces that were found to be projections of internal conflicts.[74] On the one hand, psychiatry's unqualified acceptance of a neural model, and the medications that treat it, leaves it unaware of the possibility that it is repeating its own history. On the other, psychiatry's rejection of developmental categories of gender throws its own gender up for grabs.

The former reading suggests that the change in the place of medications over time has shored up the avowed gender of psychiatry—a point that I pursue in later chapters. By this logic, medications perform the work, and the gender work, of the off-scene A-P psychiatrist while suggesting the persistence of psychoanalytic models in the face of change. The continuities between neurosis and Zoloft, or between Klerman's rejection of Freud and Klerman's position in a lineage begun by Freud, imply that the role of psychiatry as a guardian of a gender binary has in some respects expanded in the space between psychoanalysis in 1956 and Effexor XR in 2001 (because the treatment in its later iteration takes place in the offices of internists, social workers, dermatologists, and other providers of primary care). This expansion is enhanced by the fact that the treatment is effectively double-blind, denuded of the language of transference and countertransference and, thus, free to exert its normalizing effects with randomized, if uncontrolled, abandon. In each newly psychiatric setting, the potential coherence of psychiatry is reinforced by medications that act as synecdochic tools of the larger wholes of which they were once, and still are, a part. If medications became men in the 1970s, then by the end of the century medications had created a new ego ideal, a stronger, encapsulated, imagined self, representing an extension of the power of the new psychiatrist and the resilience of the models from which he emanated.

Recent work in the cultural studies of medicine and psychiatry has misperceived continuity as coherence. Specifically, scholarship based on a Foucaultian notion of power assumes that the disappearance of a corporeal form leads to new, unseen forms of regulation. For example, Lisa Cartwright argues that science has "controlled, disciplined and constructed" modern notions of the human body in ways that affect its treatment in the present day.[75] Kay Cook similarly contends that the process of "medical authoring" extends from the "physician's gaze to the medical gaze," from the empathic look of the physician to the institutionalized eye of the CT scan.[76] When extended to psychopharmacology—and once again hearing echoes of Thomas Szasz and R. D. Laing—this scholarship suggests that medications symbolize a somewhat similar form of discipline, the discipline of the mind.[77] Here, pills, as extensions of the medical establishment, demand a form of obedient control that, as Jacquelyn Zita argues, yield "a form of disciplinary expectation that goes beyond Michel Foucault's now rather quaint notions of body disciplines. . . . Pharmaceutical discipline is an expectation that calls for a psychical rearrangement of body's most intimate matter."[78] In this formulation, disappearance assumes coherence. Doctors spend less time with patients, but medications come to perform the doctor's work. Such cost-effectiveness then paves the way for the ultimate form of managed care. Prescribed, ingested, signified, and metabolized, psychotropic medications allow psychiatrists to regulate and normalize their subject from within, long after the interpersonal interaction between doctor and patient has ended.

Yet any conflation that takes at face value the ostensible power relations between old and new forms of treatment, or between disappearance and hegemony, risks overlooking the other side of this particular narrative of progress: prosthetic symbols often disguise a lack of potency rather than enhancing it. The need for a product to help the doctor help the patient carries with it the a priori assumption that the doctor has not been able to help the patient sufficiently before. From this perspective, medications can also be understood to undermine subtly the same "power structure" that they seem to uphold or to efface the psychiatry that they claim to bolster. To think this way, however, means reading the change in the position of the psychiatrist as also symbolizing a process of metonymy, a part cut off from and then standing in for a previously unified whole. This difference—between creation and augmentation or between a part of a whole and a replacement for one—then opens a space for the rethinking of panoptic notions of the gender of the powerful psychiatrist. Far from disappearing from view in the name of empowerment, the suddenly passive, anything but coherent psychiatrist might be in the process of becoming objectified within an order that threatens to render him expendable at the same time as he himself is in danger of being replaced by a less costly provider.

If this is so, then ironically Oedipal notions of development help explain how surfaces demanding to be read in the present are often also projections of the experiences of the past. Like a lost love, longings for the "real" doctor-patient relationship—a time when psychiatrists spent more time with patients, were the agents and not augmentors of their own destinies, or had the ultimate power to divide women from men without chemical assistance—are based as much in nostalgia as in reality.[79] Meanwhile, in a profession that by its own admission became more biological and objectifiable, the power vested in medications ironically becomes more abstract that actual over time since the power located in the trained body of man evolved into a power inherent in a symbol. Through this process in the *AJP* did the shift from a talking cure to a capsule, and from the language of psychotherapy to the symbolic order of psychopharmacology, become condensed into the phallic symbol of medication.

The construction of psychotropic medications as phallic is, of course, not surprising, if for no other reason than that the "potency" of medications is an explicit form of currency.[80] As I argue in chapters 3 and 4, popular magazine articles and pharmaceutical advertisements reveal numerous examples of the ways in which potency was recuperated, with the help of medications, through classic tropes of heteronormative sexual conquest. In popular magazines in the 1950s, for example, medications restore men's virility while rendering women amenable to their husbands' advances. In the *AJP*, however, the potency of medications is clearly the same potency once located in the psychiatrist himself. Articles and advertisements subtly suggest the increasing perspective of medications and at the same time trace the slow demise of the psychiatrist's own privileged spectator position. Medications grew ever larger and more active while relegating the human form to invisibility, implying the possibility that physicians were suddenly the bearers rather than the makers of meaning. Being the phallus had in the 1960s meant not seeing the phallus. But, relegated to the role of anything but coherent observers, these same diagnosticians were asked to recognize a power and a relationship to power that increasingly would not be theirs in the decades to come. "The phallus," Rosalind Minsky writes, "is a sign of power in patriarchal societies

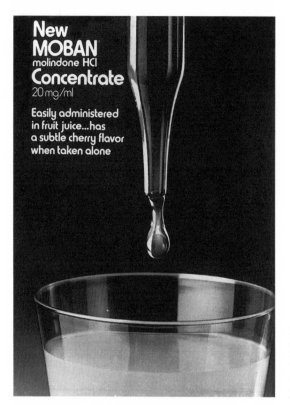

10. Promoting
pharmaceutical potency:
Moban advertisement
(*Archives of General
Psychiatry* 37 [1980]: 996).

that symbolizes a division between the sexes . . . and that those who 'have'
rather than 'lack' it are privileged."[81] What the shift in the position of the
doctor suggests, however, is the contextual nature of this binary. Doctors
who had the phallus one day might be in a position of looking compliantly
at it the next, while the prescription writing often assumed to be an extension of power and privilege can also be seen to represent the ambivalence
of power's unsteady ground.[82] In the context of the threat of a demise in
professional status, this rapid demotion then suggests an inversion of the
hierarchy set up by A-P psychoanalysis. In direct relation to the rise in power
of medications, these particular "men" were, thus, cast as "women."[83]

However, this reexamination of the psychiatrist cannot remain on the
stable ground of an inverted heterosexual binary. Quite clearly, the awareness of the possibility of lack opens a space for identification within the self-
enclosed spectrum between nostalgia and narcissism. In the former, nos-

talgic position, the subject realizes the power of pure loss, fueled by the evanescent if illusory memory of the unity, the desire for that self once imagined and then rendered conceptually impossible by the ever-shifting flow of competencies. But, in the latter narcissistic position, again thinking of the Wolf Man, one may have never lost at all. Between the 1950s and the year 2002, psychiatry was in the process of objectifying its explanations of identification, arguing that desire, object choice, and identity itself were the result of biological absolutes rather than contextual contingencies. Yet, when traced though time, the seemingly fixed position of doctor presents a startling, almost tectonic shift in the ways in which that identification was presented. Looking in from the outside, in this most negative reading of Oedipus complexes, psychiatry was asked, not to be the phallus, but to want it.

Poised in indecision between accepting and rejecting symbolic castration, or between projection and ingestion, lies the possibility that psychiatry's professional crisis was an identity crisis as well.[84] To be sure, pharmaceuticals provided a system in which prescription writing offered a means of recuperation, an externally imposed superego for a profession whose unconscious threatened to drag it into bankruptcy. At the same time, the specific manner of resolution both flipped the binary and called it into question. In so doing, in the discursive lineage of the *AJP*, medications then suggested a means for briefly stepping outside the compulsory heterosexuality—and its implicit connections to notions of progress—deeply ingrained in pharmaceutical discourse while still remaining within the system. As Freud and Gerald Klerman both seem to agree, the desire repressed in the formation of the unconscious involves a connection with both parents. In this sense, the medications that I describe in the next chapter as "mother's little helpers" represent the remnants of fathers as well. Psychotropic drugs hint at the ways in which resolution was not merely contained by, or recuperated through, the sense of loss insisted on by pharmaceutical advertisements, if not by psychiatry itself. Playing on the instability between positive and negative, diagnosis and prescription, losing and never having given up, or sadism and narcissism, psychotropic medications found a space from which to treat many concurrent psychodynamics. In the process, the assumptions at play in a system where men are doctors, women are patients, and medications help them both play the part begin to break down. Biology's medications then suggest new possibilities of identification and new markets of desire.

Chapter Three

ANXIETY, THE CRISIS OF PSYCHOANALYSIS,

AND THE MILTOWN RESOLUTION, 1955–60

*I*n the 1960s and 1970s, psychotropic medications seemed to burst onto the American scene. Popularized and problematized in the notion that these drugs were "mother's little helpers," the pills became known as the treatments of choice for the pressures of motherhood, singlehood, and other historically specific forms of essentialized womanhood. "Doctor please / Some more of these," sang the Rolling Stones.[1] Jacqueline Susann's *Valley of the Dolls* suggested that psychotropics were the treatment of choice for dealing with the pressures of working in a man's world, while Barbara Gordon's *I'm Dancing as Fast as I Can* informed "millions of Americans" about the untoward effects of a woman's addiction to and withdrawal from Valium.[2] And, most important, nearly all the research supporting the notion that psychotropic medications were overprescribed to women was conducted during the benzodiazepine craze that took place between 1965 and 1979.[3]

It is wholly understandable, then, that many social scientists, cultural critics, and historians of medicine assume mother's little helpers to be a 1960s and 1970s phenomenon. For example, Ruth Cooperstock's studies of medical communication trace the propensity for women to be "far more likely than men to describe their problems in psychological or social terms" (and thus "more frequently diagnosed with psychoneurosis, anxiety, and other

mental instabilities") to the wide availability of Valium and the other benzodiazepines in the 1970s.[4] In *Blaming the Brain,* Eliot Valenstein similarly
locates the problem in the 1970s, arguing that "there is no doubt, as in the
Rolling Stones song 'Mother's Little Helper,' far too many women had the
habit of 'running for the shelter' of the pill that would help them get through
their day."[5] And, in *Small Comfort,* Mickey Smith's analysis of pharmaceutical trends begins in the mid-1960s because, according to Smith, few data
exist supporting the argument that "tranquilizers and other anxiolytics were
overprescribed to women in the 1950s," in the way of outcome studies, cost-
benefit analyses, or other means by which gender-imbalanced prescription
patterns would later be assessed.[6]

Emphasis on the Valium craze of the 1970s, however, has caused many
scholars to overlook the 1950s as a decade in which key links were forged between "mothers" and psychopharmaceutical medications. During the 1950s,
the notion that the newly discovered tranquilizers for outpatient psychological problems treated existing concerns about a host of specifically maternal conditions entered the American cultural imagination. Whether or
not this association between mothers and medications took place in clinical interactions,[7] it clearly did in the popular print sources that are my focus
in this chapter. Between the years 1955 and 1960, articles about pharmaceutical miracle cures filled leading mass-circulation newsmagazines (*Newsweek,
Time, Science Digest*) and women's magazines (*Cosmopolitan, Ladies' Home
Journal*). These magazines reached vast audiences and were immensely influential in presenting a new type of doctor-patient prescription interaction
to middle-class America.[8] Health columns such as Henry Safford's regular
"Tell me Doctor" section in the *Ladies' Home Journal* and Walter Alvarez's
"Ask the Doctor" in *Cosmopolitan* explained how, thanks to psychopharmacology, "emotional" problems could be cured simply by visiting a doctor,
obtaining a prescription, and taking a pill. Invariably, these problems ranged
from a woman's frigidity, to a bride's uncertainty, to a wife's infidelity. The
predominance of such conditions suggests how psychopharmaceuticals came
of age in a postwar consumer culture intimately concerned with the role of
mothers in maintaining individual and communal peace of mind. As a result,
the 1950s set precedents connecting women and psychopharmaceuticals that
would play out in the 1960s, 1970s, and beyond.

In what follows, I explore this marriage of mothers and medications
through the rhetoric surrounding Miltown (meprobamate), the "miracle

cure for anxiety" that became America's first psychopharmacological wonder drug. Miltown was brought to the market in 1955, and the demand for it and related "minor" tranquilizers (Equanil, reserpine) soon surpassed that for any medication ever marketed in the United States.[9] Patients flooded doctors' offices demanding the drug.[10] Unable to keep up with requests, pharmacies hung window signs reading "Out of Miltown" and "More Miltown Tomorrow."[11] By the end of 1956, according to the magazine *Consumer Reports,* one in twenty Americans was taking Miltown or another tranquilizer in a given month, and, by 1957, "the number of prescriptions written for these drugs totaled 35 million—a rate of one prescription every second throughout the year."[12] "More than a billion tablets have been sold," added the January 1957 *Scientific American,* "and the monthly production of 50 tons falls far short of the demand."[13]

Ironically, many scientific sources of the 1950s claimed that Miltown's success disproved the psychoanalytic notion that character (both normal and pathological) was shaped by early-life, mother-child interactions. Instead, numerous medical-journal articles, scientific proceedings, and laboratory reports contended that the success of Miltown (and other important psychotropic drugs introduced in the 1950s)[14] catalyzed the realization that psychiatric symptoms were actually somatic phenomena resulting from aberrant electrical and chemical impulses. Such impulses could then be treated, not by an arduous progression of fifty-minute hours, but by quick, chemical interventions.[15] For instance, Hendley et al. wrote in a collection published by the American Academy for the Advancement of Science that Miltown "depresses multi-neuronal reflexes but does not significantly affect monosynaptic reflexes" and "has a selective action on the thalamus."[16] Kletzin and Berger's article in the *Proceedings of the Society for Experimental Biology and Medicine* described how Miltown affected the limbic system, which was thought to be the center of human emotion.[17] "Meprobamate," its inventor Frank Berger wrote in the *Journal of Pharmacological and Experimental Therapies* in December 1954, "has selective action on those specific areas of the brain that represent the biological substrate of anxiety."[18] Berger would later argue that, "if anxiety is indeed caused by repressed, subconscious conflicts, a feeling of helplessness, or by a disturbance of interpersonal relationships, it is difficult to see how tranquilizers would be useful in treatment."[19] These and other findings laid the foundation for Valenstein's description of psychiatry's eventual shift "from blaming the mother to blaming the brain."[20]

Through examining popular representation, however, I show how Miltown, and a seemingly gender-blind science of the 1950s, did, indeed, blame mothers in ways that helped shape psychopharmacology's mass appeal (despite the obvious fact that many fathers were among the one in twenty treated Americans). In my reading, the popular press constructed Miltown as a treatment for biological symptoms and also for the symptoms of a middle-class American culture facing a fundamental change in gender roles. The articles that I examine share a common perception that white, middle-class, heterosexual "mothers" voiced growing unrest with social pressures urging a return to the home or with the constraints of a new femininity. Many articles explicitly state that this unrest destabilized middle-class American masculinity. As Miltown's amazing success grew, a novel biological modality can be seen to posit a wondrous treatment for these concerns. The mothers in these magazines are overtly assumed to reject their maternal duties and spread a pathology that threatens to disrupt the well-being of their husbands and sons. Before medication, symptoms diagnosed in these mothers caused loneliness and suffering in men. Yet, after taking "the drug," as *Cosmopolitan* explained in January 1956, "frigid women who abhorred marital relations reported they responded more readily to their husbands' advances."[21]

In my analysis, this slippage between biological treatments and perceived social problems resulted from the ways psychopharmaceuticals were shaped by the very psychoanalysis that biological psychiatry disavowed. This is because, in American popular culture in the 1950s, psychoanalysis enabled the perception—indeed, the misperception—that women's unrest led to symptoms in men. In the first part of the chapter, I show how, in spite of biology's gains, Freudian psychoanalysis enjoyed near-hegemonic influence in defining popular notions of anxiety, depression, and other mental illnesses in American popular culture in the mid-1950s.[22] Many popular articles praised the talking cure, and many more used psychoanalytic concepts and language to describe a host of larger, cultural issues. Key for my purposes is the wide acceptance of the central analytic notion that psychiatric symptoms were the result of early-life experiences with mothers. Specifically, the belief that desire for one's mother was repressed in the formation of the unconscious, only to return as anxiety and neurosis in adult life, provided a ready language for talking about (but not treating) the inquietude experienced by men when interacting with the mother figures in their lives. As I explain at length below, the psychoanalytic binaries of "women" and "men" were easily adapted to the oversimplified gender binaries in popular representation and worked to efface many mental illnesses that had little to do with the role of women in civilization. The sources that I examine focus these often-ambiguous social anxieties onto women, during an era when a host of social, political, and economic issues combined to create the perception of what the historian Mari Jo Buhle and other scholars describe as a "crisis in patriarchal authority" in postwar America.[23]

I then provide a close textual reading of a *Newsweek* magazine cover article from 24 October 1955, "The Mind: Science's Search for a Guide to Sanity," which claims to celebrate the "progress" made by Freudian psychoanalysis in combating mental anguish. Appearing during an era commonly assumed to be the "golden age" of psychoanalytic influence in American popular culture, the piece readily calls on psychoanalytic methodologies to decry the American national neurosis during an "age of anxiety." Yet the use of Freud in this article, and in others of the same period, reveals an important difference from earlier psychoanalytically based cultural critiques: while psychoanalysis is lauded, it is also shown to be ineffective in treating the maternal anxiety that it has seemingly produced.

I next turn to popular and medical articles announcing the arrival of Miltown and other tranquilizers. To be sure, the scientific press claimed the discovery of a chemical treatment whose actions were not dependent on motherhood, daughterhood, or other developmental constructs. In stark opposition to prevailing psychoanalytic theories that assumed mental illness to have developed from repressed early life interactions, early proponents of biological psychiatry redefined character and its pathologies as chemical rather than developmental in nature, observable through newly evolving electromyelographic technology, and then treatable with psychotropic medications. In the popular press, however, the gender implications of this scientific progress narrative are revealed by the fact that, in nearly all the articles, exposés, and advice columns that I cite below (and many that I leave out), the patients in need of tranquilizers are women—frigid women, wanton women, unmarried women, and other dangerous elements who threatened to keep their wartime jobs, neglect their duties in nuclear households, or reject their husbands' amorous advances. Using language directly from psychoanalysis, these articles describe women as threatening, intimidating, dyspareunic, and other Freudian-inflected diagnoses suddenly amenable to pharmaceutical intervention.

I conclude by arguing that the overlap of psychoanalytic mothers and biological treatments complicates the notion that biological paradigms replaced psychoanalytic ones. The medical sociologist Loyd Rogler might describe the "biological revolution" as a process whereby diagnostic presuppositions and treatment options became "largely discontinuous with previous formulations."[24] Yet biology's seeming rejection of psychoanalysis is called into question by popular representations, which employ a hybridity of methods and assumptions regarding the role of women in maintaining individual and communal well-being. I thus describe the women in Miltown articles as *Freudian mothers,* by which I mean to suggest that the mother helped by mother's little helper had Freudian origins that shaped the construction of psychopharmacological medications in mainstream print culture in the 1950s. These representations illustrate the ways in which Miltown, and, indeed, biological psychiatry, came of age during a period in which psychoanalysis was deeply ingrained in the mode of sense making that governed how relations between women and men were written about, read about, and, likely, understood. Psychoanalysis aptly described a man's anxiety but was unable to provide a cure. As a result, psychotropic medications were, from their point of origin in American popular culture, often posited as treatments for a uniquely psychoanalytic condition: the disease of motherhood that disrupted the happiness, stability, and productivity of men.[25]

A great many factors contributed to the Miltown phenomenon in the 1950s, and it is not my intention to provide an exhaustive analysis of the transformation from unknown compound to cultural icon. Instead, I provide close readings of key articles describing popular sentiments about psychoanalysis, the physiological effects of meprobamate, and the success of Miltown and other tranquilizers. In the process, I uncover a deep resonance — one might even call it *transference* — between the popular appeal of psychoanalysis and the social construction of the tranquilizers. Biological psychiatry posited a new, corporeal definition of anxiety and introduced a new, pharmaceutical cure — discoveries widely argued to render psychoanalysis obsolete. But, in *Newsweek, Science Digest, Cosmopolitan,* and other magazines, this replacement is complicated by the fact that biological treatments were often presented as cures for frigidity, vaginismus, spinsterhood, momism, and a host of other ailments that were diagnosed and treated in mothers but of which fathers and sons were conceived to be the ultimate victims. At their point of origin, the agents thought to replace Freud can, thus, also be seen to participate in encapsulating and dispensing Freud's most problematic assumptions through time. By so doing, popular culture both portends the demise of psychoanalysis that would later take place in the *AJP* and situates the clinical narrative related in chapter 2 within a broader context.

Psychoanalytic Anxiety and the Crisis of Psychoanalysis

Psychoanalysis was not a uniform theory of practice in the United States in 1955. Deep divides between schools of thought, based on often incommensurate conceptual and political differences, often balkanized clinicians and critics alike. Ego psychologists split from Sullivanians, who in turn rejected Rankians and Adlerians. In American popular culture, however, psychoanalysis often meant Freud.[26] Ernest Jones's voluminous biography, *Sigmund Freud: Life and Work,* was a surprising addition to the best-seller list in 1955.[27] Movies, Broadway plays, and the popular press were so dominated by positive depictions of Freudian analysis that the historian Nathan Hale calls 1955 the beginning of the "Golden Age of psychoanalytic representation" in the United States—a phrase repeated by Mari Jo Buhle, who argues that psychoanalysis "walked hand in hand with mass culture through its Golden Age": "Its celebrity among intellectuals not only accompanied but nourished the rapid expansion of commercialized mass media."[28] Similarly, Glen and Krin Gabbard's *Psychiatry and the Cinema* describes the period between 1955 and 1960 as a brief "Golden Age" of cinema. Calling on the work of John Burnham, Gabbard and Gabbard argue that Freudian psychoanalysts represented popular culture's "authoritative voices of reason" in popular films and that analysts were regularly engaged in providing a "defense of traditional civilization."[29] As Walter Cronkite later explained on the popular television program *You Are There,* "Freud's ideas have penetrated the intellectual life of civilization. His words and ideas have become commonplace in literature, law, and medicine."[30]

In this section, I argue that, much as it was in clinical psychiatry, Freud's wide influence in popular culture was in part the result of the ways in which his theories justified a notion of heterosexuality based on structural imbalances between women and men. However, Freud–as–cultural model was not performing this very function in mass-circulation magazines at the moment that Miltown became a national phenomenon. The first point is far from revolutionary. In and of themselves, Freud's later theories posit a direct correlation between the development of the male individual and the development of civilization. Freud's definition of *anxiety* provides an important example because his use of the term directly implicates the maternal repressed as the cause of symptoms in the rational male subject and in the world where he lives and works. In *Inhibitions, Symptoms, and Anxiety, anxiety* is defined as an uncanny alarm reaction, often the result of an external danger, that causes a subject to reexperience briefly the apperception of vulnerability first realized in the Oedipal crisis.[31] Before Oedipus, the male child is a narcissistic fortress, unable to connect threats external with threats to the individual. Freud argues that, in retrospect, one (mis)realizes that this pre-Oedipal state represents the supreme position of power and that, during this state, the boundaries of the world are unquestionably and unconscionably clear: the self is unified, and those forces causing repose or insecurity are relegated, en masse, outside the boundaries of the pure relationship between a boy and his mother.

In chapter 2, I explained the ways in which the resolution of the Oedipal crisis, and specifically the identification with the father, led to the formation of a "moral" superego that allowed for individual entry in adult life. The division of a superego/father and an unconscious/mother constitutes the working order, not just of the individual, but of the larger environment in which he lives and works. According to Freud, the (male) superego's authority provides, not only the rules that allow the child to live in culture, but also the rules that organize culture itself. In *Civilization and Its Discontents,* Freud describes "the similarity between the process of civilization and the libidinal development of the individual." When the child becomes "civilized," Freud argues, he learns to assume his place in a like-structured civilization while contributing to the process whereby "civilization is built upon the renunciation of instinct." By *instinct,* Freud meant the child's acceptance and internalization of the father's moral authority and, specifically, the prohibition of desire for the mother.[32] The renunciation-by-repression of the mother qua instinct is, in other words, the foundation on which human "civilization" is built.[33] As a summation of individual identities, cultural identity depends on a painful act of repression in which the desire for the mother is pushed into an unconscious that is realized, as it were, only by the return of the repressed: slips of the tongue, jokes, sudden moments of anxiety, and other seemingly irrational symptoms come to signify remnants of the desire for the mother, returned from the underworld to rupture the individual and civilizational pursuit of progress.

Critics of Freud rightly point out that this notion of civilization, embedded in a readily neurotic conflation of individual and cultural pathologies, both requires and justifies institutional imbalances between women and men. Luce Irigaray, as one example, exposes the ways in which, in its very construction, "the social order that determines psychoanalysis rests on the unacknowledged and incorporated mother" and argues that civilization is built on a necessary "symbolic matricide." The mother needs to be repressed, in other words, in order to form the unconscious. Only with her symbolic death can the unconscious become separate from the conscious. This then allows the conscious, structured as the laws of the superego, to build a civilization. When, as Irigaray argues, the "maternal" returns and progress halts, "man turns away from his fears and projects them onto the woman."[34]

Yet these same assumptions go a long way in explaining Freud's mass appeal in the 1950s, a time when the notion that civilization was a man's world built on repressed desire for a mother whose return caused symptoms disrupting generative productivity resonated deeply with many prevailing gender tensions. The decade reverberated with the implications of fundamental shifts in gender roles manifest by a backlash against the ambitions of mothers.[35] For instance, public discourse concerning women's employment often focused on the notion that women's return to work was bad for the American economy. In the 1940s, according to a prevailing stereotype, many men had gone off to war; women meanwhile had learned to rivet in their stead. Women worked in factories in unprecedented numbers—but they also held a host of other jobs traditionally held by men, including engineer, chemist, journalist, and lawyer. Many women sought to keep their employment in the postwar period, even when men returned from the war and sought to return to work. Eighty percent of women surveyed by one major study responded that they wished to continue working after being laid off from their wartime jobs.[36] Academics such as Georgine Seward, writing in the *Journal of Social Psychology,* argued that women's employment was vital to the economy: "In the world beyond the home, women are needed as well as men for the tremendous task of reconstruction."[37] Finally, in the 1940s and 1950s, women workers were married as often as they were single, in contrast to the 1920s and 1930s—decades that saw mass employment for single women but not for married women, most of whom remained at home.[38] According to Buhle, "By 1952, the number of wives at work was triple the number in 1940; and women with children under eighteen represented one-quarter of the female work force. As a report from the 1952 Women's Bureau noted, the United States was approaching a period when 'for women to work is an act of conformism.'"[39]

Yet the 1950s were also marked by rhetoric urging women to return to their prewar roles. U.S. Senator Charles O. Andrews of Florida mirrored popular sentiment in urging Congress to "force wives and mothers back to the kitchen" in order to "ensure jobs for the millions of veterans" who had returned from the war.[40] Often-overwhelming social pressure sought to have women give up their jobs and return to their positions as happy, reproductive homemakers. Popular culture extolled a "new femininity"—really an old maternity—typified, not by the woman with her sleeves rolled up, ready to work, but rather by the woman in the Donna Reed housedress at home with her children. One might say, thinking of *Civilization and Its Discontents,* that a sudden onslaught of cultural pressure sought to return the repressed, married, and out-of-work woman back to the home as a mother. Magazines glorified the domestic sphere above all others—at least when it came to women and their interests. Articles told women, "Have babies while you're young." They asked them, "Are you training your daughter to be a wife?" They informed their readers that "really a man's world is politics" and that life was fulfilled by "the business of running a home."[41] In 1956, an often-cited *Look* magazine article celebrated the housewife as "this wondrous creature" who "marries younger than ever, bears more babies, and looks and acts far more feminine than the emancipated girls of the 1920s or even the 30s. . . . [S]he works rather casually . . . as a way of filling a hope chest or buying a new home freezer. . . . [S]he gracefully concedes the top job rungs to men."[42]

This climate made for an easy marriage between psychoanalytic theory and the concerns of what Rosalind Minsky calls *masculine identity in patriarchal culture.*[43] The conflation in psychoanalysis of individual and cultural anxiety provided a ready means for validating middle-class masculine inquietude in mainstream American culture—a connection fostered by analysts, psychologists, and social critics who called on psychoanalytic methods to decry the American "national neurosis" during an "age of anxiety" beginning in the late 1930s.[44] By the mid-1940s, Freudian ideas were used to justify an entirely domestic femininity and to mark a woman's ambition as a symptom of mental illness. The notion that in neurosis mankind was destabilized by the uncivilized presence of women thus proved an enormously popular conceptual weapon. For example, single women, working women, and other "nonfeminine" women who rejected their maternal duties were pathologized in the popular book *Modern Woman: The Lost Sex* by Marynia Farnham and Ferdinand Lunberg. Farnham and Lunberg used psychoanalytic methods to attack women's desire to leave the home as "a deep illness that encouraged women to assume the male traits of aggression, dominance, independence and power."[45] Benjamin Spock mixed Freudian techniques with his own version of American ego psychology in order to instruct new mothers to address themselves full-time to the needs of their developing children.[46] Finally, the term *momism* became common parlance in the 1940s and 1950s. Momism lay the blame for a vast array of psychological and social problems squarely on a single group of culprits: American mothers. In the hugely successful book *Generation of Vipers,* Philip Wylie blamed pathologically empowered women for the emasculation of men. Wylie attacked the domineering American mother as a "domestic powerhouse . . . who spends several hundred dollars a year on permanents and transformations, pomades, cleansers, rouges, lipsticks and the like." She "ruled" over her husband and children with "sharp heels and a hard backhand." Mothers, Wylie argued, had assumed "domestic authority" through "aggression" and "oppression." The result was a dynamic that "robbed men of their virility." As such he blamed mothers for an incredible array of maladies in men, from thumb sucking to premature ejaculation. And, since Wylie called on Freud to conflate the ills of the individual with those of civilization ("the philosophy of the state is only a magnification of the philosophy of the person"), he blamed mothers for dismembering the country as well, creating an apathetic, "sick society."[47]

Thus, in implicit and explicit ways, the notion that civilization was built on a repressed desire for a mother whose return caused symptoms disrupting productivity resonated deeply with many prevailing gender tensions of the 1950s, as given voice through the interrelation between Freudian psychoanalysis and Wylie's misogyny, Spock's traditional maternity, and Farnham and Lunberg's propriety. At the same time, when one looks at popular-magazine articles in the years surrounding the Miltown phenomenon, it be-

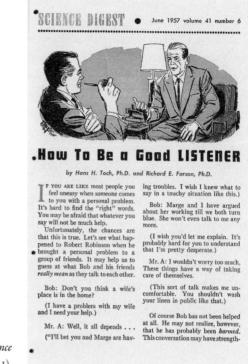

11. Learning to listen (*Science Digest*, June 1957, 1).

comes clear that psychoanalysis was not controlling the very symptoms of male neurosis that it described. Mothers still caused problems, and men suffered the consequences. As a result, numerous articles in the popular press between 1954 and 1958 reveal that America's lovefest with psychoanalysis was not entirely what it appeared to be. Although analysts were often portrayed in a favorable light and depictions of miracle cures were commonplace, analytic "words and ideas" used to describe social relations, and specifically relations between women and men, failed to defend civilization, at least in the Freudian sense. Civilization is, once again, built on repression, and that which is repressed always threatens to return as a symptom, a joke, a slip of the tongue, or the sensation of anxiety. Yet, in many popular representations of psychoanalysis, psychoanalytic treatments, or psychoanalytically influenced conditions such as momism, anxiety ran rampant.

Numerous articles in which psychoanalytically influenced talking cures are mentioned suggest that the conditions of men suffering from what can be described only as *social conditions* did not improve. In the June 1957 *Science Digest* article "How to Be a Good Listener," for example, Hans H. Toch and Richard E. Farson instruct readers about how to say the right thing "when someone comes to you with a personal problem." The trick, the authors explain, is to think psychoanalytically: "Let's see what happened to Robert Robinson when he brought a personal problem to a group of friends. It might help to guess at what Bob and his friends *really mean* when they talk to each other." Although the article proceeds to describe "the psychotherapist's tools of listening," several key points identify its psychoanalytic intentions. Differentiating between what Bob and friends say and what they "*really mean,*" for example, suggests a disconnect between manifest content and latent intent. The article also suggests that "Bob begin[s] to achieve some insight into himself" as a result of this interaction. Most important, however, is the "personal problem" that Robert Robinson describes:

> *Bob:* Don't you think a wife's place is in the home? (I have a problem with my wife and I need your help.)
>
> *Mr. A:* Well, it all depends. . . . (I'll bet you and Marge are having troubles. I wish I knew what to say in a touchy situation like this.)
>
> *Bob:* Marge and I have argued about her working till we both turn blue. She won't even talk to me any more. (I wish you'd let me explain. It's probably hard for you to understand that I'm pretty desperate.)
>
> *Mr. A:* I wouldn't worry too much. These things have a way of taking care of themselves. (This sort of talk makes me uncomfortable. You shouldn't wash your linen in public like that.)

In this rich excerpt, the personal problems are caused by a woman/wife and suffered by a man/husband. Marge's desire to work outside the home is presented as the problem and, thus, the cause of a troubled emotional state, but Bob suffers the consequences. His conscious/spoken claim that he and Marge have "argued . . . till we both turn blue" is undone by his parenthesized/unconscious admission of desperation. This emasculation, we are later told, keeps "Bob from behaving effectively or from fully experiencing personal satisfactions" and from being promoted at work. Moreover, "Bob's experience is by no means unique" but is generalizable to the multitudes of men who "suffer" similar complaints.[48]

The "treatment" described by the article then centers on helping Bob understand himself better and learning how he might better "express how he feels about something and observe what his motives are," which then helps him "re-evaluate his attitudes and his behavior."[49] In other words, Bob is asked to change himself internally, not to change his external environment. Yet such an approach clearly has no effect whatsoever on the source of the real problem: nothing at all is done to curb Marge's desire to work outside the home. Not surprisingly, at the end of the article Bob remains symptomatic and unhappy, in spite of these interventions. He may understand his problem better, but such understanding cannot neutralize the problem's maternal etiology.

The inability of psychoanalysis to treat the *real* problem, resulting in untreated symptoms afflicting a man's well-being, is a theme in many articles of the mid-1950s. *Cosmopolitan*'s "Motherhood Breakdowns, Single or Double Beds, and Office Collections," published in December 1955, follows "eight cases of women who had mental breakdowns after the birth of a child." The article diagnoses the problem as the realization that "some wives may destroy their husbands' 'masculinity,' just as some husbands may destroy their wives 'femininity.'" Either way, the result was a rampant case of "motherhood breakdown," treated by the realization that "the husband must be encouraged to build up his 'masculinity.'"[50] Similarly, in Henry Safford's September 1956 "Tell me Doctor" column in the *Ladies' Home Journal,* a newlywed husband complains, "My wife and I have been married for three months— yet it still seems impossible for us to have satisfactory marital relations."[51] Dr. Safford, a psychoanalytically attuned gynecologist and the noted author of such books as *Tell me Doctor: Frank Advice on the Intimate Problems of Women,* dispensed monthly advice concerning the "many questions which women would like to ask a trusted physician," specifically, the questions that "there is not always the opportunity" to ask. The "case of dyspareunia," however, represented something of a departure from the doctor's usual practice:

> The doctor nodded pleasantly to the couple seated in his waiting room, noting the serious expression upon their good-looking young faces. Indicating by a wave of the hand the door to the consulting room, he was slightly surprised to see the man rising to follow him. Closing the door, he pointed out a chair.
> "Your wife is not the patient?" he began.
> "Honestly, I'm not sure, Doctor," was the reply. "We have been mar-

ried for three months now and—well, it seems impossible for us to have marital relations with any satisfaction whatsoever. Every such episode has ended disastrously since our wedding night. It's gotten so that we both dread even attempting it. Both of us want a family. . . ."

"I can understand that. A satisfying sexual relationship is essential to any happy marriage."

"But what is a man to do, Doctor, when even at the beginning of each attempt she has a real spasm—and I mean an actual convolution?"

"It might create a psychological barrier that could never be surmounted. You were wise to come to me."

Only three paragraphs into the interaction, the doctor realizes that the young couple's problem is caused by a single pathogen. "Now I'm going to ask you to step into the waiting room for a few moments," Dr. Safford explains to the anxious husband, "while I talk with your wife." For the remainder of the three-page, five-column article, the wife is then described as "the patient."[52]

"It is clear that you are suffering from *dyspareunia*," Dr. Safford explains to his patient, "which means painful or difficult intercourse. This condition is commonly accompanied by *vaginismus,* which means spasm of the constrictor muscles that surround the vagina." In true psychoanalytic fashion, however, the problem is ultimately revealed to be of unconscious etiology. Vaginismus, Dr. Safford explains, results from "subconscious and involuntary contraction of these constrictor muscles." And although the dyspareunia is initially diagnosed as having a "physical cause [that] consists of a rather tough hymen," it is similarly discovered to originate in the depths of the mind:

> "Now the psychosomatic impediments are three in number, as I see them—fear of pregnancy, as inculcated by your mother, the feeling of inferiority in being female, and the childhood dogmas against sex as something sinful—"
>
> "Oh, but I don't feel that way, Doctor."
>
> "Your intellect tells you that you do not, but I fear there remain the interdictions of the subconscious mind, which are difficult to override. They are at work even when you are not thinking. But once you have developed a clearer picture of the problems in your mind, you will be able to conquer them—I am positive of that."[53]

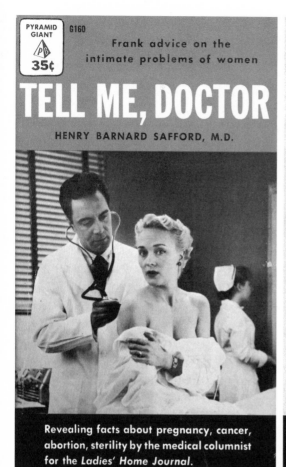

12. Dr. Safford reveals important facts
(Safford, *Tell me, Doctor* [1955], front and
back covers).

Volumes have been written about the psychoanalytic origins of frigidity called on in this passage. In *Feminine Psychology,* to take but one example, Karen Horney defined *frigidity* as a means of women's emancipation. She saw frigidity as a "determined rejection of the female role" and a "weapon expressing women's inner bitterness against the male as the privileged one—similar to the concealed hostility of the worker against his boss."[54] Within the context of Dr. Safford's column, however, the man is neither privileged nor a boss. Instead, he is sitting in the waiting room, suffering from a condition otherwise located entirely in the body of his wife. The husband, to recall, is the initial patient in the article. He describes the illness ("My wife and I . . ."), steps into the office, and earnestly asks, "What is a man to do, Doctor?" Thinking psychoanalytically, the doctor realizes that, in spite of the husband's protestations to the contrary, the wife is the patient and that her symptoms are inflicting pain on the man.[55] As such, the husband never reenters the examination room and never reappears in the text after the first paragraphs. Meanwhile, the wife's frigidity remains a potent weapon (even if the vector of illness was the mother of an "inferior female") for the simple reason that the husband's complaints remain unacknowledged, unanswered, and insufficiently addressed. Psychoanalysis may have focused its gaze disproportionately on the mother. But, in so doing, in Dr. Safford's office at least, it paid insufficient attention to the complaints of the father, who was left out in the cold both by his wife's symptoms and by the diagnostic system that defined them.

More important for my purposes is the fact that these clinical interactions represent a dynamic taking place well beyond the doctor's office or the clinic waiting room. Following Freud, the problems caused by women and suffered by men plagued civilization as well. *Cosmopolitan's* "Bigger Mamas, Bigger Babies," for example, warned that momism was an uncontrolled genetic disease of entirely maternal transfer that would live on well beyond Wylie's generation: "Birth weights of babies tend to be related to their mothers' heights, report Dr. R. H. Crawley, Dr. Thomas McKeown, and Dr. R. G. Record (England). There was little relationship to fathers' heights, indicating that it is the prenatal environment provided by the mother that counts."[56] (The accompanying piece, "Marriage Crises," then explains that "men who feel they are failures often blame their wives.")[57] Even *Science Digest's* "What's on Your Mind"—an article that explains that "all women want to be bossed" and that "it is in woman's nature to be so, and the wise man, whether her business supervisor or her husband, capitalizes on that fact of femininity"—reveals that men pay a high price for their manly role: the same "wise" men who boss their women ultimately fall prey to lost wages, "ulcer-breeding," unending "risks," and "life-shortening pursuits."[58]

The most high-profile example suggesting that male culture suffered from psychoanalytic conditions caused by mothers is a *Newsweek* "special section" that does not overtly mention mothers at all. While convention usually dictated that lead articles were but one of three or four other articles advertised on the cover, the front cover of the 24 October 1955 issue of the magazine was dominated by one story alone: "The Mind: Science's Search for a Guide to Sanity," a title illustrated by the disembodied, segmented bust of a lone male form. By all outward appearances, the eight-page article reads as an exhaustive, high-profile paean to psychoanalysis and, as such, further proof of the wide influence of psychoanalysis on the American imagination during the 1950s. For example, the article boasts that "the gist of Freudian discoveries—that the adult is in no small measure a slave to the instincts of sexuality and aggression, which become hidden in a million ways as the infant matures—has permeated in pure or distorted form almost every avenue of American thought and activity." In language strikingly similar to that used by Gabbard and Gabbard, Hale, and Buhle, the article explains that "in this day theater, the movies, and TV have almost drowned themselves in psychoanalytic plots and prose." Psychoanalysts' offices have "taken over entire sections of the nation's largest cities," including the area around Central Park in New York and a two-block stretch of North Bedford Drive in Beverly Hills known as "Libido Lane, Nightmare Alley, or Freud Boulevard." The influence of psychoanalysis has also spread to everyday life, where American mothers and American schoolteachers instruct "the young" guided by Freudian principles of childrearing. Finally, subheadings such as "The Progress," "The Treatment," and "The Hope" describe cures performed by miracle workers—most notably the deans of American psychoanalysis, Carl, William, and C. F. Menninger, who offer treatments that begin "where Freud left off." The Menningers are pictured in a quarter-page photograph in front of their bastion of psychoanalysis, the Menninger Hospital and Clinic. Patients come "from across the country" seeking palliation for otherwise untreatable conditions. Readily conflating *Freud* and *psychoanalysis* (and even *psychiatry*) the article lauds the clinical progress of the talking cure.[59]

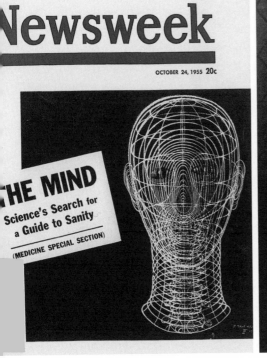

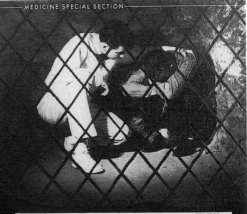

MEDICINE SPECIAL SECTION

William Campbell

THE MIND

Science's Search for a Guide to Sanity

At the most powerful and prosperous moment in their history, Americans are a notably tense people. Setting aside even the ominous mass of statistics—some 10 million suffering from mental ailments or disturbances—there is the important fact that almost every American, in one form or another, is complaining, or echoing complaints about the pressures of his time—pressures on the mind, if not the soul.

Every age has had its own pressures—the threat of the H-bomb to Americans in 1955 is probably no more horrible than the threat of the Hunnish invasion was to Romans in 455. What distinguishes this one, probably, is the totality of the change within it. The nation's

social ways, its manner of living, its way of thinking are being transformed. All this is done *without* violent outer upheaval—a fact which intensifies its people's inner burdens.

The direct reflection of this inner tenseness is the effort now lavished on exploring the mind's problems. The U.S. is without doubt the most psychologically oriented, or psychiatrically oriented nation in the world. The search into the mind's problems now goes on in the nation's art, in its schools, in its politics, even in its religion.

In this Special Section, NEWSWEEK reports on the American search for sanity—its extent, its progress, and what hope it holds.

13. The mind, ca. October 1955
(*Newsweek*, 24 October 1955, front cover).

14. Crisis in an era of prosperity
(*Newsweek*, 24 October 1955, 59).

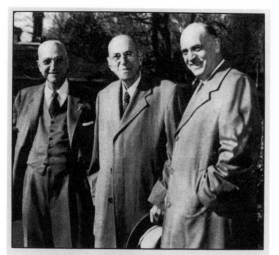

The Menningers, Drs. Karl, C.F., Bill: Papa knew first

15. Where Freud left off (*Newsweek,* 24 October 1955, 59).

At the same time, the article expresses a subtext of discontent with the ability of psychoanalysis to treat social tensions. While the text supports Walter Cronkite's notion that psychoanalysis had "penetrated the intellectual life of civilization," the article's content enters into a specific critique: in spite of the gains of psychoanalysis, white men suffer from an intractable sense of anxiety. An article that maps a Freudian model of the psyche onto America then defines *America* as floridly neurotic as a result. For example, a photograph of two white men appears above an abstract summary of the article on the special-section title page. In the photograph, a posed clinical encounter shot through a chain-link sanitarium fence, one of the men sits dejectedly in a corner with his head buried in his arms. A second man crouches above him, extending his arm around his shoulders. The second man's orderly-white uniform, combined with his open, comforting body posture, designates him as a caregiver. Set in opposition, the first man then becomes a patient—although, curiously, he appears to be wearing business clothes instead of the hospital outfits that characterized mental patients in the 1950s. Furthermore, the patient appears to be young, healthy, well groomed, and even well dressed. His hair is short and well kept. His shirt is tucked in. Yet he is the picture of despair, shamed in posture, crouched in a corner, faceless and anonymous.

The image is rendered even more discordant by the abstract below, which,

while the article glorifies the successful dissemination of psychoanalytic theories and practices, describes a virtual epidemic of anxiety spreading across
America: "At the most powerful and prosperous moment in their history,
Americans are a notably tense people. Setting aside even the ominous mass
of statistics—some 10 million suffering from mental ailments or disturbances
—there is an important fact that almost every American, in one form or another, is complaining, or echoing complaints, of the pressures of his time—
pressures of the mind, if not the soul." The subsequent paragraph of the
abstract then explains this widespread pressure by specifically differentiating between external and internal stressors. The former might be thought
to cause a state of autonomic arousal owing to an outside threat or an act
of aggression, such as a bomb or a military invasion. In 1955, however, that
Americans are "notably tense" represents a response to a threat of a different
kind, that of an enemy who is entirely within: "Every age has had its own
pressures—the threat of the H-bomb to the Americans in 1955 is probably no
more horrible than the threat of the Hunnish invasion was to the Romans
in 455. What distinguishes this one, probably, is the totality of the change
within it. The nation's social ways, its manner of living, its way of thinking
are being transformed. All of this done *without* violent outer upheaval—a
fact which intensifies its people's inner burdens."[60]

A final site of disruption in the presentation of psychoanalytic progress
occurs along the bottom of the second and third pages of the article, where a
series of *New Yorker* cartoons appears beneath the columns of text. Each cartoon depicts farcical scenes of psychoanalytic treatments in which white male
analysts interact with white male patients. The analysts appear in business
suits, are middle-aged, and are alopecic—strikingly similar in appearance, in
other words, to the Menningers. Moreover, the interactions between doctors and patients presented in each cartoon form mocking contrasts to those
"astonishing" alliances described as taking place at the Menninger Clinic. In
the text, the Menningers forge "successful" and "skilled" clinical relationships with those in need. But, in the jokes presented below the text, the relationship is based on antipathy and greed. In one cartoon, an analyst blurts
to a startled patient in repartee, "Why, you swine!" In another, an older man
nervously bemoans missed stock purchases, while, in a third, the analyst asks
a smug patient, "When did you first discover you were the salt of the earth?"

These moments of discord make no sense sociologically. By many leading
indicators, the era was as prosperous for white men as it was for psycho-

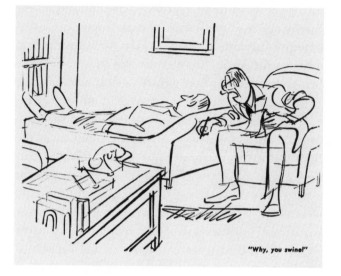

"Why, you swine!"

16. Undercutting the message (*Newsweek,*
24 October 1955, 60–61).

analysis. The country was in the midst of a period of unprecedented economic growth and, save for the Korean War, relative political calm. The Second World War was finally over. Marshal Plan America was in the process of becoming a world power. Ozzie and Harriet Nelson showed the new television audience the happiness of family life. Real-life Americans, too, shunned the conflicts that had dominated the social climate in the decades before and, according to many social scientists, focused instead on matters closer to home.[61] In other words, there was little reason for what the sociologist Emile Durkheim described as *anomie:* disturbances in the "collective order" of society in times of disorganization and upheaval.[62] According to Durkheim, periods of economic and social instability (recessions, economic depressions[63]—although, notably, not warfare) engender widespread feelings of disconnectedness and despair, leading to anxiety. Anxiety then becomes quantifiable, measured by such variables as the divorce rate, the crime rate, and the suicide rate.

By these standards, the 1950s were not a time of mass anomie. Many baseline indicators of well-being had steadily improved since the end of the war. It was widely believed that brightening economic conditions led to stable rates of employment and to generalized "optimism."[64] Suicide, central to

Durkheim's formulations, remained mostly stable throughout the decade, and divorce rates would not begin to rise until the 1960s.[65] In spite of the cold war, research indicating widespread feelings of prosperity and satisfaction, as in the satisfaction required to produce and reproduce, led many scholars in subsequent years to conclude that the 1950s were a decade of social stability and that anxiety was at an all-time low as a result.[66]

A second reason why the disjunction between prosperity and anxiety in *Newsweek*'s search for sanity does not make sense is that it is entirely unexplained by the article.[67] The "notably tense" Americans and "the pressures of his time" might have implied racial tensions during an era in which the civil rights movement was just beginning to take shape—in October 1955, for example, Martin Luther King was preparing to lead a boycott of the Montgomery bus system. Fighting a "change within" could have referenced fascism, Japanese internments, Red scares, or other examples of enemies discovered to have infiltrated the sanctity of Troy.[68] Or the tensions could have been caused by a rapidly changing postwar consumer culture in which, in the last week of October 1955, the Coca-Cola Company introduced the name *Coke* and the Tappan Company of Mansfield, Ohio, introduced the world's first microwave oven (able to cook eggs in just minutes—at a price of only $1,200). Well-dressed white men, missed stock opportunities, and "Why, you swine!" could have implied the class tensions of a psychoanalysis that would in the years to come increasingly be thought of as a treatment by the rich for the rich.[69] My point, however, is that one cannot know the cause of *Newsweek*'s anxiety because these generative moments are not qualified, substantiated, or even referenced by the article—even though nearly all the subsequent points that it makes are described in detail that would surely have been elaborate by the conventions of the mass media at the time. Readers learn, for example, that "106 young men and women from more than ten countries" trained at Menninger Memorial Hospital in 1955, that the new hospital wing contained 113 new beds, and that, "at 62, Karl Menninger has taken on much of the benign, paternalistic temperament of his father": "He is a vigorous, youthful man, whose speech crackles with homely epigrams. With his pretty, dark haired second wife, the former Jeanetta Lyle, and his young daughter, Rosemary, Karl lives in a comfortable white Colonial house in North Topeka."[70] Yet the article's main point—the picture of the two men accompanied by an abstract describing a national sense of malaise—serves as the benighted front surface of an article whose depth seems to go in an entirely different direction. Moreover, the text inside is undone by the cartoons below, as if ruptured by jokes or slips of the tongue in an otherwise coherent narrative.

But the search for sanity makes psychoanalytic sense, in so much as the condition that it describes is a sense of unease in the present as well as a metaphor for an ill-defined set of prior events. Reading the article psychoanalytically helps explain its inconsistencies. Ironically, it also illustrates how widespread symptoms of pressure and tension experienced by an America gendered as male and depicted entirely by white men are as much *caused* by psychoanalysis as they are treated by it. Placing a psychoanalytic grid over the problems of the nation, the article that lauds Freud is, thus, also an article that posits, and then critiques, specifically Freudian definitions of the maternal repressed as the cause of cultural pathology in October 1955—even though mothers are not manifestly mentioned in the exposé.

In reading the article in this way, it is important to notice the differentiation between external and internal stimuli—the "H-bomb" or a "Hunnish invasion" as opposed to a "people's inner burdens." In *Inhibitions, Symptoms, and Anxiety,* Freud separates two responses to the threat of an approaching danger in the present that can trigger a mobilization of the ego's defenses.[71] When the danger is external and, thus, directly felt, such as a bomb or a military assault, this signal is called *fear.* But, when the ego reacts to an internal stimulus—a response, not to a present stimulus, but rather to an "unconsciously or automatically controlled past, fearful state"—then the result is called *anxiety.*[72] This notion of anxiety is intimately tied to the resolution of the Oedipal crisis, a requisite event in male psychical development. For Freud, the events of the Oedipal crisis lead to the internalization of the once-rivaled father—an awareness that becomes part of the self through the formation of a superego that is at once a guide for interacting in civilization and an always-critical internal voice—and the repression of desire for the mother into the unconscious.

So, too, an unquestioned sense of unity rendered *Newsweek's* postwar America able to deal with military threats precisely because these were perceived as functioning outside the boundaries of self or nation—"the threat of the H-bomb to the Americans in 1955 is probably no more horrible than the threat of the Hunnish invasion was to the Romans in 455." Americans have only recently become aware of their country's lack of unity, their own inner burdens: growth at "the most powerful and prosperous moment in their history" is always and already tainted by the fact that, like the crumpled man in the corner, they are beset by vulnerability. Prosperity begets development, but development is called into question by the souvenir, the lost love, the return of the maternal repressed. Her vindictiveness is experienced by American civilization—in an America assumed in images, cartoons, and text to be communally male—as pressures of the mind, if not of the soul. Thus, in the 1950s, America suddenly discovers that 10 million are suffering from mental ailments or disturbances, and almost every American is echoing complaints of "the pressures of his time." The result is the symptom often undetectable by physical exam yet imbricated in social vignettes: ways of living, ways of thinking, and other examples of traumatic encryption.

Of course the maternal repressed is not the same as a real mother. Neither *Newsweek*'s reference to the disruptive unconscious, nor *Cosmopolitan*'s "bigger mamas" and their "bigger babies" or its "eight cases" of "motherhood breakdown," nor the mothers whom Congress tried to "force . . . back to the kitchen" can be mapped onto the lives of real women in the 1950s. Indeed, the voices of real women are almost never heard in the sources that I examine in this chapter. Not one woman is quoted in "The Mind," for example, and the psychiatrists pictured are all men. Robert Robinson speaks freely about his problems with Marge's need to leave the home, but Marge herself never quite makes it into the discussion. "Motherhood Breakdowns" claims to trace the problems of psychotic mothers, but the actual mothers never get to voice their delusions and hallucinations or any other first-order symptoms. And, of course, the articles were all written by men. Similarly, just as women rarely spoke on the floor of Congress, so do Henry Safford and Phillip Wylie both use quotes attributed to women but written in the author's own voice ("Oh, but I don't feel that way, Doctor"). In each case, the mother is defined through the perceptions, interpretations, and responses of someone else.

I call these *Freudian mothers,* not because Freud discovered the essential qualities of motherhood, but because he described the dynamic whereby mothers were constructed through the projected anxieties of men and, thereby, legitimated a wholly unquantifiable feeling of discontent known in 1955 as *anxiety*. The Freudian mother ruptured the progress of conscious mankind through ulcers, lost wages, or a spasmodic dyspareunia in which the woman's spasm clamps down on the man's widdler. The pain of intimacy was, in this case, a dolorous sensation realized by only one member of the interaction. And, as *Newsweek* makes abundantly clear, psychoanalysis was the only hope of treatment, the sole guide leading America in its search for sanity.

Yet my point, once again, is that psychoanalysis was not working. To be sure, psychoanalysis provided an important diagnostic model for describing, and even for exploring, the threat to men signified by the return of the maternal repressed. And the notion of neurosis allowed for a recognition that a previously unlabeled and unacknowledged discomfort in the self was, in fact, a disease in someone else. Momism, for example, shifted this discomfort from inside to outside, the anxiety over lost virility suddenly located on a familiar, if overlooked, vector, as if in a regression to the politics of the pre-Oedipal state. Generalizable, the notion that mothers were the cause of civilization's distress provided vocabulary for expressing a nonanomic despair. Diagnosis, as it often can, then became identity formation, and identity formation "permeated almost every avenue of American thought and activity," much as *Newsweek* claimed.

But it was only diagnosis. Although psychoanalysis helped name and explain the health risks that resulted when women failed to comply with their requisite repression, it offered little in the way of decisive treatment. In Wylie's formulation, apathy and despair remained out of control. Mamas kept getting bigger, and so did their babies. (Babies, meanwhile, inherited none of the genetic defects that caused their fathers to grow ever smaller in stature.) Marynia Farnham and Ferdinand Lunberg's attack on the modern woman's career intentions did not change the fact that women like Robert Robinson's wife, Marge, were about to begin returning to the labor force in numbers that would continue to grow steadily for the next half century.[73] Worst of all, an article describing the fight against mental illness at the same time enacted the very illness that it claimed to treat. The surface conveyed the progress of psychoanalysis, but this same progress was undone by the joke, the unrelenting inner burden, the "ominous" statistic revealing that Americans were still "notably tense." In *Newsweek* at least, psychoanalysis was symbolically castrated by the symptoms returned from its own repressed. The text insisted on the Menningers' clinical prowess, but the Menningers were ultimately undone by the cartoons below. For, although psychoanalysis may well have insisted on a symbolic matricide, the mother was far from dead. Psychoanalysis was, instead, unable to treat the neurosis that it had invented—a vital consideration, I will soon turn to argue, for understanding how Miltown became the first mother's little helper in the American popular press.

American popular culture in the 1950s thus *foreshadowed* the demise of psychoanalysis that by many accounts did not begin for another decade while at the same time providing a larger context for the undertones of inefficacy of analytic treatment in the Glueck's "Psychodynamic Patterns in the Homosexual Sex Offender" and other *AJP* articles in the 1950s. Like the mother's little helper, the fall of psychoanalysis from influence in American psychiatry is often located in the 1960s and 1970s, as the result of its failure to provide evidence of clinical efficacy. Leslie Prioleau and his colleagues, for example, found wide acceptance in 1973 for the notion that "we are still not aware of a convincing demonstration that the benefits of psychotherapy exceed those of placebos for real patients."[74] And Gerald Klerman's influential critiques, begun in the mid-1970s, cite "the lack of Randomized Control Trials": "Psychotherapy and psychoanalysis were consuming ever larger amounts of the health budget, with little evidence that they worked for anything in particular."[75] In these and other instances, psychoanalysis was attacked for providing a treatment that consisted of nothing more than diagnosis. No doubt it offered compelling, if often competing, formulations of pathology. But an ever-growing number of critics argued that the treatments were anything but cost effective, that they extended for indeterminate and unending periods of time, and, worst of all, that they had not yet been shown to work in clinical settings.

Yet it can also be argued that all conditions may not be clinical and that outcome studies may have more variables than those for which they can control—especially when the clinical model also purports to understand the cultures in which the clinic functions. Psychoanalysis may have been called into question in this larger arena first. *Newsweek, Generation of Vipers,* "How to Be a Good Listener," "Motherhood Breakdowns," Dr. Safford's column, and the other sources that I cite suggest ways in which psychoanalysis may not have been *working* in the most structural sense: the cultural ego was not protecting the well-being of the national individual.[76] Like dreams, the symptoms were not well defined and were always open to interpretation. But their continued presence could not be disputed because the patient compulsively remained symptomatic. Freud might have understood and beautifully diagnosed this problem in American popular culture in the 1950s, but he was not able to provide the cure. Worse yet, an understanding of the diagnosis was a tacit acknowledgment of complicity in the system, experienced as an uncontrolled "change within," a confusing, immobilized reaction to a strangely familiar sense of anxiety.

Meprobamate, Biological Anxiety, and the Scientific Press

It seems ironic that Miltown was associated with mothers at all; Miltown emerged from a biological science that sought to eliminate the mother from the conversation. Dreams, slips of the tongue, and other referents of the unconscious were no longer considered valid sources of information for the diagnosis of anxiety. Instead, and in rejection of the psychoanalytic model, anxiety was supposed to be a wholly rational phenomenon.

At least this was the assumption when a series of scientific research reports announced the early success of meprobamate. At the same time that psychoanalysis enjoyed near hegemony in dictating how anxiety was understood in many facets of American psychiatry, biological evidence quietly suggested that anxiety did not result from inner conflicts and frustrated drives but was, instead, caused by aberrations of physiology, neurochemistry, and other body functions uncovered by the illumination of microscopes and electrical nerve tracings and then treated by the administration of medication.[77] Before turning to the matter of popular representation, I briefly examine how the scientific community's embrace of Miltown was, in large part, the result of the ways in which Miltown's "new" science reconceptualized illnesses that were previously the domain of psychoanalysis.

It is well-known, in retrospect, that the 1950s were an important time in the history of neuropsychopharmacology, even though, at the time, many important developments received scant attention in the *AJP* or other analytic and psychological (A-P) journals. In 1949, lithium, an alkali metal isolated from stone, was reported to exert a "calming effect" on the manic phase of manic-depression.[78] Chlorpromazine, a compound whose "mechanism of action was both as an antihistamine and a sedative," was found in 1952 to demonstrate previously unimaginable efficacy against the "psychotic agitation, aggressiveness and delusive conditions of schizophrenia" in institutionalized psychiatric patients.[79] In 1956, minor tranquilizers were discovered to provide new treatments for "outpatient" anxiety, even though the psychoanalytic establishment was openly resistant to the notion of medical treatments for neurotic illnesses.[80] And, in 1957, the first "antidepressant" medications, both tricyclics and monoamine oxidase inhibitors, were marketed in the United States.[81]

Meprobamate was promoted as a "uniquely mild" tranquilizer that relaxed skeletal muscle without causing sedation, a marked improvement over other chemical treatments for nervousness such as the barbiturates or neuroleptics.[82] These medications were frequently far too sedating to be used by many noninstitutionalized psychiatric patients. Meprobamate, however, was argued to selectively depress only certain areas of the brain responsible for emotions—the so-called biological substrate of anxiety—without causing a more generalized cortical depression.[83] Further, meprobamate did not interfere with "intellectual functions" or with "motor performance."[84] The medication could be taken, not merely by patients confined to psychiatric hospitals and institutions, but by those in the "real world" as well.[85] "Miltown," wrote its inventor, Frank Berger, in December 1954, "possessed a muscle relaxant and sedative action of an unusual kind. It depressed multineuronal reflexes but did not significantly affect monosynaptic reflexes. It was readily absorbed from the gastrointestinal canal. It also had a taming effect."[86] Hendley et al. reported that Miltown "has a selective action on the thalamus."[87] Kletzin and Berger described how Miltown affected the limbic system as well.[88]

Of course, the idea of a chemical treatment for anxiety was not entirely a new phenomenon. The concept can arguably be traced back as far as 400 B.C., when Hippocrates cured emotional worries with black hellebore.[89] At the turn of the twentieth century, the American scientific community briefly focused on "localizing" mental illnesses to specific "brain lesions," which were treatable by a mix of electric currents, diet, rest, and heavily sedating medications. Neural explanations for emotional illnesses were given new life in the mid-1950s, however, by state-of-the-art electrophysiological research that exposed anxiety as an alteration of impulses emitted by a certain area of the brain or between areas of the brain. Specifically, the thalamus and the hippocampus were shown to emit spontaneous and most unwelcome electrical and chemical signals during "anxiety states." These signals caused hyperexcitable or hyperirritable interneuronal conduction and, ultimately, the clinically observable sensations of sweating, tremor, palpitations, and other "body discomforts."[90]

The notion of a neurophysiologically based, chemically treated anxiety spread rapidly throughout the neuroscientific community. And, as this notion spread, *anxiety* became a much broader diagnostic term than it had been when confined to the secrecy of an analyst's office. In fact, it became a term of redaction. Numerous scientific journal articles between the mid-1950s and the early 1960s demonstrated Miltown's broad, unqualified success in treating the corporeal manifestations of anxiety. Dickel et al. gave Miltown to a group of "tense, anxious, and fatigued working people" and found a "definite" improvement in coordination and the ability to perform tasks on command.[91] Rickels et al. found that Miltown effectively relieved the "insomnia and GI [gastrointestinal] symptoms of anxiety."[92] Dixon reported a "strikingly good response" in 86 percent of 104 anxious patients with tension headache.[93] Pennington discovered that 78 percent of patients suffering from "headache and nervousness" and "abdominal distention" found relief with Miltown.[94] Agitated children responded to Miltown.[95] The "anxious, emotional component" of allergic asthma responded to Miltown.[96] Dogs with the seemingly conflicting presentations of "car sickness, hyperexcitability, viciousness, and shyness" responded to one to four hundred milligrams of Miltown, orally supplied.[97] Anxiety, suddenly treatable, was suddenly everywhere.

These examples suggest that much more than the treatment of anxiety was at stake with the development of the new medication—so was the very definition of *anxiety*. As we have just seen, the prevailing psychoanalytic model conceptualized anxiety as a conscious manifestation of unconscious symptoms. Unease in the present was always and already linked to past traumatic events. Yet the science behind meprobamate boldly suggested that anxiety was not a somatic remembrance of things past but instead merely somatic. Anxiety was not a deep conflict; it was a physical condition, a brain-mediated medical state, manifest and quantifiable by headache, asthma, tremor, and a host of other physical symptoms. Whereas psychoanalysis posited that anxiety resulted from early-life developments with mothers and fathers, developments later mapped onto husbands and wives, meprobamate worked on the thalamus, the substrate, the alimentary tract, and other sexed structures that functioned independently of gender. Whereas psychoanalysis assumed the unseen, biological psychiatry demanded the observable, the tremorous, the pulsatile. And, whereas a psychoanalytic diagnosis implicated context and, ultimately, culture, a biological diagnosis remained fixated on the symptoms at hand, either under the microscope or within the examination room.

The argument that Miltown revealed a biological substrate of anxiety, a finding that then unhinged psychoanalysis from its point of capitation, became a common theme among early biological psychiatrists. Miltown was said to herald the replacement of outdated, gender-obsessed constructs with a paradigm that saw beneath gender differences to the level of chemical imbalances and neurochemicals. Frank Berger claimed that "the drug most needed is one that would liberate our minds from their primitive and outdated ways. Meprobamate may be the first substance of this type."[98] Berger later argued that the success of the tranquilizers bought home the realization that "no psychoanalytic ideas can be evaluated by direct experiments, so it is difficult to assess their merit."[99] Behind reports of a "selective action on the thalamus" and proof of limbic system involvement lay the notion that the new science of the mind allowed for a praxis that was more scientific, and ultimately more effective, than a primitive, untestable theory.

Miltown's success also shifted the class implications of anxiety because, when anxiety became a motor phenomenon, it became an egalitarian condition experienced by everyman. The "tense, anxious, and fatigued working people" described in Dickel et al.'s study were neither neurotic CEOs nor their wealthy wives; they were, instead, the previously unseen and unaddressed proletariat. Symptoms described by Rickels et al. as "insomnia and GI" effects, if not Pennington's headache, nervousness, and abdominal distention, were experienced by those with too little time on their hands, not those who could digest the implications of their existence in an endless stream of fifty-minute hours. Finally, these problems could be diagnosed by anyman's doctor, not only by the specially trained, ivory-tower, A-P Menninger psychoanalysts. Elitist interpersonal training was rendered moot, in other words, when the precision of treatment had already been titrated—by a directive and organic practitioner no doubt—at a response dose of four hundred milligrams, orally supplied.[100]

This is in no way to say that Miltown threatened the existence of talking cures, either psychotherapeutic or psychoanalytic. To recall, many psychoanalysts in the 1950s actively pursued biological understandings, a seemingly natural outgrowth of Freud's own insistence on biological absolutes, and, again, Miltown was often touted as a facilitator of, rather than a threat to, the analytic notion of self-exploration.[101] *The Physicians' Reference Manual* claims that, "on Miltown therapy, alertness is maintained and psychotherapy is facilitated."[102] Numerous studies reflected this overlap. Dixon's "Meprobamate, a Clinical Evaluation" examined forty-nine patients whose "anxiety tension states" were linked to "immaturity reactions, particularly those of emotional instability and passive dependency." The "most significant gains" were found when Miltown was coupled with psychotherapy.[103]

Yet I remind readers that such ambiguity is often effaced in the *AJP* as well as in work by historians who argue that the biological revolution in psychiatry was, much like the mother's little helper, a phenomenon that took place in the 1970s. Recall that both Spitzer, Endicott, and Robins and Klerman argue that the 1970s transformed psychiatry from a set of illusive and illusory theories into an investigative science concerned with proof claims and, as Klerman puts it, "the importance of getting the diagnosis right." This transformation culminated in 1980 in the *DSM-III,* which represented, according to Klerman, a "victory for science" in psychiatry.[104] The same narrative is taken up by Mitchell Wilson, who argues that the events of the 1970s and early 1980s transformed psychiatry from a profession that saw presenting symptoms as conduits to earlier, traumatic events to one that saw with the precision of science, laying the groundwork for the changes that would take place over the remainder of the twentieth century and beyond.[105] And Loyd Rogler describes the 1970s as a decade in which psychiatry's new diagnostic presuppositions and treatment options became "largely discontinuous with previous formulations."[106] In each case, the 1970s are partially misidentified as the time when psychiatry "pitched out" the notion of the unconscious in a manner that then altered psychiatric practices, at the same time splitting the profession into two minds, one that spoke in talking cures, another that prescribed medications.

Biological Anxiety and the Popular Press

Scientific sources alone cannot adequately explain the less-revolutionary aspects of the story: the ways in which Miltown set the stage for psychotropic medications to become known as *mother's little helpers,* possibly overprescribed to women, and surely considered cures for "women's" discontent. This unseemly aspect of psychotropic medication was not a property forged in the laboratory. Rather, the connection of mothers and helpers is a mechanism of action developed in the popular cultures and cultural contexts of which the laboratory was but a part. To address this point, I now more fully explore articles announcing the arrival of Miltown in the American popular press. I argue two things: first, that the timeliness of a quick, easy, and precise treatment for anxiety drove the discourse of "Miltown-mania" in popular literature much as it did in scientific journals; and, second, that, at the same time, the notion of a revolution-by-precision does not account for the possibility that precision was not the only problem with psychoanalysis in the 1950s. Biological psychiatrists may well have announced a new formulation of anxiety, couched in the rejection of the unconscious and the replacement of a cultural model with a scientific one. But, in popular print culture, this formulation was called into question by depictions of the new tranquilizers in *Newsweek, Time, Science Digest, Cosmopolitan,* and other sites where pharmaceuticals were posited as treatments for marriage phobia, women's frigidity, castrating mothers, and other psychoanalytically inflected conditions.

It is important first to note that many complicated factors are involved when products become the objects of popular frenzy. Supply, for example, is often limited at first, creating an aura of demand. Demand soon follows, stretching the limits of the supply. Possession of the product, when the product is most appealing, comes to divide those who have from those who want to have. The havers define themselves as such, for a while at least, and see those who lack as lacking. In time, however, supply exceeds demand in the politics of identification. Those who have find something new or realize that they were better off before. Those who want suddenly do not want quite as much. A fall from grace ensues, until the process begins again. Predicting when this process will occur is a science of tremendous retrospective and prospective analysis. Marketing, consumer preference, competition, availability, and many other variables all play a part. And, often, selecting the latest, greatest new thing simply comes down to happenstance, in the seemingly random chasm dividing a Pokemon toy from an Olestra potato chip.

Many such quantitative and qualitative forces were at play in constructing Miltown in American popular culture in the mid-1950s. Initially reported in obscure journals, Miltown became the public marker of the new science of the mind. In the language of popular magazines, Miltown represented new relationships and new progress and a time when Americans began to understand the tensions of peacetime, a healthy economy, and the pleasures of home. Consumers within a suddenly consumer society, obsessed with brand-name appliances, discovered an appliance for the mind, a fetish that cured their fetish, a brand-named cure for a newly brand-named illness.

Yet I suggest that much more than consumerism was at stake when, in the 1950s, Miltown became a popular icon overnight. Miltown was not merely a commodity—it was the very commodity that threatened to replace Freud. Before Miltown, the possibility that everyday emotions and anxieties were electrical or chemical would have seemed like a brave new world, the idea that these could be cured by an ingested substance even more far-reaching. Talking cures cornered the market on neurosis. Yet beginning in 1955—to recall, also the height of the psychoanalytic golden age—the same magazines that lauded Freud also entered what *Newsweek* exuberantly described as the "new era in mental health."[107] Hundreds of articles appearing in popular magazines between 1955 and 1960 informed their readers of the basic tenets of biological psychiatry: that anxiety, and, indeed, all personality, was in some way biologically based and that the treatment for it lay in understanding the precise mechanism of chemical alteration demonstrated by Miltown and other tranquilizers. The July 1956 issue of *Science Digest,* for example, presented scientists engaged in a "search for new 'mental chemicals.'" These "psychochemists" worked at the intersection of "psychiatry and the laboratory" in a "search for . . . sanity." *Sanity,* however, was a term of a different composition than that sought by *Newsweek* nine months earlier. Synthesized in the laboratory, the "incredible" tranquilizers were shown to work by "decreasing the production of serotonin, the hormone-like compound in the body that can block the 'nerve switchboards' in the brain and central nervous system, stopping the transmission of messages. It is an imbalance of serotonin—an excess of this chemical—that may well be the cause of mental imbalance."[108] Subsequent articles in *Science Digest*—"Truth about the Tranquilizers" and "New Clues about Mental Illness"—described the "dramatic" and "amazing treatment of states of excitation and increased tension."[109] Meanwhile, the 7 March 1955 *Time* exposé "Pills for the Mind" explored a "revolution" in the "treatment of mental illness," tranquilizers that "improved sleep" and "rendered anxious patients quieter and calmer"—the same points made by Dickel et al., Rickels et al., Pennington, and other biological scientists.[110] Similarly, *Cosmopolitan's* January 1956 article "The New Nerve Pills and Your Health" stated that the "revolutionary drugs" such as Miltown were so effective that "a number of 'anxious' cerebral palsied children improved . . . to such a degree that muscle function was notably improved": "One twelve year old boy gained enough confidence to walk for the first time."[111]

Even *Newsweek* jumped on the biological bandwagon. The 21 May 1956 "special article" "Pills vs. Worries" explained that medications had "revolutionized the treatment of mental and emotional patients": "The pills are harmless. They are not habit forming. . . . When you have 600 drugstores and only 400 bottles of Miltown, how can you ration them?" The article presents Miltown with almost unquestioned enthusiasm, an enthusiasm based both on the merits of medication and on the notion that tranquillity could be attained with minimal need for introspection: "News of the 'wonder drugs' that offer peace of mind without the necessity of going to a psychiatrist or even reading a book has so raised the hopes of the emotionally ill that over-the-counter sales of these prescription drugs are inevitable."[112] Finally, the 24 December 1956 *Newsweek* article "How Tranquilizers Work" raised the question "How do these new drugs act on the nervous system?" and then answered it in definitively biological fashion: "The tranquilizers seem to affect the globus pallidus . . . which in turn influences motor movements."[113]

Yet these same articles clearly suggest that something else drove this discourse, something having as much to do with anxieties about relationships between men and women as with enthusiasm over a new form of treatment. Biology may have introduced an anxiety that saw a person as a globus pallidus, a thalamus, or some other structure that functioned beneath the level of gender—insomuch as these neuroanatomic regions were thought to be largely the same in men and in women. At the same time, however, the same gender themes at play in articles about psychoanalysis also appeared in the articles that introduced biological principles to mass audiences.

Like many information articles of the day, for example, *Cosmopolitan's* "The New Nerve Pills and Your Health" calls on "expert opinion" to describe the effects of the wondrous new treatment for everyday worries. Readers learned about the research of Dr. Frank Ayd, a "leading pioneer" in pharmaceutical innovation and development. *Cosmopolitan,* however, reveals aspects of Ayd's research left out of his numerous scientific citations and important treatises concerning the history of psychopharmacology: "Among the one hundred psychiatric patients given relaxant drugs for various conditions by Frank Ayd, Jr. of Baltimore, Maryland were a number of frigid women. After taking the drug, 'frigid women who abhorred marital relations reported they responded more readily to their husbands' advances.'"[114]

In *Cosmopolitan's* "Live with Your Nerves and Like It," Dr. Walter Alvarez, a "famous doctor," describes cases such as "an unmarried buyer of forty" "who was frantic when examiners found nothing wrong with her" despite repeated headaches. "What she did not know was that such headaches always come out of a sensitive place in the brain." Yet, on closer examination, Dr. Alvarez diagnoses the "terrible strain" that resulted from her "love life." "She was in love with an attractive man who was begging her to marry him," he reports. "When I insisted that she make a decision immediately"—and, of course, through treatment with psychotropic medication—"she showed marked improvement" and, ultimately, wed her suitor.[115]

And *Time* magazine's "Pills for the Mind" begins with the following statements: "The treatment of mental illness is in the throes of a revolution. For the first time in history, pills are enabling some psychiatrists to nip in the bud some burgeoning outbreaks of emotional illness, and treat many current cases far more effectively. When Cincinnati's Dr. Douglas Goldman told fellow psychiatrists that 'the revolution is at hand,' some doctors scoffed, and most were skeptical. But at two recent meetings, psychiatrists packed the halls to hear dozens of papers reporting almost identical successes." Yet, at the bottom of the very same page on which these statements appear, the article proceeds to explain that the very "revolutionary pills" that "improved sleep" and "rendered anxious patients quieter and calmer" also magically restored maternity, fidelity, and sexual compliance all at once. Here appeared the case study of "a petite blonde, 36, wife of a journeyman carpenter":

> In her hallucinations, she heard voices: . . . her own daughter calling "Mummy," and finally a woman telling her that her husband was unfaithful and she should leave him. She had left him many times, only to end up in hospitals, where electric shock made her outwardly calmer but with no normal ebb and flow of emotional responses. . . . After [medications], and with no more help from the psychiatrist than she had always had, the woman went home on a maintenance dose of one pill a day. Her husband had only one complaint: she had become so demanding in her newfound love for him he wondered whether the doctors could make the pills a bit smaller.[116]

The husband could surely be a journeyman. But, given her propensity to ebb and flow, a woman's place was in the home, ebbing and flowing with her husband.

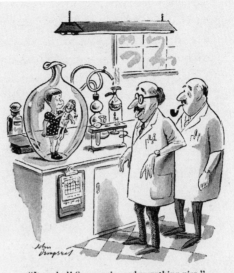

17. "It worked!": the promise of laboratory science (*Cosmopolitan*, January 1956, 74).

"It worked! Sugar, spice and everything nice."

Most obviously, these articles suggest that Miltown and the tranquilizers offered a treatment for the crisis of masculinity described above. These drugs were products of the same cultural milieu that produced momism, arguments about a mother's return to the home, male anxiety about women's work, and Dr. Safford's fear of dyspareunia. As such, *Science Digest*'s "Truth about the Tranquilizers," *Newsweek*'s "How Tranquilizers Work," *Cosmopolitan*'s "The New Nerve Pills and Your Health," and other articles about tranquilizers responded directly to the concerns described in "Bigger Mamas, Bigger Babies," "A Woman's Place Is in the Home," and "Have Babies While You're Young."[117] While "How to Be a Good Listener" asked the pressing question "Do you think a wife's place is in the home?" tranquilizers answered the question with the precision of science, restoring a 1950s version of marital love while returning the mother to her rightful place in the home and in bed as if a conjugal-strength Mickey Finn. And, while the young husband in "Tell me Doctor" complained of dyspareunia, the husband in "Pills for the Mind" had more pareunia than he knew what to do with. In the process, tranquilizers promised to restore a man's mastery of his own home and his sense of tranquillity within it. Karen Horney may well have described frigidity as a potent weapon in defiance of patriarchy, but, armed with the tranquilizers, as a cartoon (fig. 17) embedded in "The New Nerve Pills and Your Health"

less than subtly suggests, patriarchy fought back. In a historical sense, tranquilizers thus became treatments for clearly psychoanalytic problems.

These articles suggest that Miltown did not merely come of age alongside psychoanalysis; it also posited a treatment for the larger, philosophical
anxiety that psychoanalysis defined but could not control. To recall the argument made above, Freud's model of civilization divided the world into a pro-
gressive conscious realm and an unseen, repressed unconscious below. While
this model proved an immensely popular means of justifying an era-specific
notion of heterosexuality in the 1950s, pathologizing a woman's desire to
work outside the home, for example, it proved unable to stop the perception that many symptoms returned from the repressed. Not only, however,
did the notion of a bodily anxiety ablate the possibility that symptoms could
return from the repressed—it ablated the repressed altogether. As it came
to be defined in the popular press, and, once again, well before similar arguments appeared in the *AJP,* biological psychiatry treated the symptoms
and deconstructed the diagnostic system that defined them. If anxiety was
of the body, observable by electroencephalogram and quantifiable by laboratory assay, then the fallacy of the unconscious-conscious dichotomy was
exposed by science.

For example, the May 1957 *Science Digest* article "Mirror in the Brain" reported Dr. Wilder Penfield's discovery that "under certain circumstances a
person may be possessed of two consciousnesses—one of the immediate surroundings and circumstances, and one of the circumstances of something
subconsciously remembered." Dr. Penfield, the director of the Montreal
Neurological Institute, had realized this finding during surgical procedures
for intractable epilepsy, "when the cerebral cortex that covers one of the
temporal lobes of the brain is stimulated with a wire during surgical operations."[118] Nearly seventy years earlier, in the famous case of Anna O.—later
published by Freud and Josef Breuer as *Studies in Hysteria*—a young Freud
had reached something of a similar conclusion regarding a secret part of
the mind that could be unlocked by the doctor's stimulation.[119] Freud and
Breuer theorized that Anna's hysterical deafness resulted from the guilt that
she experienced as a result of listening to music while caring for her dying
father. These "unacceptable" sentiments were blocked, repressed into her unconscious, until they were released by the talking cure. In "Mirror in the
Brain," however, not only is Dr. Penfield able to unlock the passion of ca-
tharsis; he is able to reproduce it again and again: "Here is one of several

Mirror in the Brain

There is a mirror of one's past in one's brain.

Under certain circumstances a person may be possessed of two consciousnesses — one of the immediate surroundings and circumstances, and one of the circumstances of something subconsciously remembered. The phenomenon amounts to a "doubling of consciousness."

This weird condition is reported by Dr. Wilder Penfield, director of the Montreal Neurological Institute, in a report to the Smithsonian Institution.

The condition arises, Dr. Penfield reports, when the cerebral cortex that covers one of the temporal lobes of the brain is stimulated with a gentle electrical current applied through a wire needle during surgical operations. Such surgery on the cortex lying just above one ear is performed under local anesthesia for a certain type of epilepsy. The patient remains conscious and free from pain throughout.

Here is one of several instances reported by Dr. Penfield:

"A young woman heard music when a certain point in the cortex was stimulated. She said she heard an orchestra playing a song. The same song was forced into her consciousness over and over again by re-stimulation at the same spot . . ."

There were many other examples of patients hearing music.

"If the individual was asked later to recall the song he might be able to sing it, but he might not be able to recall the circumstances of any one previous hearing," said Dr. Penfield.

Doctor Penfield advances a possible explanation of the phenomenon. Apparently every sensory experience is carried by the appropriate nerves to a specific part of the cortex. There it is coordinated with other sensory impressions to make up a total pattern of experience. This pattern is recorded, although it may pass completely out of conscious memory.

In some way, electrical stimulation of the temporal cortex reactivates one of the permanently recorded experience-patterns, and nerve pathways act as a mirror, a reflection of the former experience. Thus the doubled consciousness results.

MAY 1957

SCIENCE DIGEST

18. A mirror in the brain (*Science Digest,*
May 1957, back cover).

instances reported by Dr. Penfield: 'A young woman heard music when a certain point in the cortex is stimulated. She said she heard an orchestra playing a song. The same song was forced into her consciousness over and over again by restimulation of the same spot.'" Dr. Penfield explains that the woman's awareness of music does not represent evidence of the unconscious, of repression, or of other hysterical truths unearthed by Freud. Instead, this is evidence of "double consciousness," two parallel conscious states whose mere presence disproves the unconscious altogether: "Doctor Penfield advances a possible explanation of the phenomenon. Apparently every sensory experience is carried by the appropriate nerves to a specific part of the cortex. There it is coordinated with other sensory impressions to make up a total pattern of experience. . . . In some way, electrical stimulation of the temporal cortex reactivates one of the permanently recorded experience-patterns, and nerve pathways act as a mirror, a reflection of the former experience. Thus the double consciousness results."[120]

The *Newsweek* article "How Tranquilizers Work" is another example of how the construction of biology denatured the more troubling philosophical aspects of psychoanalysis. In explaining the mechanism of action of the tranquilizers, the article uncovers the biological substrate of desire: "The possible source of psychic energy (including the energy of the erotic instincts, which Freud calls libido) is the basal ganglia, a group of structures at the base of the brain. The tranquilizers seem to effect the globus pallidus, the most primitive of these structures."[121] Even the deepest and most troubling impulses are rendered rational and knowable, in other words, when the conditionality of *possible* ("possible source of psychic energy") is negated by the certainty of *is* ("is the basal ganglia"). In this description, the article connects biological and psychoanalytic assumptions that the unseen can be made visible and rational through the act of uncovering, whether by verbal interaction or by newly emerging technology. But, unlike psychoanalysis, biology uncovers the "fact" that these unseen entities had been in mankind's purview all along; only the correct machinery to see them had been lacking. Erotic instincts, for example, are localized to their anatomic points of origin, the basal ganglia, in much the same way that Dr. Penfield discovered music in the temporal cortex. And, if all the repressed is visible and knowable, then, by extension, the very idea of the unconscious—and, with it, the notion of repressed conflict—is false.

Popular print sources thus suggest that the rejection of psychoanalysis, and the embrace of Miltown, in magazines such as *Newsweek, Time,* and *Cosmopolitan,* was based on something more than one clinical model replacing another. Also at stake, and even more so in these articles, was the embrace of a new model for talking about a specifically gendered perception of "cultural" problems. Of course, this is the very point disavowed by early biological psychiatrists, who argued for a hermetically clinical, scientifically driven psychiatric language. Yet these articles suggest that, from its point of origin, biology was made to reject psychoanalysis on a cultural level as well—and, in the process, presented a new means of justifying what Rosalind Minsky might call *patriarchal* unrest. In the popular press, biology rendered mental processes and "repressed, subconscious conflicts" as being, quite literally, biological: of the body and on the body; observable, controllable, and reproducible. As *Science Digest* explains in "Search for New 'Mental Chemicals,'" "Today, psychiatry and the laboratory have joined hands in *psychochemistry,* the science of chemically-induced behavioral change" (emphasis added).[122] Chemical change then brought housewives in from the cold and rendered psychotic mothers suddenly able to perform their motherly duties. And, if there was no unconscious, then anxiety could not have been a narrative of return. Anxiety as non–depth model was, in fact, an aberration of chemicals and electrical impulses from the basal ganglia, having been corporeal all along.[123]

By replacing context with text, the production of biology not only demystified anxiety by making it entirely conscious and, thus, entirely predictable; it also made it a wholly civilized narrative. Offering a replacement for psychoanalysis both as a clinical mode of treatment and as a discursive system, biology thus posited a ready response to the social crisis implied in *Newsweek*'s search for sanity. The article, to recall, described an epidemic of maternally based, psychoanalytic anxiety that threatened to rupture the social structure of America. Psychoanalysis offered a beautifully conceptualized diagnosis without hope of immediate alleviation. In psychopharmacology, however, *Newsweek* found its cure.[124]

Finally, biology as it came to be defined in the popular press solved the crisis of the failure of psychoanalysis in the most fundamental way possible: it worked. *Newsweek*'s America, to recall, was in crisis because psychoanalysis was unable to arrest the very condition that it described. Mothers grew larger and gave birth to ever bigger babies. Husbands and wives slept in separate beds. Change, accompanied by the phobic pain of dissemination, threatened the stability of such pillar institutions as family and marriage. These threats cut off productivity, uncoupled progress, and ruptured the power structure of civilization. However, the new science, and Miltown specifically, demonstrated a cultural potency that Walter Cronkite attributed to psychoanalysis but that psychoanalysis could not deliver. "The tranquilizing drugs interrupt overstimulating nerve impulses," *Cosmopolitan* reported in January 1956, "in amazingly chemical ways."[125] Miltown selectively acted on the parts of the brain representing the biological substrate of anxiety. The result was, as reported, a decrease in symptoms. Muscles relaxed. Palsied children walked. Nerve impulses interrupted. Hyperexcitable conduction was delayed and possibly even arrested. Frigid mothers came home and came back to bed. Even "neurotic mice" were treated by the new drugs, once it was discovered that their symptoms could be explained by the response to "four-ring phenyl structures with flat benzine rings."[126] Scientific precision returned the phallus to its rightful owner, enacting the victory of man over nature, of civilization over barbarism. Miltown may or may not have treated mothers in real life. But, in popular magazines at least, it was a highly effective means of sedating the Freudian mother left unsedated by Freud. Acting on the very substrate of anxiety, order was restored.

Married People Live Longer: 24 December 1956

Change, once again, occurs for many complicated reasons, some having to do with group psychology, many more the result of everything else in the world. Yet psychoanalysis does teach something quite useful about the types of change described by Thomas Kuhn:[127] at the level of perception, change often takes place only when there is a desire for change. Progress and innovation are very often responses to a painful present and the illusory hope of a less-painful future. This is especially so in the case of illness, where new treatments bring the promise of more meaningful lives. When they are well, people can consider the future and, with it, plans for marriage, generativity, security, and everything else that is fundamentally threatened when disease enters a narrative. To be sure, a substantial part of my project involves considering the ways in which terms such as *illness* and *health,* or *abnormal* and *normal,* are not essentialized categories but rather mediated through power, culture, and context. It is important to remember, however, that even within the most pernicious change—which the rise of tranquilizers was not—lies a desire for palliation. Such sentiments were certainly at play in the excitement surrounding the discovery of medications for everyday worries in the 1950s. Many readers of journals and magazines, practitioners and patients alike, surely felt excluded from treatment. A new science, embodied in a new medication, offered the possibility of a new level of access and, with it, the hope of a better future.

Problems arise, however, when this enthusiasm translates into disavowal. Ayd's claim that "it is difficult to see" how the old paradigm was in any way valid implies, not only a new answer, but also a reformation of the old problem. What may have troubled you in the past, in other words, need not be a matter of concern in the present; all your worries can be dealt with simply by taking a pill. In the process, old bodies and old concerns are brushed away in the plasticity of the moment. But psychoanalysis has something to say about these claims as well and specifically about how declarations of certainty must be met with quiet skepticism. Psychoanalysis contends that no innovation, however revelatory, arises from a blank template, that no replacement is ever wholly complete. Those who forget the concerns of the past learn that the past always returns as a symptom. No replacement should be assessed by its surface when repression is involved. The most absolute replacement is the replacement least trusted.

Throughout this chapter, I have suggested that the clean break of biology from psychoanalysis is complicated by the historical fact that the release of Miltown took place concomitantly with psychoanalysis' golden age, or, rather, its "golden crisis," in American popular culture. During this time, psychoanalytic theories affected every avenue of American popular culture—including, it seems, the popular construction of Miltown. I now conclude by expanding the notion that this overlap was not only historical but functional as well: psychotropic drugs can be seen to perform the cultural work once assumed by Freudian psychoanalysis—treating the regulation of gender norms and modulating gender-based discontent.[128]

I begin my explanation of this concept by pointing out that women are absent from articles about Miltown in much the same ways as they were absent from articles about psychoanalysis. The voices of real women never appear in the magazines and journals announcing Miltown's early success. Articles in women's magazines such as *Cosmopolitan* (which, like the *Ladies' Home Journal,* had an almost all-male editorial board) were written by men such as Donald Cooley and Walter Alvarez. Even articles supposedly "told" by women and providing perspective on men's anxiety—*Cosmopolitan*'s "My Husband Came Home" or "I Had My Husband Committed," for example— were actually written by men who put on a skirt, so to speak.[129] To be sure, this fact reflects a convention of the magazines that I read in this chapter— but this is, in part, my point.[130] Because of these conventions, the specifics of what women's anxiety was really about are never revealed. Perhaps it was frustration about work opportunities, or a desire to leave the nuclear home, or unhappiness about social policy, or even anxiety caused by biological pathogens. Any, all, or none of these could have been true, for the simple reason that, in the sources that I examine, it is impossible to tell. Instead, and by design, the threat remains illusory and illusive, never directly cited and never overtly explained. What does remain constant, however, are the ways in which the description of a woman's anxiety is always mediated by men and destabilizes a specific, 1950s notion of heteronormativity. And, most important, this destabilization is almost globally perceived as causing symptoms— in men.

The anxiety caused by women and experienced by men is, once again, the anxiety that biology claimed to replace: there could be no return of the repressed if there was no unconscious. Yet, as the popular sources that I examine make clear, Miltown posited a cure for psychoanalytic anxiety as well. A woman's frigidity, itself a historically psychoanalytic category, caused a breakdown of the family unit. A woman's psychosis threatened a man's place as the master of the home. A woman's waywardness ruptured a man's sense of progress. These were the conditions for which Freud became known as Freud. And, as *Newsweek, Time,* and *Cosmopolitan* all seem to agree, these were the same conditions diagnosed and treated by the new science of the mind as well. At these times, the notion that biology reconceptualized anxiety was called into question by the fact that biology treated psychoanalytic conditions. The symptom remained the same, even as the language describing it underwent radical revision—a new diagnosis, itself diagnosed as a preexisting condition.

The trope of marriage provides an important illustration of this point. Marriage, and specifically the causal link between a stable marriage and a husband's well-being, has been a recurrent theme in many of the articles cited thus far. Walter Alvarez's "Live with Your Nerves and Like It," Frank Ayd's research, and the case study of the petite, blonde housewife in *Time*'s "Pills for the Mind" are but a few examples of the ways in which psychotropic drugs represented the restoration of a specific, 1950s-style conjugal home. In beginning my transition to chapter 4, I want to suggest that the complicated overlap between marriage and psychopharmacology in the 1950s lets us more fully understand the ways in which psychotropic medications not only accrued remnants of psychoanalysis from popular culture but often behaved the way they did specifically because of this act of incorporation.

Consider, for example, the interesting relation between psychotropic drugs and a psychoanalytic approach to marriage that played out in the *Newsweek* medicine section on 24 December 1956. This is the same section in which the article "How Tranquilizers Work" explains the mechanism of "biological anxiety" and its treatment with tranquilizers and then posits a scientific explanation for psychoanalytic "erotic instincts": "The possible source of psychic energy (including the energy of the erotic instincts, which Freud calls libido) is the basal ganglia, a group of structures at the base of the brain." Another brief article appears on the same page, directly beneath "How Tranquilizers Work," this one entitled "Why People Don't Marry." The second article describes how a threat to the institution of marriage is sweeping the land. "One out of every three Americans does not marry," it reveals. A plague-like scourge, the rejection of marriage has the potential to cause financial and personal ruin if not treated. And, while both "masculine" and "feminine" explanations are presented, the article makes it clear that men are the victims of this illness. For example, the article's "star patient," a thirty-one-year-old law clerk, failed the bar examination five times: "He was unable to concentrate and suffered from severe headaches. For four years, he had had an affair with a divorced woman whom he could not marry because of religious differences." What was wrong? In the text, an expert psychoanalyst, Dr. Jacob H. Friedman, the director of psychiatric service of Fordham Hospital, diagnoses the man's fear of matrimony as an "unconscious wish to keep himself poor," manifest by an aversion to conjugal bliss—a clear-cut case, in other words, of marriage phobia.[131]

However, the story ends with successful narrative closure after the patient is psychoanalytically diagnosed and treated. His unconscious block is realized and brought to consciousness, and, after a year of intensive psychotherapy, "the man began to associate with eligible girls": "His symptoms vanished and he married happily. Passed the bar exams, too."[132]

Just as in "The Mind" of fourteen months prior, however, the successful resolution of the psychoanalytic narrative is called into question by a

How Tranquilizers Work

A new victory for the widely used tranquilizing drugs, chlorpromazine and reserpine was chalked up last week by the Veterans Administration. Dr. Ivan F. Bennett, chief of the VA psychiatric research in Washington, D.C., announced that electric- and insulin-shock treatment for mental illness had been reduced by 90 per cent in VA hospitals throughout the country where the drugs were used. Like the older shock therapies, the tranquilizers are not a cure for mental illness. They simply make psychotherapy possible with patients who otherwise are too disturbed to be treated, and hasten the patient's discharge, at a cost much cheaper than insulin, Dr. Bennett said.

Psychic Energy: How do these new drugs act on the human nervous system? Partial answers to this question came last week at a meeting in New York of the American Psychoanalytic Association. Dr. Mortimer Ostow of the Albert Einstein College of Medicine in New York and Dr. Nathan S. Kline of Rockland (N.Y.) State Mental Hospital have ascertained that chlorpromazine and reserpine, the oldest of the tranquilizers, reduce the symptoms of mental illness by cutting down the quantity of "psychic energy" which would otherwise break through the repressive forces holding them back. In this way, the patient's "aggressive, assaultive, and destructive" behavior is controlled; he is less absorbed in filling his psychotic and neurotic needs and is better able to react to psychotherapy.

Drs. Ostow and Kline believe that the possible source of psychic energy (including the energy of the erotic instincts, which Freud calls libido) is the basal ganglia, a group of structures at the base of the brain. The tranquilizers seem to affect the globus pallidus, the most primitive of these structures, which in turn influences motor movements.

This idea is significant. If it is proved, it may be possible for the first time to measure the quantity of man's psychic energy, which up to now has existed only in theory.

Why People Don't Marry

One out of every three Americans does not marry. The why of this statistic led Dr. Jacob H. Friedman, director of the psychiatric service of Fordham Hospital, on a complicated chase. Last week he reported his finding: Most unmarried men and women give reasons plausible not only to themselves but to outsiders; actually, they are single because of unrecognized phobias about matrimony.

Among the masculine rationalizations, all "irrelevant," listed by Dr. Friedman: (1) Marriage entails too much responsibility; (2) it means loss of liberty; (3) deceived by one woman, they feel that "all women are no good"; (4) aggression against mother ("women are too maternal"); (5) women are promiscuous and untrustworthy; (6) marriage is too much of a gamble ("look at the divorce rate"); (7) wives are too demanding.

Feminine "false reasons" for not marrying: (1) Fear of pregnancy; (2) parental attachment; (3) fear of infidelity of the future husband; (4) guilt in relation to childhood sex activity; (5) fear of marital relations; (6) fear that the husband will have the undesirable traits of a father or brother; (7) jilted by one man, they claim that "all men are brutes"; (8) desire for a wealthy husband.

Dr. Friedman described the plight of twenty men and women patients who suffered from various marriage phobias. When they were shown the kind of defense mechanisms they were using to avoid marriage, they gained insight and, with psychotherapy, all twenty lost their complexes and married.

Lawyer Barred: A star patient, a 31-year-old law clerk, was referred to Dr. Friedman after he had failed his bar examinations five times. He was unable to concentrate, suffered from insomnia and severe headaches. For four years, he had had an affair with a divorced woman whom he could not marry because of religious differences.

The repeated failures in his tests, Dr.

Friedman reported, were due to the man's unconscious wish to keep himself poor, financially unable to support a wife. The wish was traced to his family. His parents had been unhappily married; all his aunts (one of whom raised him) and uncles were single. He was one of five brothers, none of whom was married.

After a year of psychotherapy, the man began to associate with eligible girls. His symptoms vanished and he married happily. Passed the bar exams, too.

Blood Test's End?

The value of state laws requiring premarital blood tests (mandatory in 41 states) was challenged last week by Dr. Adele C. Shepard, chief of the bureau of venereal-disease control of the New Jersey State Department of Health. Dr. Shepard's laboratories perform about 45,000 premarital tests annually at a cost of more than $17,000, excluding overhead. Last year 310 persons were referred for follow-up tests in New Jersey. One-third were brought up for treatment for syphilis for the first time or were returned for further treatment.

"Only eighteen were diagnosed as having early syphilis, and only one of these had degenerative syphilis," said Dr. Shepard. "I question whether a case-finding yield of this magnitude justifies the continuance of the premarital law."

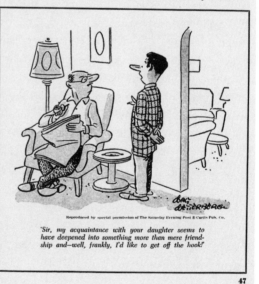

Reproduced by special permission of The Saturday Evening Post © Curtis Pub. Co.

'Sir, my acquaintance with your daughter seems to have deepened into something more than mere friendship and—well, frankly, I'd like to get off the hook!'

19. Illustrating how tranquilizers work
(*Newsweek*, 24 December 1956, 47).

cartoon. In "The Mind," to recall, cartoons of farcical therapeutic alliances served to undo a text describing the Menningers' authority. In the case at hand, a cartoon, similarly embedded in the article's text, depicts a young, well-dressed man speaking to an older, fatherly man. This scene, too, directly enacts and then mocks the anxiety that the article purports to treat. While the text describes Dr. Friedman's successful treatment, the young man in the cartoon exclaims, "Sir, my acquaintance with your daughter seems to have deepened into something more than mere friendship and—well, frankly, I'd like to get off the hook!"

When read together, "Why People Don't Marry" and the cartoon below display a cultural logic of anxiety similar in structure to that presented in "The Mind." Much like the earlier article, "Why People Don't Marry" reveals a plague sweeping the land, affecting the way of life of one of three Americans. An aberration threatens to rupture, not only the stability of a way of life, but also the progress needed for its perpetuation: it should be, the article seems to say, a world in which every "star patient" passes his exams, gets the job and the girl, and lives happily ever after. Marriage is presented as the assurance that this will take place. A threat to marriage is a threat to this sense of progress, just as, in "The Mind," a "change within" was a threat to progress. Here as well, the threat is not caused by an external force—a world war, say, or an economic depression, which would have been known causes for a drop in the marriage rate (and also the birth rate) in the decades preceding the 1950s. Instead, at this time of prosperity, the threat to the progress narrative is presented as a phobic, uncanny fear inside America, or, rather, inside Americans. The article's Americans needed to be protected, not from invaders, but from themselves.

It is known with some certainty (i.e., from Census Bureau data) that the marriage rate did not go down for the readers of *Newsweek* in the 1950s—and specifically for the white men and women depicted in every image of every magazine that I discuss in this chapter. Rather, it was at its highest point in the twentieth century, peaking in 1956. At that time, nearly half the women who would ever marry would do so before age twenty. The annual birth rate reached its highest point in 1957. The divorce rate, meanwhile, had taken its sharpest drop at any time since such statistics were recorded in the United States.[133] There seemed little to be phobic about, in other words, when it came to the institution of marriage.

"Why People Don't Marry" thus worried about marriage when all the ways of counteracting senile psychoses might well be one result of these investigations.

Of course, the laboratory approach to mental illness is but one of many: scientists are also studying such things as the mother-baby relationship, adolescent environment, and other psychological factors in the complex picture of mental illness.

Nevertheless, a main benefit of such approaches as psychochemistry, is that they bring exact measurement to an intricate field. Two mental diseases have already received such an approach:

One disease with marked mental symptoms, pellagra, once accounted for 10 percent of all mental patients in the U.S.'s South. Biochemists found that it was caused by lack of nicotinic acid in the diet, and wiped it out with proper nutrition.

Another, general paresis, was formerly as widespread and baffling as schizophrenia is today. Chemotherapists traced it to syphilis, and by curing syphilis, physicians hope soon to eliminate paresis once and for all.

Interestingly enough, two Chicago physicians have come up this past year with what may well be a laboratory test for schizophrenia! It involves adding insulin to the blood sample, removing the white cells by centrifugation, breaking down the red cells, then measuring the tendency of the resulting red cell "cream" to form enzymes. Blood from patients with schizophrenia is consistently deficient in enzyme formation.

This "biochemical test" for schizophrenia, if perfected, would be no small achievement — furnishing a concrete "specification" for one of man's most elusive and destructive ills.

● ● ●

U. S. Women Now Mothers at Younger Age

American women today are marrying and becoming mothers at a younger age.

These two facts are the reasons for the increase in the number of the nation's children during the last ten years, and not the popular belief that large families are back in fashion, P. K. Whelpton, director of the Scripps Foundation for Research in Population Problems at Miami University, Oxford, Ohio, reports.

About 50 percent of the women reaching ages 20 to 24 had already married in 1915, as compared to 60 percent for the same age group in 1945, and 70 percent last year (1955).

Among these married women, Mr. Whelpton reports, the percentage childless declined from about 27 in 1945 to 17 in 1955. This decrease, he states, was almost exactly balanced by an increase in the percentage of women with 2 children—from about 20 in 1945 to 29 in 1955.

The picture is very similar for married women aged 25 to 29, Mr. Whelpton states. Whereas one-fifth of these women were childless in 1945 the figure has dropped to one-tenth today. One-child families have also decreased — from one-third of all families in 1945 to one-fourth at present.

In most cases these changes mean a shift to 2- or 3-child families. There has been little increase in those with 5 or 6 children.

20. "Search for New 'Mental Chemicals'" and "U.S. Women Now Mothers at Younger Age" (*Science Digest,* July 1956, 86).

evidence in the world pointed to the prosperity of marriage. The article displays an anxiety that is not rational, is not conscious in the most Freudian sense: it has little to do with the tale as it is told. Anxiety, rather, is, as "The Mind" revealed, the result of something unrecognized and unrecognizable yet uncannily destabilizing to the structure of life, a terror that might grip the nation, adversely affecting productivity and spreading disease, an irrational fear that might cause a man to fail the bar yet again.[134]

By itself, "Why People Don't Marry" thus offers further evidence that psychoanalysis as cultural metaphor did not work in the reification of a psychoanalytic notion of civilization during an era commonly referred to as *the psychoanalytic golden age*. The article touts the effectiveness of "treating" marriage phobia, but its effectiveness is immediately undone by the joke, the slip of the tongue, the cartoon. The cartoon, in other words, functions as the symptom, returned from the unconscious to reveal that repression (unlike oppression) is always incomplete. The cartoon's presence on the page reveals that, even though the unconscious phobia is made conscious by a year of psychotherapy, the anxiety to get off the hook remains. Just as psychoanalysis did not cure the marriage phobia (according to the article, one in three Americans remained unmarried), the search for sanity did not stop insanity (a lack of productivity, a generalized anxiety) from sweeping the country. And, as long as the symptom persists, the progress narrative remains in jeopardy.[135]

Yet the important difference here is that an article explaining the mechanism of the tranquilizers appears directly above an article voicing concerns about marriage, propagation, and the longevity of mankind. This arrangement is uncannily replayed in each of the other articles mentioned at the beginning of this section. In *Science Digest,* "Search for New 'Mental Chemicals'" ("Today, psychiatry and the laboratory have joined hands in psychochemistry, the science of chemically-induced behavioral change") sat above "U.S. Women Now Mothers at Younger Age" ("About 50 per cent of women reaching ages 20 to 24 had already married in 1915, compared to 70 per cent last year [1955]. . . . [T]he percentage of childless women declined from about 27 in 1945 to 17 in 1955").[136] The article "New Drug for Mental Patients" appeared above "Want a Long Life? Get Married," that explains how "married people live longer." Replaying a familiar theme, the "married people" whose mortality is at stake represent a clearly male population: "Statisticians at the Metropolitan Life Insurance Company report the married have an advantage as to mortality all through life, particularly before 45. At ages 20–44, for example, the death rate for the married man is only about half that for the single. The difference is not so marked among females, and it is only recently that married women have had a lower mortality than the unmarried."[137] Finally, *Time* magazine's "Pills for the Mind" begins with a description of a "biological revolution," placed directly over the case study of "a petite blonde" whose marriage was saved by tranquilizers.

I use these examples to suggest that the notion that the biological paradigm provided a definition of *anxiety* that functioned free of prevailing concerns about women's role in civilization is inaccurate. Rather, at the very moment when the notion of a drug treatment for anxiety entered mainstream consciousness, biology provided a new component within a preexisting narrative form. To be sure, the texts of "How Tranquilizers Work" and other "scientific" articles promise that psychoanalysis will be rendered obsolete when the science of psychiatry provides a logical explanation for the notion of the unconscious. And the psychoanalytic notion of anxiety in "Why People Don't Marry"—in which stability is ruptured by unconscious, maternal symptoms—is the very same anxiety that is negated by the explanation in "How Tranquilizers Work" that the unconscious no longer exists.

But, by their configuration on the page, these two articles undermine the certainty of the argument that biology civilized psychoanalysis. Instead, in *Newsweek* at least, the article announcing the death of psychoanalysis visually participates in re-creating the basic structure of the psychoanalytic model of anxiety that it sought to replace. The upper article, "How Tranquilizers Work," represents the post-Oedipal, superegoic realm in which the rules of rationality—"the tranquilizers seem to affect the globus pallidus, the most primitive of these structures"—exert order and define progress. This top realm, however, has meaning only through its placement above an earlier desire, an anxiety once known, represented by that which is below, "Why People Don't Marry." Herein lies the threat of the repressed, the dyspareunic bride, the maternal threat as described by Dr. Friedman. And, together on the page, conscious and unconscious, the articles reconstruct the psychological apparatus of civilization.[138]

Rendering all as conscious, in other words, could not prevent worries about the security of the economy of marriage, of reproduction, and of the stability of social order, in spite of the fact that America was reproducing exceedingly well. These tensions, like the repressed, formed the underside of

THE MILTOWN RESOLUTION * 121

the surface on the page. The performativity of "How Tranquilizers Work" could not function free of its context in relation to "Why People Don't Marry." Over time, the discourse of the upper article expanded, while the lower component was relegated to an uninsured position outside the system of care. As a result, a conversation demanding to be heard only on the surface developed a depth.

At this early point in the popular construction of biological psychiatry, the new science of the mind functions in much the same way as did the old psychoanalysis when anxieties about women were the subject of concern: both participate in the construction of a binary in which the underside of progress is assumed to be the site where *woman* resides. In both paradigms, *woman* implies the threat of lack, the anxiety that scientific precision might not be all it appears.[139] *Newsweek* thus shares with psychoanalysis the assumption of who is rupturing whose progress narrative. The "star patient" is a man. Only when he figures out his woman problem does he pass the bar and go on to a successful career. Unmarried, especially before age forty-five, he risks death.

We might think again of Irigaray's critique that, in its very construction, "the social order that determines psychoanalysis rests on the unacknowledged and incorporated mother." Irigaray argues that such construction is built on a necessary symbolic matricide in an avoidance of a certain pain. The mother *needs* to be repressed, in other words, in order to form the unconscious. Only with her symbolic death can the unconscious become separate from the conscious. This, then, allows the conscious, structured as the laws of the superego, to build a civilization. When the maternal returns and progress halts, as Irigaray argues at the end of *Speculum*, man turns away from his fears and projects them onto the woman. These concerns are brought to life in American popular culture in the 1950s, where the white, often middle-class housewife with psychotic designs on a better life and the single yet ineligible woman who (because of religious differences or object choice) will not allow passage of the bar exam are both constructed as the disease.[140] The symptom may have been defined as outside civilization, even hospitalized and, as Joel Braslow argues, electroconvulsively shocked.[141] But, by the nature of the construct, the symptom finds its way back, the myth of the eternal feminine suddenly situated as the not-in-any-way-good-enough mother, she who forever ruptures Frank Ayd's notion of innovation and spoils his implicit claims of disavowal.[142]

In response, perhaps, is Freud's notion in *Inhibitions, Symptoms, and Anxiety* that the effective neutralization of anxiety is an activity—indeed, a requisite activity in the neurotic state—that the psyche attempts to accomplish by itself, without chemical assistance. In times of tension, the id battles with the superego over the expression of drives. While the former seeks to enact instinctual desires, the latter works—through the voice of the parent and, later, through the voice of culture—to block this fulfillment for the greater good of society. The result of this well-conditioned immune response is the awareness of an internal state of unease called *anxiety*. Freud believed that, in times of anxiety, the ego stands as gatekeeper between these opposing forces, concomitantly perceiving the overwhelming excitation from the id and the threat of punishment from the superego. The unconscious ego's actions in the face of this inquietude are taken with one goal in mind: to protect the psyche from the painful awareness that the very notion of "coherence and sufficiency" is itself a fragile construct.[143] So, in the face of the threat of competition, or the possibility of loneliness, or the potential of the loss of power, comes the defense of repression. Repression, as a defense mechanism, is an attempt to "bind" anxiety.[144]

By *binding*, Freud means that the ego takes these perceived threats to livelihood, wraps them up through the act of repression, and submerges them beneath the radar of consciousness. To bind these emotions is to neutralize and disempower the threat that they represent. This is accomplished by a joining, a pairing, a coming together of valences. Coupling in this sense brings together that which needs to repress and that which needs to be repressed. The latter is a remembrance of things past, the former an identification and a plan for the future. And, together, person and nation are able to go forward in life.[145]

Binding seems to be enacted in the rhetoric around Miltown in the 1950s. In many of the articles that I cite, women are depicted as free radicals, floating threats to stability and generativity. A frigid woman who does not respond to her husband's advances, or a single woman who does not assume her role as mother, or a working woman who threatens to keep a man's job, or an improper woman who does not marry—that woman elicits a certain kind of anxiety within popular discourse. Marriage in this world of signification is not only the blissful union of, it was always assumed, man and mother. Marriage marks the response to the "change within" and a symbolic act of repression in the most literal sense. Marriage also works as a discursive reduction, a way of dealing with a not entirely rational threat. Marriage, in this sense, is a binding, a union and a placement, and, at the same time, a way of talking about anxiety. Out of sight and, if well bound (younger, less educated, more gravid), out of mind. Marriage maintains the requisite components of a structure of order, in the face of constant, psychoneurotic reminders such as jokes, and slips of the tongue, and the one in three Americans who remained unwed at the risk of his own mortality.

Miltown the metaphor was a superb binder. By providing exogenous relief for anxiety, it helped the psyche when the psyche was unable to cope. It bound when psychoanalysis or marriage could not. An adjunct to therapy then became a potent remedy for a "change within." Seven, eight, or nine of ten anxious patients, one in twenty Americans, and countless dogs and cats felt calm after Miltown. Petite blonde women warmed to the touch after Miltown. Mothers came home full of love after Miltown. Spasms quelled after Miltown. What is interesting in the case of Miltown is not that it illustrated a problem that we already knew about—in which women were constructed as the idealized and feared other—but rather that it solved the problem in such seemingly absolute ways. Article after article recounts the claims of amazing efficacy described by the *Physicians' Reference Manual:* "There is perhaps no other drug introduced in recent years which has had such a broad clinical spectrum as meprobamate. . . . The primary indication for Miltown is in anxiety states, in which 70–90 percent of patients are reported as recovered or improved."[146] Unlike psychoanalysis, Miltown offered a discourse of the absolute. It worked. Not vaguely, or with slippage.[147] But completely. It was man's VE day, his Marshal Plan. Miltown, progenitor of Valium and of Prozac, visually and textually accomplished what analysis could not, achieving placebo-controlled, chemically induced resolution in the battle against the repressed. And, as such, Miltown came to embody a system of treatment that upped the ante on Luce Irigaray's diagnostic critique of psychoanalysis. It was, as she might have predicted, a discourse in which the anxiety of patriarchy was inscribed on the symbol of woman. But, taking it a step further, Miltown offered the effective treatment as well. Bound, progress continued.

And thus did Miltown set the stage for future discussions connecting a man's anxiety about change and a woman's name on a prescription pad that would soon become known as a mother's little helper. This because, from its interdisciplinary origins, Miltown provided ready relief for the two types of anxiety that can often function in an examination room—a topic that I explore in chapter 4, where I trace the ways in which themes from popular culture in the 1950s returned to the pages of medical journals in subsequent decades in the guise of pharmaceutical advertisements for later generations of wonder drugs. On the one hand, Miltown was the first in a line of increasingly effective medications for the anxiety suffered by the patient. But, at the same time, Miltown set a precedent for treating the anxiety that had little to do with the patient and a great deal to do with the doctor. Anxiety was the pressure of keeping intact the structure in which the doctor prescribes and the patient ingests. Actual changes in the structure of the doctor-patient relationship would not take place in the medical system for quite some time. But the analogy in this case is accurate. The doctor spoke of the need to keep things as they were. The patient, likely unknowingly, threatened change. The result of their interaction, when acts of diagnosis and treatment followed the transference-countertransference dialectic set forth by Miltown, was anxiety.

In this sense, at stake in the paradigm shift from psychoanalysis to biology is not entirely a new relationship to the symptom. This despite some very real innovation, betterment, and change. Also at stake, as the biological approach to the mind begins to expand in influence in the 1960s, and as data begin to accumulate documenting the untoward effects of biology, is the way in which the symptom is talked about. Psychoanalysis, an elusive and elitist discourse flawed in many regards, gave a language with which to discuss its participation in a process. Countertransference forced a recognition of complicity, at the very least. The change in nosology and treatment brought about by the biological revolution, however, threatened to erase awareness of the power imbalance still inherent in the clinical interaction. As countertransference began to give way to diagnosis and an often-encapsulated treatment, a clinician's awareness of involvement in a process was replaced by an often-prescribed response. The former is on some level an awareness that culture is built on an autobiography of personal and communal repression; the latter, meanwhile, is an experts' inscription, pen and pad firmly in hand.

What was lost in the move to precision and reproducibility was, in other words, not the language to describe the interaction with the woman who had just come to your office seeking treatment. She may well have been in need, and the treatment that you offered her may well have provided relief from her despair. Lost, rather, was the language with which to describe how the context of this interaction may still have been a problem in many ways: a recognition of how an act of prescription can also be an act of resolution and how a narrative seemingly about replacement can at the same time be a narrative about the fear of return.

Chapter Four

THE GENDERED PSYCHODYNAMICS OF

PHARMACEUTICAL ADVERTISING, 1964–97

Women are uniquely vulnerable to institutional pressures toward defining their problems in medical terms.—C. Nathanson, "Social Roles and Health Status among Women"

Pharmaceutical marketing is the last element of an information continuum, where research concepts are transformed into practical therapeutic tools and where information is progressively layered and made more useful to the health care system.—Richard Levy, "The Role and Value of Pharmaceutical Marketing"

*L*ike so many other advertisements, print advertisements for prescription psychotropic medications in professional journals translate existing passions about women into the promotion of specific products. And, like many other types of advertisements, print advertisements for psychopharmaceuticals engage in "masterly manipulations" of gender stereotypes to create consumer identification, followed by identificatory consumption.[1] However, in this chapter, I argue that print advertisements for psychotropic medications, which introduce and promote brand-name psychotropic medications in the pages of nearly all American psychiatric journals, are unlike other advertisements. Pharmaceutical advertisements are unique because of their history of representing women patients in particular ways and because of the specific, psychoanalytic his-

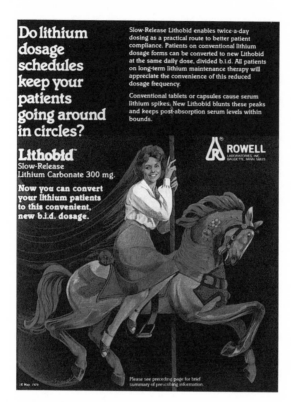

21. A woman rides a horse: Lithobid advertisement (*Archives of General Psychiatry* 36 [1979]: 697).

tory of wonder drugs in which these promotional representations are embedded.[2]

To be sure, representations of women in pharmaceutical advertisements have been sources of controversy for much of the past thirty years. Feminist scholars in the social sciences have shown that the representations of women utilized in these ads give the impression that many more women visit psychiatrists and other health professionals than actually do.[3] Clinicians and health-policy experts have, meanwhile, connected such ads to the prescribing patterns of physicians, suggesting that the overrepresentation of women in them may work to expand epidemiological norms.[4] In building on this work, I want to explore the ways in which the problem is as much historical and visual as it is clinical and quantifiable. Over the time period that I trace, 1964–97, a representational system evolves in long-running, front- or back-cover promotions for Deprol, Valium, Librium, Prozac, and other medications for outpatient conditions in the *American Journal of Psychiatry*

(*AJP*) and the *Archives of General Psychiatry,* arguably the two most influential American psychiatric journals of the past half century.[5] Here, by means of positioning and symbolic consistency, the visual construction of *patienthood* implicitly connects a woman's sanity with her marital status. Manipulations of perspective are also used to paint women's illnesses as threats to a specific notion of *doctorhood,* defined by convention as male, despite the fact that women were entering the profession of psychiatry in increasing numbers.[6] And, most troubling, since the purpose of these images was to enhance sales, the visual relationships between these patients and doctors are shamelessly—indeed, erotically—mediated through psychotropic medications.

This coding system was not invented by an advertising agency or a marketing firm, although the producers of pharmaceutical advertisements clearly benefited from the traditionally lax regulation by the FDA of visual images (the texts of ads, however, were closely monitored to ensure "accuracy").[7] Instead, the advertisements build on the correlation, begun in the 1950s, between specifically gendered notions of anxiety and the promise of pharmacochemical restoration. Reading against psychiatry's own claim to represent a more biologically "objectifiable," gender-neutral classification system, these ads offer an endless stream of enlarged, castrating mothers, colorfully frigid daughters, and shrunken, emasculated sons.[8] Tropes of marriage and motherhood arising directly out of the 1950s provide successful marketing strategies, strategies based on the time-honored assumption that mental health is attained through the pharmaceutical "binding" of women, whose free-radicalized status threatens the ego functioning of men. Once again, the notion that psychopharmaceuticals were treatments for the ills of civilization had imminently psychoanalytic origins, born of the influence of Freudian psychoanalysis on the construction of biological treatments in American popular culture in the 1950s. Pharmaceutical advertisements posit a specific means of discharge (prescription) by which such concerns can be dealt with while attesting to the mutability of this methodology in the face of change. As such, I argue that the ads both convey information about pharmaceutical products and ironically perpetuate what I have called *Freudian* assumptions about symptoms within the pages of journals that were increasingly hostile to psychoanalysis in general and psychoanalytic notions of gender in particular. Providing further evidence for my contention that psychoanalysis formed the unconscious of biological psychiatry, the ads offer a visible forum in which psychotropic drugs argued to treat individual, bio-

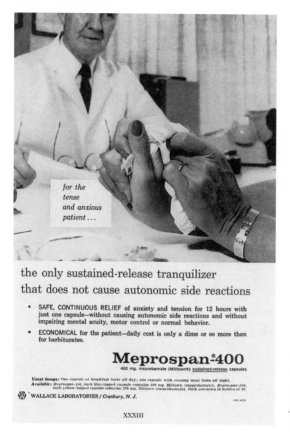

22. A prescription for worried hands: Meprosan advertisement (*American Journal of Psychiatry* 118 [1961]: xiv).

logical illnesses were shown to respond to social problems and specifically problems posed by women at different points in time.

In *Couching Resistance,* Janet Walker argues that feminist attacks on the American psychoanalytic establishment in the latter half of the twentieth century helped change hegemonic notions of gender within psychiatry. Citing Betty Friedan's *Feminine Mystique* and Simone de Beauvoir's *The Second Sex,* Walker claims that "the major challenge to rigid psychiatric notions of femininity came, of course, from the women's movement of the 1960s," which called into question "the second-class status of women perpetuated by aspects of psychoanalysis."[9] Walker rightly points out that such attacks were furthered by scholar-activists in latter decades, including Kate Millett (*Sexual Politics*), Phyllis Chesler (*Women and Madness*), and P. Susan Penfold and Gillian Walker (*Women and the Psychiatric Paradox*). These are but a few of the works that, according to Walker, illuminated the ways in which psychiatric treatments "reproduce the female experience in the family, in which men are dominant," as well as a diagnostic system in which "girls feel and are inferior" and "maternity is the final (and only) step to mature normal femininity."[10] Meanwhile, such standard psychoanalytic concepts as *castration anxiety* and *penis envy* came under specific condemnation owing to their underlying, "phallocentric" assumptions (thus suggesting a certain confluence between feminist and biological projects).[11] The result of these and other critiques was, Walker concludes, an increasingly fractured and decreasingly influential psychiatry, forced to grapple with more complex definitions of the "female role."[12]

Yet this is the exact notion of change called into question in pharmaceutical advertisements, which base their visual appeals on reformulating and rearticulating over time the male-female system exposed by feminist critics and critiqued by biological psychiatrists. Thus, an important context for my reading of the advertisements is provided by "feminism"—a term that I bracket because it is not feminism per se that appears in the images but, rather, mainstream concerns about feminist protests. That is, the ads reflect the threat that these protests seemed to pose to marriage, maternity, femininity, normality, and other indicators that were defined differently at different points in time yet were statically perceived as being in flux. Following the discourse of Miltown, the advertisements then merged popular anxiety about the "female role"—and specifically that role once defined and guarded by psychoanalysis—with emerging information about new forms of chemical, biological treatment while unsubtly presenting their products as cures for wholly social problems. A point of connection between medical and cultural representation systems, the ads thus place the identity crisis taking place in psychiatry within the context of larger conversations about women and men and suggest yet another way in which American culture helped shape biological notions of psychopathology and its chemical treatments.

First, I trace the tensions at play in tranquilizer advertisements from the 1960s, where the still-momist ambitions of married women and the early protests of the second wave of feminism combine to destabilize the smooth running of civilization. Then I turn to a series of Valium advertisements from the 1970s in which radical feminism blatantly plays a similar role. I conclude with an analysis of selective serotonin reuptake inhibitor (SSRI) images from the late 1990s, in which seemingly innocuous depictions of working women wearing wedding rings reveals a parlance between contemporary advertisements and prior waves of psychopharmacology. In each image, mental illness is predictably presented as a threat to the nuclear family, a condition that requires treatment with pharmaceuticals instead of the talking cure. The persistence of this connection allows me to historicize the advertisements and to argue that their history evolves out of the analytic logic that they perpetuate: that anxieties undiagnosed and untreated in women are the cause of anxieties in men.

Of course, nearly all advertisements work through this conflation of transference and countertransference. Successful advertisements, Susan Josephson argues in *From Idolatry to Advertising,* create a broadly understood point of conflict—an ellipsis, an empty space, a feeling of need—that leads to a realization of "anxiety, in the form of an inadequacy or fault that the product can cure." An advertisement acts best, according to Josephson, as "a reminder," "a memory image that viewers can think of when they feel a desire that needs to be filled."[13] As such, advertisements are not so much full of information as they are empty or loose. Advertisements create anxiety and then provide their viewers the relevant information with which to construct a narrative that resolves the anxiety with an understanding of—to be followed, it is hoped, by the consumption of—the brand-named object being promoted.

Another key difference here, however, is that pharmaceutical advertisements from professional journals require a slightly more complicated notion of the relational aspects of anxiety because a prescription interaction is involved. Unlike their direct-to-the-consumer (DTC) descendants in the popular media, advertisements from professional journals ask their target audience, primarily physicians, to locate anxiety in someone else.[14] Pharmaceutical advertisements from the *AJP,* the *Archives,* and other psychiatric publications ask their viewers, not to become aware of an "inadequacy or fault" in themselves, but rather to use their diagnostic powers to ascribe an inadequacy or fault to someone whom they will view at a later point in time. It then follows that the products that cure this fault do so, not in the doctor, but in the patient. Pharmaceutical advertisements could, thus, be said to create anxiety by the transitive property: while most advertisements seek to establish a direct correlation between point a (the viewer) and point c (the product), pharmaceutical advertisements must account for, and, indeed, appeal to, an intermediate point b (the doctor) along the way.

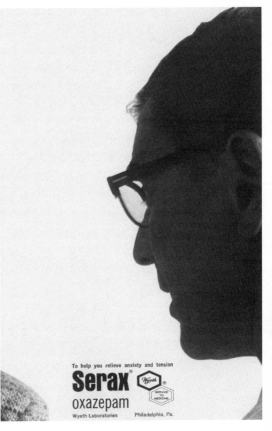

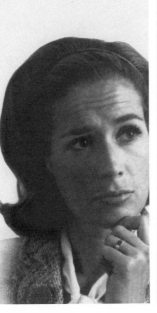

In managing tense, anxious patients here's one combination that makes sense: your understanding counsel and Serax®

oxazepam, Wyeth

Precautions: Hypotensive reactions are rare, but use with caution where complications could ensue from a fall in blood pressure, especially in the elderly. One patient exhibiting drug dependency by taking a chronic overdose developed upon cessation questionable withdrawal symptoms. Carefully supervise dose and amounts prescribed, especially for patients prone to overdose; excessive, prolonged use in susceptible patients (alcoholics, ex-addicts, etc.) may result in dependence or habituation. Reduce dosage gradually after prolonged excessive dosage to avoid possible epileptiform seizures. Caution patients against driving or operating machinery until absence of drowsiness or dizziness is ascertained. Warn patients of possible reduction in alcohol tolerance. Safety for use in pregnancy has not been established.

Not indicated in children under 6 years, absolute dosage for 6 to 12 year-olds not established.

Side Effects: Therapy-interrupting side effects are rare. Transient mild drowsiness is common initially; if persistent, reduce dosage. Dizziness, vertigo and headache have also occurred infrequently; syncope, rarely. Mild paradoxical reactions (excitement, stimulation of affect) are reported in psychiatric patients. Minor diffuse rashes (morbilliform, urticarial and maculopapular) are rare. Nausea, lethargy, edema, slurred speech, tremor and altered libido are rare and generally controllable by dosage reduction. Although rare, leukopenia and hepatic dysfunction including jaundice have been reported during therapy. Periodic blood counts and liver function tests are advised. Ataxia, reported rarely, does not appear related to dose or age.

These side reactions, noted with related compounds, are not yet reported: paradoxical excitation with severe rage reactions, hallucinations, menstrual irregularities, change in EEG pattern, blood dyscrasias (including agranulocytosis), blurred vision, diplopia, incontinence, stupor, disorientation, fever, euphoria and dysmetria.

Contraindications: History of previous hypersensitivity to oxazepam. Oxazepam is not indicated in psychoses.

Availability: Capsules of 10, 15 and 30 mg. oxazepam.

Photograph posed by professional models.

To help you relieve anxiety and tension

Serax® oxazepam

Wyeth Laboratories   Philadelphia, Pa.

23. When a doctor's understanding counsel is not enough: Serax advertisement (*American Journal of Psychiatry* 123 [1966]: 372–73).

That these advertisements often successfully negotiate this algebra is a point that I take as given. While in no way do I mean to imply a causal relation between image and action, I support (and take as a central problematic of this chapter) the contention made in Thompson's "Sexual Bias in Drug Advertisements" that "drug companies, of course, believe their advertising sells drugs, or they would not be spending millions of dollars annually on drug advertising": "If experience did not show beyond doubt that a great many physicians are splendidly responsive to current advertising, new techniques would be devised in short order."[15] Moreover, it is important to note that many people, and many more women than men, visit physicians seeking treatment for problems that are in many cases successfully treated with psychotropic medications.[16] However, pharmaceutical advertisements have historically amplified the frequency of this interaction by translating oversimplified markers of women's gender, race, and class into a visual language. The result has been a highly successful marketing strategy, one based on the destabilization of the selfsame biological anxiety that the medications were purported to treat. Blurring the line between marriage, maternity, and mental illness, the advertisements then ask doctors to look at certain women from predetermined spectator positions, view them as patients, and treat them as such.

Deprol, 1964: Psychopharmacological Momism

In many pharmaceutical advertisements of the early 1960s, the white, middle-class married woman was, not only the victim of mental illness, but once again the cause of it as well. A back-cover advertisement for the tranquilizer Deprol, which ran in the *AJP* for six months in 1964, asked doctors to make a diagnosis that illustrates my point all too well.

Deprol was the direct pharmaceutical descendant of Miltown. A modified minor tranquilizer that combined four hundred milligrams of meprobamate with one milligram of the anticholinergic drug benatyzine hydrochloride, Deprol was argued to better control the corporeal symptoms of anxiety by providing additional sedation and muscle relaxation. Yet the advertisement suggests that much more than chemical composition connected Deprol with its famous forefather.[17]

The advertisement enters a scene likely familiar to many *AJP* readers in the mid-1960s: a clinical interaction between a white physician and a middle-aged white woman. By depicting a medical encounter at the moment of assessment, before the treatment has begun, the advertisement invites its viewers to join with the doctor in the act of diagnosis. Here, these viewers would have had no trouble locating what Josephson terms the "inadequacy or fault that the product can cure"—it surely exists on the woman marked as patient in the foreground of the image. Situated to the left of the doctor, the clearly unmedicated woman demonstrates the conventions of psychoneurotic distress. Her brow, for example, is markedly furrowed, her gaze is nervous and indirect, and her hand clutches her heart is if in the throes of a painful emotion. Few viewing this image would have needed to reference the *DSM-I* to ascertain that the woman suffers from a textbook case of anxiety.[18]

Similarly, many of the visual markers in the image point to a power imbalance between doctor and patient, which is assumed requisite for a clinical interaction to take place. The physician's authority is vested in his white coat, in much the same way that it was on the cover of Henry Safford's *Tell me Doctor* (see chapter 2), and further sanctioned by his framed license on the wall. From his position behind the desk, the physician gazes at the patient with what the art historian Tamar Garb calls the "socially legitimated, historically specific, socially and psychically produced look, the non-innocent look of culture."[19] The woman patient, seemingly in the less-powerful position of object, is, therefore, defined in opposition to the doctor's medically legitimated gaze. As such, the advertisement asks its viewers to think like doctors when viewing the image: to observe the diagnosed but not-yet-treated patient in much the same way that the physician in the image does and to come to the conclusion that the diagnosis requires treatment with Deprol.

However, in contrast to the cover photograph of *Tell me Doctor* (an image in which the doctor's scopic power literally disrobes the helpless patient), the advertisement destabilizes the hierarchy of the clinical interaction through a subtle manipulation of the system in which doctors have power and women lack it. This difference can best be understood by considering the implications of the large wedding ring appearing on the fourth finger of the woman's left hand. While in *Tell me Doctor* the ring connotes modesty—the woman uses her ringed hand to hold up her falling gown—here the ring suggests a host of confrontational meanings.

Certainly, in the 1960s, the trope of a middle-aged woman wearing a wedding ring still implied normativity, stability, and adherence to social mores. According to *Gender Advertisements,* Irving Goffman's classic book

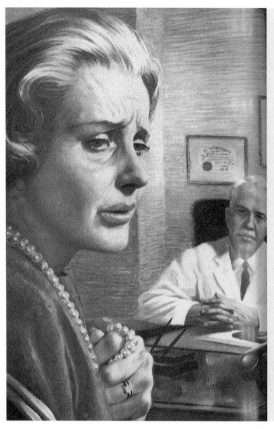

To relieve symptoms of depression and associated anxiety

helps release normal aggression

In neurotic depressive reactions, 'Deprol' helps relieve oppressive despondency and reduce self-hostility. Psychotherapy can then more readily guide the patient's aggressions into more normal and acceptable channels.

helps calm related anxiety

'Deprol' is particularly useful in reducing the anxiety associated with depression and thereby promoting restful sleep.

helps relieve depressive rumination

'Deprol' can often relieve depressive rumination and help the patient function better at home, social and business environments while more lasting gains are being sought through psychotherapy.

Deprol®

meprobamate 400 mg. + benactyzine hydrochloride 1 mg.

Ⓦ WALLACE LABORATORIES/Cranbury, N. J.   CS-5171

24. Viewers are invited to join with the white-coated doctor in the act of diagnosis: Deprol advertisement (*American Journal of Psychiatry* 120 [1964]: xviii–xix).

examining advertisements of the 1960s and 1970s, "Women more than men are pictured using their hands in advertisements." That wedding rings feature prominently on these hands shores up a woman's place in a cosmology where the coherence of "the nuclear family as a basic unit of social organization" was primary.[20] Wedding rings thus locate the women in advertisements, and the products they represent, within the larger narrative structure in which marriage implies narrative resolution. According to Laura Mulvey, such strategies also pervade Western cinema, marriage at the end of a movie implying "symbolic social integration" into the patriarchal structure of narrative (a point that Mulvey accesses through the work of Vladimir Propp, who traces similar tropes in cultural modes of storytelling, arguing that marriage often is an important convention in the narrative closure of folk tales).[21]

The wedding ring in the Deprol advertisement, however, has the opposite narrative effect: rather than being a symbol of closure and resolution, it is a locus of ambiguity, opening up the possibility of two equally plausible readings or, more accurately, two possible notions of psychopathology. First, the ring implies that the married woman is the source of a mental illness that threatens both the "basic unit of social organization," the family, and the civilization of which this unit is a part. But, second, it suggests that, rather than the married woman causing the pathology in civilization, civilization could also be the cause of the pathology in the married woman. The first reading is the one supported by the advertisement's accompanying text: "depression and associated anxiety," "oppressive despondency," and "self-hostility" cause the aggression and anxiety that render the patient unable to "function" at "home," that is, as a mother and wife. Society suffers as a result. One need only consider the obvious manipulation of perspective to understand how such a reading is borne out by the image. Visually foregrounding the unmedicated woman serves both phantasmagorically to dwarf the suddenly small doctor and not so subtly to invert the site of anxiety in the advertisement.[22] As Goffman indicates in describing advertisements in which the "social weight of power, authority, rank," do not fall along traditional gender lines: "On the very occasions where women are pictured larger than men, the men seem almost always to be not only subordinated in social class status, but also thoroughly consumed as craft-bound servitors."[23] In the Deprol advertisement, however, the inversion of the status relationship serves to shift the anxiety from the patient to the doctor, thereby complicating Goffman's notion of servitude.[24] The licensed, white-coated physician is marked as the

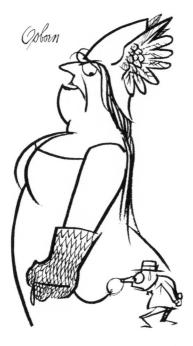

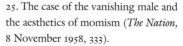

25. The case of the vanishing male and
the aesthetics of momism (*The Nation*,
8 November 1958, 333).

bearer of authority, rank, and office, yet his authority is visually subverted by
the untreated patient, whose size and potential for aggression and hostility
present her as a threat, not only to the doctor, but to the very structure of
the medical interaction.

Presenting an oversized, married woman as a threat to the authority of
men is a message that would still have carried a great deal of cultural valence
in the early 1960s, following the sociopathology of the "momism" of earlier
decades (see chapter 3). To recall, Philip Wylie's *Generation of Vipers* cited
women's "ambitious rage" and the "collective aspects of marriage" as causes
of the emasculation of men, who were "made into slobby onans" and "carica-
tures of themselves by reversed ontogeny."[25] Momism is also important for
my purposes here because it carried a visual as well as a textual threat. Taking
their cue from Wylie (who claimed to take his cue from Freud), depictions
of large, intimidating women and resultantly microscopic men appeared in
images ranging from the cartoons of James Thurber, to representations on
the cover of *Look* magazine, to the Osborn cartoon from Eve Merriam's 1958
satire in the *Nation* entitled "The Matriarchal Myth; or, The Case of the Vanishing Male."[26] In each case, the constructed threat of woman—much like

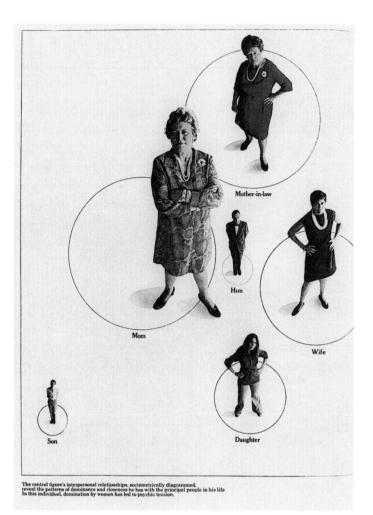

The central figure's interpersonal relationships, sociometrically diagrammed, reveal the patterns of dominance and closeness he has with the principal people in his life. In this individual, domination by women has led to psychic tension.

26. Domination by women leads to psychic tension in men: Librium advertisement (*Archives of General Psychiatry* 24 [1971]: 290).

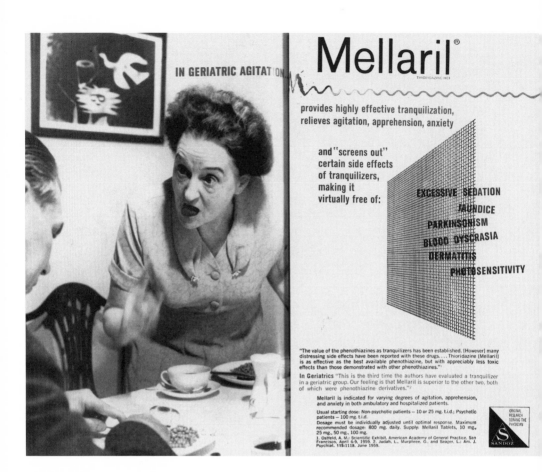

27. Let me eat my peas: Mellaril
advertisement (*American Journal of
Psychiatry* 117 [1960–61]: xii–xiii).

the inverted power relationship between a large, well-manicured patient and a relatively shrunken clinician—is presented as destabilizing the structure of society.

Such a configuration appeared in numerous pharmaceutical ads throughout the era, each suggesting that the uncontrolled, married woman was as much of a threat to the white-coated biologist of the 1960s as she had been to the psychoanalyst of the 1950s.[27] As an inside-front-cover Librium advertisement from the *Archives of General Psychiatry* well illustrates, the visual trope of the threat of the married woman to a man's virility lived on in the conservative pages of psychiatric journals well after the notion of momism had fallen out of popular discourse.[28] Implicitly, the threat that this woman presents is cast as her direct confrontation of male power and privilege.

The second implication suggested by the wedding ring in the Deprol advertisement, and by the many other advertisements of the mid-1960s that connect visual markers of marriage with the symptoms of mental illness, is that, rather than the married woman causing the pathology in civilization, civilization could also have been the cause of the pathology in the married woman. By this reading, marriage is not an institution that empowers women to become domestic superwomen; it is an arrangement that drives middle-aged white women to visit psychiatrists. In this case, the ring implies a mother's dissatisfaction, and even despair, with the structure of marriage and, by extension, with the structure of society. Correlatively, while momism enjoyed its final, senescent days in the sun, mothers were beginning to voice their unhappiness with an American culture that was, to refigure the language of the advertisement slightly, despondently oppressive.

For example, Friedan's *The Feminine Mystique,* published in the same year that the Deprol advertisement appeared, articulated the discontent of a generation of women. Often described as the turning point in the second wave of feminism, Friedan's book traces a shift in the female image from the "Madonna/whore" binary that traditionally characterized "men's representations of women" to the "split" between "the feminine woman, whose goodness includes the desires of the flesh," and "the career woman, whose evil includes every desire of the separate self." Such stereotypes are intimately connected with psychotherapeutic narratives. The "bright, well educated career woman" is so "masculinized by her career that her castrated, passive, impotent husband is indifferent to her sexually," and, therefore, she seeks "help from a psychiatrist."[29] That Friedan gave voice to the discontent felt by many

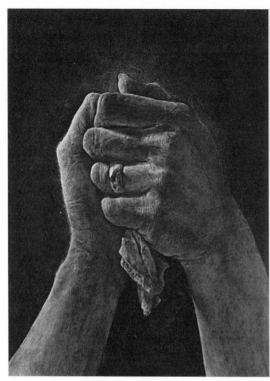

The emotional symptoms that go hand in hand...

Diagnosed psychoneurotic anxiety and depression.

Increasingly, physicians have come to recognize that, "Patients seldom, if ever, appear with depression or anxiety alone; more often they have both in varying degrees."[1]

Clearly, this poses a problem in the patient treated with a tranquilizer or an antidepressant alone: "The combination of anxiety and depressive states often makes the diagnosis confusing. Some apparent anxiety neurotic states merge into clear-cut psychotic depressions. When the patient recovers from the depressive episode, he is left with residual anxiety states. The anxious neurotic background may predispose to a psychotic depression. It is important to recognize the predominant affective reaction in order to give proper therapy."[2]

Since psychoneurotic anxiety and depression may coexist, there is often a place for Sinequan (doxepin HCl).

Because Sinequan is the first *single* agent effective against a broad range of symptoms of both anxiety and depression.

Its marked activity against the common symptoms of *both* anxiety and depression—apprehension, insomnia, fatigue, functional complaints—may often eliminate the need for fixed combinations or admixtures of agents, with their inherent potential for two sets of adverse reactions.

And, although Sinequan itself is a potent antidepressant and tranquilizing agent, clinical experience has shown it to be well tolerated—even in the elderly. The nature and incidence of side effects compare favorably with those of other psychotropic drugs, the most common reactions being drowsiness and symptoms due to anticholinergic activity.

The frequent association and the difficulty in recognizing depression underlying anxiety make Sinequan a prime candidate in the choice of a drug to be employed routinely in the office management of diagnosed psychoneurotic anxiety, especially when depression may suppress therapeutic response?

1. Claghorn, J.: Psychosomatics Supplement 11:438, Sept.-Oct., 1970.
2. Bennett, A.E.: G.P. 27:101, May, 1963.
3. McLaughlin, B.: Psychosomatics Supplement 10:28, May-June, 1969.

because psychoneurotic anxiety and depression often coexist

Sinequan®
DOXEPIN HCl

Starting dosage
25 mg. t.i.d.
for mild to moderate
symptomatology

©1971, PFIZER INC.   Please see following page for adverse reactions, contraindications, warnings and precautions.

28. The hands of emotion: Sinequan advertisement (*Archives of General Psychiatry* 27 [1972]: 346–47). *Note:* Rather than the married woman causing the pathology in civilization, civilization could also have been the cause of the pathology in the married woman.

of the housewives she described is a point that hardly needs to be argued. As Susan Douglas writes, "The real tip-off that many of our mothers hated their assigned positions, weren't sure whether to hate themselves or the men around them, and were tired of straddling the untenable contradictions in their lives was the eagerness with which thousands of them ran out to buy *The Feminine Mystique.*"[30]

Advertisements, like Rorschach tests, are texts that ultimately profit by ambiguity, and pharmaceutical ads of the 1960s are no different. It is impossible to discern which reading of the ring was "intended" (this is, of course, the point), and, anyway, such information would reveal little about the ring's role in the advertisement's reception. Clearly, however, the success of the ads is due in part to their ability to reflect the tensions inherent in the moment in which they were produced. In an ambiguous symbol, pharmaceutical advertisements connected the concerns of Wylie's and Friedan's books and, more important, of the social movements that they represented. In the space between the decade before and the decade to come or between the threatening mom of momism and, as I discuss next, the protesting mom of feminism, the wedding ring translated the concerns of both women and men, patients and doctors, into the language of illness and its brand-named, chemical cure.

Valium, 1970s: Jan's Feminism

As we have seen, as a result of its massive overprescription to married, middle-class women in the 1970s, Valium became known as *mother's little helper.*[31] However, judging by subtle differences between the two seemingly similar inside-front-cover *Archives of General Psychiatry* advertisements to be discussed in this section, Valium might have been intended for daughters as well as mothers.

When in the late 1960s and early 1970s the women's liberation movement burst onto the national stage, American popular culture turned its attention to the next generation of women. "Many of the new feminists are surprisingly violent in mood," *Time* magazine's November 1969 article "The New Feminists" reported, complete with photo exposés of "angry young women" who "hate men" and "learn karate" and descriptions of the legions of women who "burn their brassieres."[32] In March 1970, *Newsweek's* "Special Report: Women in Revolt" contended that "women's lib groups have multiplied like freaked-out amoebas . . . spreading a hostility that is gravely

infectious."[33] Kate Millett was featured on the cover of *Time* in August
1970: an accompanying article condemned her argument in *Sexual Politics*
that women's oppression originates in men's "sexual power over women"
and is institutionalized through the "political economy of patriarchy" inherent in the institutions—such as "marriage" and the "male-female role system"—that they imply.[34] Ti-Grace Atkinson explained to a national television audience that "marriage means rape."[35] Importantly, in its coverage of
the debates within the women's movement about female orgasm and lesbian-
ism, the mainstream press zeroed in on the notion that women may not need
men—a point derived from, among many sources, Jill Johnson's claim that
"a true political revolution would not occur" until "all women are lesbians"
and Anne Koedt's essays.[36] Psychoanalysis, and Freud specifically, became a
target in the ensuing debates about biology as destiny and biology as determinism. "Freud," Millett wrote, "is the strongest counterrevolutionary force
in the ideology of sexual politics."[37]

Far from the national glare, a biology claiming to work at a more fundamental level than anatomy or destiny grew in stature in psychiatry. Double-
blind, placebo-controlled research methods allowed investigators to control for transference, countertransference, and other "subjective biases" of
human interaction, in the project of objectively determining the effectiveness
of new drugs.[38] Split-brain research, evoked potentials, and the discovery of
neural pathways and neurotransmitters moved psychiatry farther away from
the consideration of the links between gender, culture, and identity formation. Instead, the profession turned its focus to biological substrates: brains,
pathways, and peptides that were described as largely the same in women
and men, wives and husbands. To recall the *AJP* (see chapter 2), a crisis was
averted when psychiatry was found to be "primarily a medical specialty" that
was "overstepping its boundaries in attempting to treat problems of living,
and was too involved with social questions."[39]

Riding the crest of this new science were the next miracle treatments in
the fight against the anxiety of everyday life, the benzodiazepines, of which
Valium was the most famous. Approved by the FDA in 1964, Valium was
shown in 1967 to "reduce the activity of serotonin neurons . . . and reduce
the activity of norepinephrine neurons."[40] What followed was what the *New
York Times Magazine* would aptly describe as "Valiumania."[41] In 1969, Valium
became the most widely prescribed medication in the United States, on its

way to becoming the most commercially successful drug in pharmaceutical history.[42] By the early 1970s, one in ten Americans was taking Valium for tension and nervousness. According to many credible studies, close to three-quarters of regular users were women.[43]

The makers of Valium took no chances with the ambiguity of a ring to connect mainstream anxieties about the role of women with the selling of psychopharmacology in a series of advertisements that appeared in the *Archives of General Psychiatry* in the summer of 1970. The connection was explicitly illustrated on the page. Here, Josephson's notion—that advertisements create points of tension and then provide their viewers the relevant information with which to construct a therapeutic temporality that resolves the state of tension with a brand-named product—unfolds in a narrative trajectory from top to bottom, left to right, and past to present. In the first of the two-page advertisements, which appeared in April 1970, a series of framed pictures, arranged chronologically, constructs a visual narrative of a woman named Jan.[44] The advertisement invites its viewers to "read" the story of Jan's fifteen-year history of unsuccessful heterosexual relationships after her happy childhood playing tennis with her father (top, left). But neither Tom (top, middle), nor the James Dean–like Joey (top, right), nor buff Charlie (middle, right), nor drunken, groping Bunny (bottom, left) measure up to Dad (who reappears twice): "Jan never found a man to measure up to her father," the text explains. The narrative's final photograph (bottom, right) shows Jan alone on a ship, standing next to a life preserver, looking forlorn.

In the space of six years, the single woman has replaced the married woman as the marker of pathology and abnormality. While the Deprol advertisement presented marriage as the source of anxiety, the Valium advertisement shifts the medical gaze from a woman's control of a man to her lack of one. Jan's inability to find the right man is unequivocally presented, not merely as the result of illness, but as the illness itself. As the text reveals, she is "35 and single." Drug advertisements, it seems, had negotiated the path between momism and daughterism, emerging with a new product in the fight to restore the "male-female role system."

Nonetheless, the message of the Valium advertisement presented some problems, even within the highly problematic world of pharmaceutical advertising. In pharmaceutical advertisements in general, social and cultural tensions are used to broaden existing definitions of disease, thus expanding

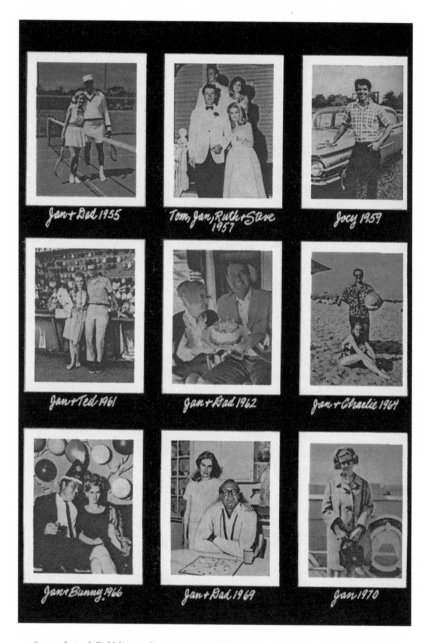

29. "35 and single": Valium advertisement (*Archives of General Psychiatry* 22 [1970]: 290–91). *Note:* In the space of six years, the single woman replaces the married woman as the marker of pathology.

the pool of potential consumers. The more an advertisement can persuade a physician-viewer to think of quotidian assumptions as pathological, the more the product in question is prescribed, bought, and sold. In the Valium advertisement as it appears in the April 1970 *Archives,* however, a line seems to have been crossed since there is no disease except for a social disease. The mental illness is put entirely under erasure, completely effaced by gender-inflected social and cultural tensions.

I make this claim for the simple reason that, when the advertisement re-appeared inside the front cover of the June 1970 *Archives of General Psychiatry,* the word *psychoneurotic* suddenly accompanied the word *single* in the head-line, perhaps to imply that Jan's visit to the psychiatrist might have some connection with psychopathology and that Jan's failure to adhere to social mores of coupling might not have been her only reason for seeking treat-ment.[45] Importantly, however, nothing else in the advertisement has been changed. The flow of images, from dad to desperation, remains intact. As such, the pictures tell the story: not merely that the diseased patient is the single patient, but that being single *is* in this case the disease—a disease that would be cured were the patient simply to get married.

Beneath this glaring change in matrimonial status, however, are sugges-tions that the Valium advertisements are points on, rather than separations from, a visual continuum developed in pharmaceutical advertisements. In the introduction to this chapter, I stated that the method of these adver-tisements remained the same, even when medications, nosological systems, and social conditions changed. Such is the case here, where attention to visual conventions reveals three important points of connection between the Deprol and the Valium advertisements.

First, like the Deprol advertisement, the Valium advertisement asks its viewers to enter into a narrative at a moment immediately prior to the initia-tion of treatment. In both images, the moment of encounter begins when the "illness" has reached its most symptomatic moment—the moment of pre-sentation to the physician. Like the woman in the Deprol advertisement, Jan comes to the physician's office when her symptoms cross the line from de-spair to disease. Here again, viewers are asked to think with the authority of doctors: to recognize the presence of psychopathology and to construct a diagnostic narrative that leads to the conclusion that the object of their gaze requires treatment with a specific brand of medication.

Second, both advertisements attempt to bolster the viewers' sense of

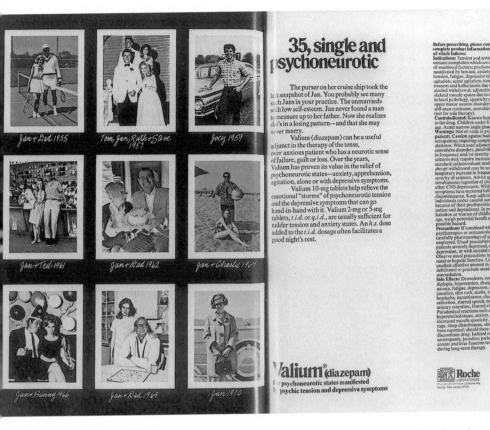

30. "35, single and psychoneurotic": Valium advertisement (*Archives of General Psychiatry* 22 [1970]: 481–82). *Note:* Three months after this ad's first appearance (see figure 29), the word *psychoneurotic* suddenly accompanies the word *single* in the headline, perhaps to imply that Jan's visit to the psychiatrist might have some connection with psychopathology.

visual authority through identification with "the name of the doctor." The Deprol ad invites the viewer to gaze along with the fatherly figure of the physician at the motherly figure of the patient. The Valium ad invites the viewer to be the father or a man of equal stature. The flow of images tells the story of Jan's search for a man who "measure[s] up to her father," a search that seems to have ended in despair. The final photograph of Jan alone near the guard rail on a cruise ship raises the possibility that her search ended with a plunge into the abyss. However, the present-tense syntax of the text reveals that Jan lived to visit the psychiatrist—"Now she realizes she's in a losing pattern—and that she may *never* marry." Lest the viewer miss the point, a glaring empty space, an ellipsis just large enough for one last photograph, appears to the immediate right of the now-penultimate image of Jan on the ship. In other words, the psychiatrist is invited to stand next to Jan in the yet-untaken photo and to provide a welcome sense of closure. The message borders on a breach of the Hippocratic oath: the psychiatrist is implicitly asked to be the next man in the narrative, the man who might finally make Jan happy, the true, Freudian father of the always histrionic, always dissatis-fied woman.[46]

Third, and finally, I argue that the gendered forms of mental illness, whether single or married, function in remarkably similar ways in both images. In the Deprol advertisement, the symptoms of the married woman were depicted as an emasculating threat to the power of the physician. The image suggested that the woman's anxiety, and specifically the possibility that her anxiety might be the result of dissatisfaction with the social order, was a component of a disease. In the Valium advertisement as well, the threat of illness is constructed as the threat of a reading outside the heteronor-mative structure framed by the image. Just as in the 1950s the ring raised the possibility of discontent with the system, so too in the 1970s does the single woman suggest a constellation of alternative symptoms and alterna-tive readings. Perhaps Jan prefers a union with another woman. Perhaps she wishes to live alone. Perhaps she needs a man like a fish needs a bicycle, or burns her bra, or is frigid or ambivalent, or reads Kate Millett, or is a vector for a gravely infectious social pathology. Each of these (overtly hysterical)[47] readings raises the possibility of a life beyond, or a life without, the doctor's control. Each broaches the prospect that the doctor's power—the power to "bind" a patient and, in so doing, bring her back into the fold—might not

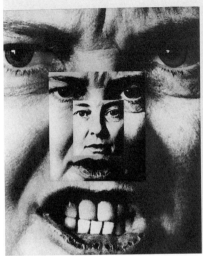

reduce psychic tension

In psychoneurotic patients who overreact to situational or emotional stresses, administration of Valium (diazepam) can help reduce mounting psychic tension with or without associated depressive symptoms and reduce distractions that sometimes interfere with psychotherapy. Moreover, Valium (diazepam) can achieve these beneficial effects even in some patients who had little or no improvement on other psychotherapeutic medications.

with associated depressive symptoms

Because symptoms of psychic tension, anxiety or depression are often intermingled and rarely appear as separate, distinct elements, certain tranquilizers which may precipitate or deepen a depression are of limited value or make additional therapy necessary in some patients. With Valium (diazepam), however, this clinical problem can usually be avoided. For, although this agent is not an antidepressant, it appears to be particularly valuable in patients with psychic tension or anxiety with associated depressive symptomatology. With adjunctive support from Valium (diazepam), patients generally find life more bearable despite continued situational problems.

in refractory patients

When Valium (diazepam) was given by psychiatrists to "difficult" patients considered refractory to other psychotropic agents, significant clinical improvement was observed in many. In numerous instances it was apparent that Valium (diazepam) was effective in controlling tension-associated symptoms such as insomnia, restlessness and other psychic and somatic complaints. It also proved valuable in helping to facilitate psychotherapy, and in enhancing the patient's ability to withstand the stress and strain of environmental pressures.

usually without complications

Valium (diazepam) is generally well tolerated. Positive results are usually seen without impair-

ment of awareness or interference with normal activities. Although side effects such as ataxia or drowsiness may occur, they are avoidable in most cases with simple adjustments in individual dosage schedules.

In prescribing: Dosage – Adults: Mild to moderate psychoneurotic reactions, 2 to 5 mg b.i.d. or t.i.d.; severe psychoneurotic reactions, 5 to 10 mg t.i.d. or q.i.d.; alcoholism, 10 mg t.i.d. or q.i.d. in first 24 hrs, then 5 mg t.i.d. or q.i.d. as needed, muscle spasm with cerebral palsy or athetosis, 2 to 10 mg t.i.d. or q.i.d. Geriatric patients: 1 or 2 mg/day initially, increase gradually as needed.

Contraindications: Infants, patients with history of convulsive disorders or glaucoma.

Warning: Not of value in the treatment of psychotic patients, and should not be employed in lieu of appropriate treatment.

Precautions: Limit dosage to smallest effective amount in elderly patients (not more than 5 mg, one or two times daily) to preclude ataxia or oversedation. Advise patients against possibly hazardous procedures until correct maintenance dosage is established; driving during therapy not recommended. In general, concurrent use with other psychotropic agents is not recommended. Warn patients of possible combined effects with alcohol. Safe use in pregnancy not established. Observe usual precautions in impaired renal or hepatic function and in patients who may be suicidal; periodic blood counts and liver function tests advisable in long-term use. Cease therapy gradually.

Side Effects: Side effects (usually dose-related) are fatigue, drowsiness and ataxia. Also reported: mild nausea, dizziness, blurred vision, diplopia, headache, incontinence, slurred speech, tremor and skin rash; paradoxical reactions (excitement, depression, stimulation, sleep disturbances and hallucinations) and changes in EEG pattern. Abrupt cessation after prolonged overdosage may produce withdrawal symptoms similar to those seen with barbiturates, meprobamate and ethchlorvynol HCl.

Supplied: Tablets, 2 mg and 5 mg; bottles of 50 and 500

now available for the greater convenience of patients on higher dosages—NEW 10-mg tablets

Valium®
(diazepam)

ROCHE LABORATORIES
Division of Hoffmann–La Roche Inc.
Nutley, N.J. 07110

31. A visually threatening, "feminist" woman is tamed, centripetally, by Valium: Valium advertisement (*American Journal of Psychiatry* 121 [1965]: xii–xiii).

be all that it seems. Each falls under the broad rubric *35 and single,* or *psychic tension,* or any of the many other formulations from the 1960s and 1970s suggesting how a woman's madness was marked by the absence of a man.[48] In each case, a patient's symptoms carry the potential of undermining the authority of the doctor and destabilizing the structure of the normative social order that he represents. And, most important for my purposes, this then destabilizes the biological notion of the complaint suffered by the patient and diagnosed by the doctor. To be sure, the symptoms constructed in the ads might appear similar to those that afflict patients. But, within the psychoanalytically informed visual systems created in images viewed by the prescribers rather than the recipients of medication, these symptoms threaten the doctor much more.

Prozac, 1997: Resolution

Almost twenty-five years later, Prozac became America's next psychotropic wonder drug. Prozac, and its class of SSRI antidepressants, was found to inhibit the brain's uptake of serotonin selectively. "We believe," the scientist David Wong and his colleagues wrote in the journal *Life Sciences* in 1974, that "the discovery of specific inhibitors of 5HT reuptake like 110140 will help in elucidating the function of 5HT in the brain and the importance of reuptake as an activating mechanism in 5HT neurotransmission."[49] The result was a medication widely believed to resolve the symptoms of mental inquietude without the risk of addiction or the danger of overdose. Released in December 1987, Prozac had by 1990 become the drug most often prescribed by psychiatrists in the United States. By 1994, Prozac was the second-best-selling drug in the United States, following only Zantac.[50] "Susan A. has spent most of her adult life fighting with people—her parents, her husband," *Newsweek*'s "The Promise of Prozac" explained in March 1990. "But within a month [of taking Prozac] Susan had given up psychotherapy in favor of school. . . . 'I feel 1,000%' she said in a handwritten note. . . . 'I actually like Mom & Dad now, and my marriage is five times better.'"[51] "Prozac is much more than a fad," *Time* similarly wrote in October 1993. "It is a medical breakthrough that has brought relief to individuals such as 'Susan,' a self described workaholic who becomes irritable around the time of her periods and once threw her wedding ring at her husband. Now the edges of her personality have been planed off a bit."[52]

Prozac catalyzed a shift from anxiety to depression (see chapter 5), and from an emotional state to a chemical imbalance, that brought the diagnosis and treatment of mental illnesses in line with widely held, epidemiologically determined gender norms. For instance, numerous studies contended that women were two to three times as likely as men to suffer from major depression—a ratio argued to result from hormonal and genetic differences between the sexes.[53] This finding correlated with prescription rates for SSRI antidepressants, where the fact that women were again two to three times more likely than men to be prescribed these medications was a vast improvement over the far-more-imbalanced numbers seen in the Valium craze.[54]

Moreover, the Prozac phenomenon played out within a cultural climate in which it was widely reported that the women's movement had fundamentally changed conditions for many women in the United States. A 1989 *Time* magazine poll reported that 77 percent of women believed that the women's movement had made life better, 94 percent said that it had helped women become more independent, and 82 percent reported that it was "still improving" the lives of women.[55] The workplace was once again the site where this success was realized, although, unlike women in the 1950s, women in the 1990s found corporate and professional employment.[56] Women, for example, were discovered by De Titta and Robinowitz to be "the future of psychiatry." In a 1991 *AJP* article, these authors examined "the changing demographic trends in psychiatry manpower" and discovered that the percentage of women had increased from 32 percent of all psychiatric residents in 1978–79 to 41 percent in 1987–88. Their conclusion, therefore, was that "gender differences that affect practice patterns and career opportunities may very well change as a function of the increasing representation of women in the profession of psychiatry, and these changes need to be taken into account in planning for future patient care and research needs."[57]

Many of these needs were, indeed, taken into account when, beginning in March 1997, an advertisement for Prozac touting the medication's success in promoting "restful nights and productive days" appeared in both the *AJP* and the *Psychiatric Times,* reappearing monthly or bimonthly for two and a half years. The image used in the widely published ad depicts the clinical narrative at a different starting point than did the advertisements for Deprol or Valium and, thus, does not overtly mark a woman as a disease. By entering the scene at a moment after the visit to the doctor has occurred and the treatment taken place, the Prozac image constructs a narrative of treatment rather than of illness or of follow-up rather than of diagnosis. The woman appears without the symptoms seen in previous images—her brow, for example, is not furrowed, unlike that of the woman in the Deprol advertisement. At the moment of encounter, the tension of illness has dissipated; the work is already done. As such, the woman in the advertisement is depicted as a generative, working member of society, holding fruitful employment in her "productive days," then sleeping soundly in her "restful nights." There seem to be no overt signs of momism, men, or misogyny in the picture; neither is there a threatened physician. The woman appears to be anything but the passive stereotype of the feminine mystique. "Prozac," to quote the popular slogan, "means progress": it restores productivity without a hint of dependence, a cultural aesthetic that Peter Kramer describes as a "drug-induced normal or near normal condition called 'hyperthymia' ": "Hyperthymics are

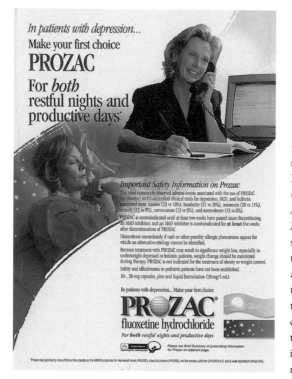

32. Constructing a narrative of treatment: Prozac advertisement (*American Journal of Psychiatry* 155 [1998]: A7). *Note:* By entering the scene at a moment after the visit to the doctor has already occurred and the treatment taken place, the Prozac image constructs a narrative of treatment rather than of illness or of follow-up rather than of diagnosis.

optimistic, decisive, quick of thought, charismatic, energetic, and confident. Hyperthymia can be an asset in business."[58]

However, the advertisement's progress narrative begins to unravel when considered within the representational continuum linking women, marriage, and the marketing of pharmaceuticals whose origin was, in fact, 1950s popular culture.[59] With this history in mind, it becomes clear that the Prozac advertisement represents a specific response to, rather than a departure from, this evolution. Most obviously, the Prozac image, like the Valium image, presents an ellipsis next to a lone woman. To the right of the sleeping woman is a potential space, covered over by the other image and by text.[60] Here, however, the image depends on a different interpretive strategy since every indication suggests that the space is occupied: the hint of a second pillow, accompanied by draped bedsheets to the right of the "restful" woman, implies that she has a partner sleeping next to her. Further, the woman in the Prozac advertisement prominently displays the fingers of her left hand both at work and in bed; and in each scene she wears a shining, gold wedding ring on the fourth finger. Indeed, the images are positioned so that the wedding ring is the visual focal point of each, and the wedding ring thus functions visually as a point of connection between the woman at work and the woman in bed. In bed, the ring appears unnaturally placed as if to highlight its presence (since people rarely sleep with their hands in such a configuration).

At first glance, this appears to be the same thin, gold wedding band worn on the hand of a middle-aged white woman in the Deprol ad three decades earlier. However, because of the different point of narrative entry, a not entirely empty space, and the familiar symbol of a ring, an important change has occurred. The presence of a wedding ring on the hand of a symptom-free woman who is likely not sleeping alone subtly implies that, unlike her long-suffering predecessors, the Prozac woman has taken her place in the social order. The ring functions, not as a marker of a momist threat, as it had in the Deprol image, but as a marker of restoration and containment, a sound night's sleep with a partner whose very presence reassures that the woman no longer suffers the ailment born of the feminist movement. And the ring indicates that what was once a threat—a symptom—has become docile and domesticated by day and by night, in work and in love.

Here, again, the distinction holds true in numerous advertisements for psychotropic medications—advertisements that appear and reappear in professional psychiatric journals throughout the late 1990s and into the twenty-first century. Ringed women smile confidently from Effexor advertisements, 1997–2002, that proclaim "I Got My Mommy Back," "I Got My Marriage Back," and "I Got My Playfulness Back." Over this same time period, Luvox images promote contented mothers holding children, while Wellbutrin and Buspar ads tout a similar return to the nuclear fold.[61] In each case, a wedding ring—and specifically a wedding ring on the finger of a white, middle-aged, middle-class woman—works to identify the cured patient as compliant, bound, and, most important, medicated.

Conclusion: Anxiety

Why is this a problem? Many types of advertisements show women wearing wedding rings very similar to the wedding rings worn by many women in real life. And, surely, all advertisements mirror social mores and cultural beliefs, the intended and unintended outcome of translating denotative prod-

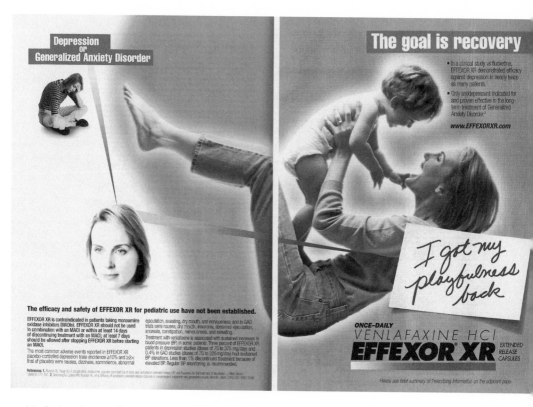

33. Motherhood is visually restored:
Effexor advertisement (*Archives of
General Psychiatry* 58, no. 4 [2001]:
368–69).

ucts into connotative promotional representations. Yet I conclude by returning to my argument that context, audience, and the connection to a very
specific history make pharmaceutical advertisements unique. As such, the
changing symbol of a wedding ring over the latter half of the twentieth century, in advertisements directed at psychiatrists, provides further evidence
for my larger claim that certain specific gender tensions continued to exist in
psychiatric diagnoses and treatments, even as psychiatric language claimed
that they did not.[62]

As I explained at the conclusion of chapter 2, real changes in nosology,
diagnosis, and systems of care separate Deprol from Prozac. Over this time
period, a therapeutic system based on the nuances of the interpersonal interaction was called into question by a system in which the relationship between
doctor and patient was thought secondary to each party's relation to medication. Shorter office visits were the result, as were caregivers trained in the
subtleties of pharmacokinetics at the expense of the kinetics of intersubjective communication. Many historians and practitioners of medicine contend
that these changes were to the benefit of the profession. Psychiatry, the argument goes, became more precise, more practical, and even more gender
blind when the object of its gaze shifted beneath the level of maternal-based
conflict to the level of serotonin. To recall Edward Shorter's argument, cited
in chapter 1, a revolution took place in psychiatry: "The biological approach
to psychiatry—treating mental illness as a genetically influenced disorder of
brain chemistry—has been a smashing success. Freud's ideas . . . are now
vanishing like the last snows of winter."[63]

To their credit, however, Freud's ideas did force a continued, if not always
comfortable, recognition of the ways in which interactions—both contrived
clinical interactions and the real-life interactions that they replicated—functioned along intersecting axes of gender and power. The perceptions of the
patient were conceptualized in conversation with the perceptions of the doctor, while medical "knowledge" was defined in interrelation with its larger
context. For every transference there was a subsequent countertransference,
for every manifestation a prior, if not entirely latent, threat. Nothing in this
system, not even the most quotidian of exchanges, could be understood free
of an often-erotic matrix of signification and exchange. A cigar, in other
words, was never really just a cigar. The biological approach to psychiatry,
meanwhile, was certainly a more precise endeavor. It rejected the nuances of
intrapsychic process and just as often eschewed (or blanched at) the embar-

rassment of penises and absences, of lust and lack. No doubt, the system of care became more efficient, more double-blind, and certainly more objectifiable as a result.

Pharmaceutical advertisements again suggest, however, that psychotropic medications do not wholly nullify the dynamic tensions identified by talking cures. Rather, these medications are also imbued with the very castration, and displacement, and erotic instincts, that the profession of psychiatry "pitched out" of its vernacular. If Shorter were to consider the possibility that biology might have accrued remnant components of psychoanalysis before it melted—after all, the last snows of winter nourish the first flowers of spring—he would surely have realized that even the most objectifiable objects are never defined in a neural vacuum. Instead, in the space between drug and wonder drug, medication and metaphor, these objects become imbued with the anxieties, gender politics, and predetermined categories at play in the larger contexts in which they are produced and metabolized. Without considering this point, psychiatry loses the capacity to understand why, even though biology might disavow the mother (without positing a viable alternative), the "mother" often returns in strange and predictable ways that are the direct result of the categories created and then disavowed by psychiatry itself. Once again does psychoanalysis form the unconscious of biological psychiatry. And, as a result of this repression, psychiatry loses the capacity to understand why its negation of cultural influence, its focus entirely on the brain, renders it less aware of the cultural categories and categorical manipulations so obviously relied on by the makers of pharmaceutical advertisements.

This, then, makes the ads all the more problematic. When read psychoanalytically, their "success" depends on a troubling slippage between transference and countertransference, conscious and unconscious. In their manifest content, the advertisements claim to present a discussion of the anxiety of women, for better and for worse. For better, because many women suffer from anxiety, depression, and other painful conditions treated by psychotropic medications. For worse, because the representations of women in the ads translate a wedding ring, the symbol of the normativization of marriage, into a symbol of the normativization of feminism and of mental illness. Yet, beneath the surface, the message of the advertisements has little to do with women at all. Instead, a discourse insisting to be about women is instead an oversimplified discussion of the anxiety of men as doctors and doctors as men looking at women. Just as in *Newsweek* in 1955, anxiety is not merely the problem described by a patient (either Jan or Susan) who may have felt unhappy in her marriage, or unhappy with her inability to find marriage, or unhappy with the politics of a system that, thinking of Chesler, marks marriage as an index of sanity.[64] Anxiety is also the inquietude in the doctor, made uneasy by the threat that these symptoms come to represent.

Again, there is nothing innovative about this diagnosis. Images of women constructed through the anxieties of men are hardly novel constructions either in medical advertisements or in medicine. The pathologization of the single woman, or the unmarried woman, or the lesbian, extends through the history of psychiatry and many years beyond (consider, e.g., hysteria and its treatments).[65] What is new, however, is a treatment that claims the potential to enhance the ego's ability to bind and, thus, to alter the trajectory of the psychoanalytic narrative. Between an image of a married, symptomatic woman in an office and a married, symptom-free woman in bed three decades later lies the implicit assumption that a crisis has been resolved and order restored. In this visual system, however, the symbol of the resolution of anxiety and the assertion of control—the wedding ring—is connected, not only to marriage, but to prescription. The images, in other words, convey a message that a man's anxiety does not represent the passive, helpless state described by Freud. Rather, following Miltown and the *AJP* itself, this state can now be assuaged by resolving a crisis—a professional crisis or an identity crisis—in someone else. In this equation, objectifiable borders closely on objectification. The woman who threatens the doctor in 1964 sleeps with Prozac in 1997, while the empty space vacated by the shrinking doctor is filled, once again, by the symbol, the prosthesis, the ring. And, in advertisements in mainstream medical journals between the years 1964 and 2000, this symbol is constructed as the symbol of psychotropic medication.

Effectively re-creating the very binary that their products were argued to replace, psychotropic advertisements thus promote the message that male doctors—so construed by looking at the ads—can react to various forms of anxiety by the act of writing a prescription. Prescription writing is, in this system of not entirely chemical imbalance and rebalance, presented as a relationally gendered, if not entirely stabile, form of power. And medications function as the agents of a form of resolution that, I now turn to argue, is once again Oedipal in the classically Freudian sense. Rising and falling as if feminism's protests and successes, the mother thus returns and re-

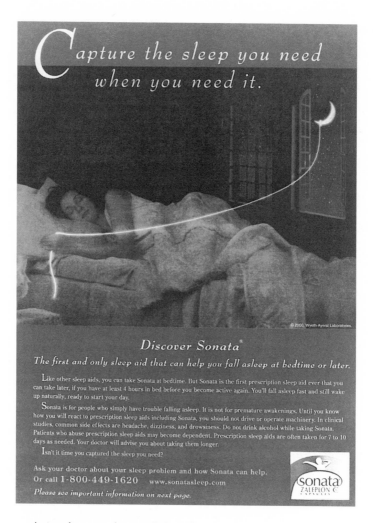

34. A ringed woman sleeps with the aid
of Sonata: Sonata advertisement (*Self*,
July 2000, 91).

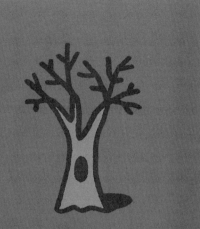

Depression isolates.

Depression can make you feel all alone in the world. Especially when you're around people who think depression is all in your head. Well, it's not. Depression is a real illness with real causes. It can appear suddenly, for no apparent reason. Or it can be triggered by stressful life events, like losing a job or having a chronic illness.

When you're clinically depressed, one thing that can happen is the level of serotonin (a chemical in your body) may drop. So you may have trouble sleeping. Feel unusually sad or irritable. Find it hard to concentrate. Lose your appetite. Lack energy. Or have trouble feeling pleasure.

These are some of the symptoms that can point to depression—especially if they last for more than a couple of weeks and if normal, everyday life feels like too much to handle.

To help bring serotonin levels closer to normal, the medicine doctors now prescribe most often is Prozac. Prozac isn't a "happy pill." It's not a tranquilizer. It won't take away your personality. Depression can do that, but Prozac can't.

Prozac has been carefully studied for nearly 10 years. Like other antidepressants, it isn't habit-forming. But some people do experience mild side effects, like upset stomach, headaches, difficulty sleeping, drowsiness, anxiety and nervousness. These tend to go away within a few

Prozac can help.

weeks of starting treatment, and usually aren't serious enough to make most people stop taking it. However, if you are concerned about a side effect, or if you develop a rash, tell your doctor right away. And don't forget to tell your doctor about any other medicines you are taking. Some people should not take Prozac, especially people on MAO inhibitors.

As you start feeling better, your doctor can suggest therapy or other means to help you work through your depression. Remember, Prozac is a prescription medicine, and it isn't right for everyone. Only your doctor can decide if Prozac is right for you—or for someone you love.

Prozac has been prescribed for more than 17 million Americans. Chances are someone you know is blossoming again because of it.

fluoxetine hydrochloride

Welcome back.

Please see important information on following page. *Lilly*
http://www.lilly.com

35. Often, popular pharmaceutical ads seem vague, caricatured, or abstract to the point of being unproblematic: Prozac advertisement (*Self,* March 1998, 19).

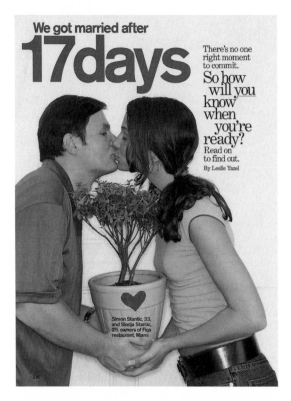

36. "We got married after 17 days" (*Glamour,* June 2002, 236).

returns to psychiatric journals, translated and, ultimately, rescripted into a more digestible narrative form.

Patients, of course, became targets of pharmaceutical advertisements in late summer 1997, when the FDA relaxed restrictions on pharmaceutical promotion. In the years hence, pharmaceutical ads have appeared, not only in professional journals, but also (and predominantly) in women's magazines such as *Cosmopolitan, Marie Claire,* and *Self,* as well as on television, the Internet, and other sites that allow pharmaceutical companies to appeal directly to the consumer. Although the empowered voice of the consumer-patient becomes my focus in chapter 5, for now suffice it to say that current DTC ads occasionally evoke themes that expose a connection with their direct-to-the-doctor progenitors—a point neatly illustrated by an advertisement for the sedative Sonata from *Health* magazine in which the word *capture* is illustrated by a golden string, leading from a bound moon directly to the ringed finger of a woman who would otherwise appear to be sleeping alone. More often, however, popular ads seem vague, caricatured, or abstract to the point of being unproblematic—such as a long-running cartoon Prozac ad from *Self* and *Marie Claire*. Except, of course, for the placement of these ads in women's magazines intimately concerned with "self-improvement," or ways to "feel more attractive," or "ways to catch a man." In this context, mental illness comes to mean the absence of these qualities—not attractive, not self-improved, and, most important, not able to attract a man. When coupled with the implicit message that drugs like Prozac might help achieve such a state, these advertisements potentially cue women readers to provide the other half of a historically developed relationship by asking them to ask the same questions that their doctors have already been prepared to hear—or, more appropriately, to see.

Chapter Five

PROZAC AND THE PHARMACOKINETICS

OF NARRATIVE FORM, 1994–2002

A breakthrough moment occurs near the end of Elizabeth Wurtzel's now-canonical memoir *Prozac Nation*. Throughout much of the narrative, Wurtzel describes her ongoing struggle with depression, experienced as a state of constant inquietude and self-criticism as well as an isolating sense of feeling "like a defective model." This condition is largely unresponsive to talk therapies. However, the author then takes Prozac, and, for an evanescent moment, realizes a sense of liberated actualization: "And then something just changed in me. . . . It happened just like that. . . . It was as if the miasma of depression had lifted off me, gone smoothly about its business, in the same way the fog in San Francisco rises as the day wears on. Was it the Prozac? No doubt. . . . It took a long time for me to get used to my contentedness. It was so hard for me to formulate a way of being and thinking in which the starting point was not depression."[1]

In this chapter, I take a closer look at the posttreatment Prozac self, the self in whom Prozac makes possible a new way of being and thinking, as it is presented in American fictional and autobiographical accounts of women suffering from mental illness in the 1990s. Wurtzel's coming to terms with a sudden lifting of an otherwise intractable depression through treatment with Prozac and her subsequent discovery of a sense of connectedness constitute a narrative convention mirrored in a number of literary works, four of which I will examine here: Lauren Slater's essay "Black Swans"; Pagan Kennedy's short story "Shrinks"; Gary Krist's short story "Medicated"; and Persimmon Blackbridge's novel *Prozac Highway*. Co-opting themes from psychiatry's biological revolution, each text embraces Prozac specifically, and biological psychiatry more generally, to treat both the symptoms of mental illness and a set of gender conventions in which that illness is embedded. At the same time, the escape that these texts celebrate, the sudden lifting of a miasma through a chemical cure, is incompletely sustained. In each case, Prozac's inability to liberate is narrated in terms of the reappearance of the previously defeated gender conventions. Mental health is, thus, undone in these stories by the reappearance of psychoanalytically defined identities and norms, now figured as the limit of Prozac's curative powers. Further, these identities and norms become all the more impervious to critique, inasmuch as they are reinstantiated through the language and the logic of biological psychiatry. Not only do Prozac narratives reproduce a psychoanalytic paradigm, but, in so doing, they risk reinforcing that paradigm's gender conventions by recontextualizing them.

This claim reads against much of the contemporary criticism concerning Prozac-inspired literature (a form so widespread it threatens to go generic along with the medication), specifically the notion that the selves discovered in these and other narratives written by or about women suffering from "mental illness" are constructs of late-twentieth-century postmodern discourse formation.[2] Critics as disparate as Jacqueline Zita, a feminist philosopher, and Edward Shorter, a medical historian, locate Prozac-related works in a cultural moment struggling to come to terms with the perceived breakdown of familiar binaries in the project of a new, more complicated framework for self-definition. For example, Zita describes the women diagnosed and treated in Peter Kramer's *Listening to Prozac* as functioning within a landscape in which "the experience of living in a postmodern body becomes more commonplace as the body loses its prior symbolic unities": "It [the body] becomes a less distinct nexus, merging boundaries of nature/culture, body/mind, self/notself."[3] Shorter, meanwhile, locates the numerous popular and medical writings about Prozac in an era in which patients rush to physicians for pharmaceutical quick fixes and "the pool of postmodern distress is enormous."[4] In these and many other critiques of Prozac, the descriptor *postmodern* is closely aligned with an understanding of the present moment—the moment of treatment or the moment of existence—as one that holds a disregard for temporality and history. Just as Prozac the medication claims to alleviate the symptoms of depression and its related illnesses without the need for retrospection, Prozac the literary genre claims liberation from a cultural discussion rooted in specific notions of the past. This liberation inaugurates what John Schilb has described as a "present widespread biological discourse" leading to "new accounts of selfhood."[5]

Yet describing Prozac literature as a "new account" of selfhood or as a sudden break from the past misses the point that Prozac-inspired fiction and autobiography both listen and talk back to two important conversations, conversations that take place at the intersection of popular and psychiatric cultures over the past half century and that form the foundation of my rereading of the psychiatric paradigm shift in this book. A consideration of these two narrative trajectories allows for a historicization of the criticism of Prozac literature and a better understanding of the gender tensions at play in the literature itself. The first of these conversations concerns the narrative trajectory of wonder drugs—psychotropic medications that become the objects (or, indeed, the subjects) of popular frenzy. As the historian of pharmacology Mickey Smith explains, the patterns of popular euphoria and disenchantment surrounding the release of prior generations of popular drugs designed to treat everyday worries—Miltown and the tranquilizers of the 1950s, Valium and the benzodiazepines of the 1970s—were governed by the three-phase "law of the wonder drug." In *phase 1*, an initial embrace, filled with high hopes and a suddenly fickle discontent with prior forms of treatment, is "encouraged by science writers and an expectant public waiting for miracles from medicine." This leads to a period of "wild enthusiasm" in which the new drug is overvalued, overrequested, and overprescribed. In the process, prior forms of treatment are deemed obsolete. In *phase 2*, "problems" are discovered, and the drug is "undervalued and overcondemned." The result is a fall from grace. Finally, in *phase 3*, "stability" is achieved with what Smith describes as "appropriate evaluation of the comparative worth of the drug." Resolution leads to a rational, if somewhat tempered, understanding of the drug's benefits, which then results in "judicious" long-term use in clinical practice.[6] The social scientist John Marks translates prescription rates during the benzodiazepine craze into the diagram shown in figure 37.[7] In my reading, this trajectory of euphoria, disenchantment, and rationalization applies, not only to broader cultural patterns of drug utilization (or to the rise and fall of anxieties in pharmaceutical advertisements), but

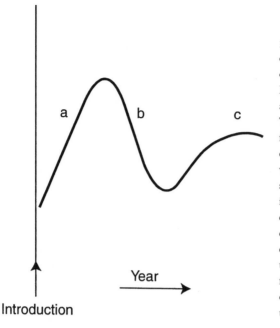

a   b   c

Year

Introduction

37. Prescription patterns during the Valium craze (Marks, "The Benzodiazepines—Use and Abuse," 84). *Note:* The curve of acceptance for a new drug can be outlined as follows: first, wild enthusiasm (the sensation that everything is cured) and no side effects (point *a*); next, devaluation, many side effects, and a decrease in use (point *b*); and, finally, the establishment of rational therapeutic use (point *c*).

also to narrative accounts of individual treatment. In the texts that I examine, characters experience immediate salvation from Prozac, then invariably claim that the drug "does nothing," and, ultimately, discover a more lasting resolution.

The second historical narrative interwoven in Prozac literature concerns the particulars of psychiatric and popular notions of selfhood. Here as well, far from representing a new mode of expression, the Prozac of literature and essay bears the mark of a specific discussion that has taken place over the past half century, although, by the time Prozac arrived, the conversation had seemingly been long over. The dynamics of this discussion—played out simultaneously in American academic psychiatry departments and treatment clinics and in the pages of popular magazines, newspapers, and other forums where the findings of neurochemistry laboratories commingled with the vernacular of public discourse—involve the politics that define how selves are treated and understood. I expand on this definition in the section that follows, but, for now, suffice it to say that the fundamental point of contention centers on different conceptualizations of time that inhere in what might be thought of as modern versus postmodern models of the mind. To recall, psychoanalysis assumed past experiences with mothers and fathers to be the foundation of present identities and posited a notion of change through reflection on patterns of behavior, thus repositioning an individual subject in relation to his or her understanding of the self constructed through prior events. Yet Prozac, and the biological psychiatry for which it often stands as a metonym, would seem to have construed identity and autobiography as a present-tense dialogue. To be sure, biological psychiatry does believe in the past—one is not just born, but also becomes, a chemical imbalance. Buoyed by advances in neurochemistry and genetics, the success of Prozac capped a shift in the discussion of selfhood away from symptoms, words, and understandings that implied prior events. In their stead, a language developed that focused on the here and now and on symptoms immediately observable and quickly treatable. Over the course of the revolution, men were replaced by medications, case studies by MRI scans, fifty-minute office visits by ten-minute evaluations, and retrospection by prescription. In the process, "I am in pain because of where I have been" became "I am in pain." And "I am because of my past" became simply "I am."

Biological psychiatry's insistence on the present tense serves a specifically feminist purpose in the works that I discuss below. In each text, the immediacy of symptoms, the real time of neuroimaging technology, the precision of neural chemicals, and even the space vacated by the disappearance of the doctor become tools with which to renarrate the gendered self. Whereas, in the 1950s, doctors—the Menningers, Dr. Safford, and other white men—were the experts whose words forged knowledge and public opinion (see chapter 3) and patients—women, persons of color, the infirm—were hardly ever allowed to speak, in these texts the voice of the doctor struggles to be heard over that of the empowered health-care consumer. "Black Swans," "Shrinks," "Medicated," and *Prozac Highway* present women protagonists or narrators in explicitly biological terms, as mediated through the literary character of Prozac. Although these texts differ in important ways, each effectively co-opts biological language in the name of ideological critiques of past structures of oppression such as psychoanalysis, literary genre, or self-narration. As Slater explains, "I was a purely chemical being, mood and personality sweeping through serotonin."[8] Breaking from prior renditions of the mental illness narrative, the women presented in these works posit notions of selfhood in which individual and individually gendered subjects —previously considered products of neurotic mothers or of neurotic civilizations—are engaged in the active construction of the terms of their own "illnesses."

At the same time, however, these texts suggest unacknowledged continuities between Prozac narratives and psychoanalytic narratives, continuities pertaining specifically to definitions of gender identity. While each narrator or protagonist overtly dismisses Freudian notions of development—as Jam explains in *Prozac Highway,* "most psychiatrists had moved into the prescription writing business, leaving Oedipus and his buddies behind"—each text reveals that Freudian concepts continued to play out in biological narratives long after Freud fell out of favor.[9] The temporal flow of impassioned embrace, horrified disavowal, and generative resolution—as phase 1 becomes phase 2 and phase 2 becomes phase 3—reenacts a specific and specifically Oedipal notion of gender development, a dynamic that is textually driven by the drug itself. Narratives that laudably reject the gender assumptions so painfully evident in psychotropic drug advertisements are nonetheless affected by these drugs' gendered effects. In highlighting these continuities, I suggest that moves either to embrace or to reject Prozac narratives as new notions of selfhood misconstrue the historicity called on—indeed, depended on—by each text. In so misconstruing, critiques that take biological presentism at face value fail to understand the ongoing relevance of psychoanalytic paradigms as cultural scripts and as social and narrative resources—the Freud of Prozac, as it were—and, thus, fail to see the salience of the gender identities to which those paradigms give shape.

In what follows, I first explain the key distinctiveness of Prozac discourse: its appeal to an atemporal, ahistorical notion of subjectivity that has, in other contexts, been described as *postmodern.* I then explore more fully the ways in which attention to the language and ideology of an always-immediate present is taken up by a literature that stakes its claims of liberation on this postmodernism. Given that, in my reading, the Prozac narrative recapitulates the psychoanalytic trajectory of the self, I ultimately argue that the insistence on a transparent present and on the death of the unconscious denies central insights of the psychoanalytic framework concerning the always-constructed, always-critical status of sexual identity. Grappling with the continuities *and* the disjunctures between past and present discourses of the self (and between literary theory and biological psychiatry) is necessary in order to avoid reinventing and rearticulating the same gender hierarchies for which psychoanalysis was widely and rightly attacked.

Prozac Selfhood

It seems easy to understand why Prozac reads as a postmodern trope. As comes to be recognized in medical and popular discourse, Prozac claims a selfhood that works by a new mechanism of action, wrapped in the promise of a new, chemically engineered neuroscience. But, more important, Prozac's mechanism of action both mirrors and helps produce a new language for representing the internal workings of human experience. Prozac represents the end point of the more than fifty-year-old argument concerning the very framework in which self-narration has been spoken and understood. Psychoanalysis, the loser in the argument, posited a world (and a cultivated self within that world) divided into realms of conscious and unconscious, into those things seen and those things realized only in the threat of dreams and slips of the tongue.[10] Biology, however, proves once and for all that, with the correct visualizing machinery, everything can be made conscious. The biological self is, as proved by state-of-the-art research in neurochemistry, endocrinology, and genetics, not concerned with the modernist plot devices of early-life experiences and unresolved conflicts. It does not narrate a beginning, a middle, and an end, read within a vortex of having and wanting to have. Neurochemical subjectivity is, instead, ahistorical. The biological self—both the abject, imbalanced, diseased self and the desired, posttreatment, healthy self—is explained by the immediacy of presenting symptoms, the impartiality of PET scans and mu-receptors, and the precision of neural chemicals.

Outpatient conditions such as anxiety and, to a lesser extent, depression were once regarded as reenactments of an earlier form of loss in which a patient's presenting symptoms were implicitly assumed to be the result of prior relationships and events.[11] By contrast, late-twentieth-century biology constructs a depression (of which anxiety itself became a symptom) in the present tense beyond even Frank Berger's wildest dreams. This is not only because of the insistence in the *DSM-IV* on defining symptoms as those aspects of disease that can be observed, and often pharmacologically treated, at the time of diagnosis but also because behind the clinical interaction functions an immortal language that is both observational and highly figural. "Major depression is due to a deficiency of available serotonin receptors in relevant brain regions," the *American Journal of Psychiatry* explained in February 1996. "The authors have developed a method for visualizing in vivo regional brain responses to serotonin release by comparing regional brain glucose metabolism after administration of the serotonin-releasing drug dl-fenfluramine, relative to placebo."[12] Biological psychiatry introduces the terminology of science, of chemical imbalances and dopamine hypotheses.[13] And it employs the observing eye of high-speed, echo planar magnetic resonance imaging and positron emission tomography, each of which frames anatomy, destiny, and cortical blood flow in the simulacrum of real time.[14]

Even the most fundamental psychoanalytic concepts of gender difference and gender identity appear sudden, chemical, and observable. The Oedipus complex had been understood within a psychoanalytic paradigm to arise from (past) childhood incestuous desires for the mother, severed and renounced in response to a child's apperception of the rivaled father. The result was the formation of the civilizing superego (present) and the evolution of identity (future) through an act of repression. Neuroscience, however, realizes the fallacy of such temporality by discovering biology beneath culture and context. This biologism was but a rumbling in 1972 when, in the midst of a revolution, Money and Erhardt discover that a child's "core gender identity is" (present) "established before the oedipal phase is thought to begin, shaped primarily by biological forces including the organizational effects of prenatal androgen."[15] By 1995, Friedman and Downey announce (in "Biology and the Oedipus Complex") that the effects of "prenatal androgens causes" (present) an "innate, biologically determined tendency," mediated by distinct biochemical pathways, for sons to feel "rivalrous," "competitive," and "aggressive toward their fathers." "Androgen induced variations" between men and women, and "not early life experiences," are shown to account for the "greater aggressiveness of males within our species."[16] "It appears, in fact," Michael Stone argues, "that male-male competitiveness subserves an adaptive function as a rehearsal of the dominance/submission relationships that are an inextricable (because they are useful!) part of human society."[17]

In this context, Prozac comes to signify conclusive evidence of the death of the unconscious, the final nail in the Freudian coffin. Colorful Prozac advertisements in the pages of popular women's magazines paint mental illness and mental "health" in a presentist syntax that claims to know nothing of the past. The depression long thought to be the result of prior, unresolved conflicts is transformed into the commodified ahistorical. "Depression Hurts: Prozac Can Help."[18] The message—reinforced by a medical system that replaced interaction with prescription—is that excavation and retrospection are not required when medication can do all the work.[19] Similarly, that self of image and representation, of desire and projection—that cultural self once defined by the psychoanalysis that gave Americans a terminology with which to define their national neurosis—often reflects this newfound presentism. "El Sayyid Nosair, the man accused of shooting Rabbi Meir Kahane, reportedly was taking the antidepressant Prozac, which has been blamed by some users for suicidal and homicidal behavior," the *Washington Post* reported on 10 November 1990, attributing Nosair's violence to a chemical rather than a developmental (or political) causality.[20] On 29 November of that same year, the *San Francisco Chronicle* proclaimed Prozac "The hottest pill of 1990."[21] Prozac soon became a national metaphor, and America became a Prozac nation. Prozac proves once and for all that mental illness—and, for that matter, personality in its entirety—is not the result of early-life experiences with gender and sex, with penises and absences. Rather, drive, temperament, and emotion are determined to be the result of neurochemicals and genes. In 1996, the *New York Times* announced the discovery that "individuals who have a slightly abbreviated version of the gene for the serotonin transporter are higher in negative thoughts and feelings than those with a relatively long rendition of the gene."[22] Prozac discourse exposes the imprecision of the analytic narrative and corrects the imbalance once and for all—and with fewer side effects.

Of key importance, Prozac selfhood is constructed in distinct opposition to that posttreatment, healthy self created by prior wonder drugs. The Prozac nation is definitively not "Valiumania" and is even farther removed from the road to Miltown. These psychotropic progenitors produced narratives of sedation and withdrawal, of tranquilizing, toning down, and tuning out. To recall, the public discourses of Valium and Miltown often constructed women like "Jan" as threats to the generativity of men. Competitiveness, assertiveness, and the desire to succeed were coded as anxiety and sedated accordingly. Prozac's, however, is a productivity narrative—and an equal-opportunity one at that. Before Prozac (and surely before Sarafem), most psychotropic medications exerted their effects on numerous neurotransmitters in the brain. Yet the singular effect of the selective serotonin reuptake inhibitors (ssris) on the indolamine system guarantees therapeutic benefit without the untoward cholinergic side effects—lethargy, constipation, sedation—that had long accompanied treatment like thorns on a rose. Ingestors feel "normal," "grounded," and "better than well," able to work, play, and live life to the fullest.[23] The Prozac hero is not Miltown's thirty-six-year-old housewife who learns to ebb and flow on drugs or Valium's strung-out Neely, who pays a heavy price for working in a man's world.[24] Rather, she is Rebecca Buck, a.k.a. Tank Girl—one of what Suzy Menkes calls "fearless heroines with looks to match"—who wears a necklace of silver-dipped Prozac.[25] Implicit in this shift is the notion that the now successfully liberated women no longer threaten men but, rather, can work alongside them in a brave new world that encourages, promotes, and rewards equality in work and in love—a point obviously picked up by Prozac advertisements.[26] As Peter Kramer explains, the Prozac aesthetic allows women to become what he calls *hyperthymic,* that is, chemically Taylorized beings whose disconnect from affective fluctuations renders them manically hyperproductive: "How might a substance like Prozac enter into the competitive world of American business? Psychiatrists have begun to recognize a normal or near-normal mental condition called 'hyperthymia,' which corresponds loosely to what the Greeks called sanguine temperament. . . . Hyperthymics are optimistic, decisive, quick of thought, charismatic, energetic, and confident. Hyperthymia can be an asset in business."[27]

Prozac Narratives

The changes brought about by Prozac, and specifically the promise of a newly presentist discourse of self, also allowed for a new telling of the woman's mental-illness narrative. Since the late nineteen century, the genre had been marked by often-tortured relationships between women and the psychiatric establishment. In texts ranging from the 1892 "The Yellow Wall-Paper" by Charlotte Perkins Gilman to the 1964 *I Never Promised You a Rose Garden* by Hannah Green (Joanne Greenberg), women were confined in the name of treatment. Often, as in Kate Millett's *The Loony Bin Trip,* they were treated against their will. Occasionally, they overcame great obstacles—as in Barbara Gordon's *I'm Dancing as Fast as I Can*—and went on to lead productive lives. In these and similar works, the treatment of women's mental illness was often depicted as synonymous with the treatment of "female emotions."

In reading these stories today, the suffering that they present seems as much a function of structural factors as of physiological ones; the protagonists' pain appears inseparable from a social context in which they are locked in attics and subjected to "rest cures" rather than the unavoidable consequence of inherent illness. The constraints placed on women in the mental-illness narrative were, however, by no means limited to the structure of psychiatric institutions. Rather, the rhetoric through which mental illness was described and communicated, and through which the internal workings of human psychological experiences were made literary, had long been supplied by a psychoanalytic vocabulary that assumed that the world separated into a familiar division of mothers and fathers and that coded threats to this binary as pathological.[28] In Lucy Freeman's autobiography *Fight against Fears,* for example, the "successfully" treated narrator comes to reproduce the psychoanalyst's contention that mental health is made manifest by heterosexual marriage and that "the happy person settles for one mate."[29] Meanwhile, Hannah Green's cure is contingent on her realizing that her "symptoms" are conscious manifestations of unconscious processes, which her psychoanalyst helpfully defines: "The symptoms and the sickness and the secrets have many reasons for being. The parts and facets sustain one another, locking in and strengthening one another. If it were not so, we could give you a nice shot of this or that drug or quick hypnosis and say, 'Craziness begone!' . . . But these symptoms are built of many needs and serve many purposes, and that is why getting them away makes so much suffering."[30]

Three decades later, Prozac becomes such a drug. Embedded in the shift from a language of long-suffering neurosis and its discontents to a language of neutral, scientific precision lies the possibility of a narrative free of the problematic gender implications that have permeated discussions of mental illness and mental wellness. This is the case in the Slater, Kennedy, Krist, and Blackbridge texts, which present their protagonists in explicitly biological terms, mediated through the literary character of Prozac. To be sure, important differences in form and content separate these four works. "Black Swans," the template for Slater's later best-selling *Prozac Diary,* is an autobiographical essay about the then twenty-something graduate student author's coming to terms with the diagnosis of depression and obsessive-compulsive disorder. In it, Slater outlines a long and difficult process of seeking treatment and the effects of such treatment on the course of her life. After numerous unsuccessful therapies, she finds temporary relief from "the Prozac Doctor."[31] Kennedy's "Shrinks" and Krist's "Medicated" are fictional short stories about women involved in various relationships with medications. In "Shrinks," Sara, a thirty-year-old graduate student, searches for an illusory

Prozac prescription and an equally illusory notion of happiness. Prozac had worked wonders for Sara's mother, who, "before Prozac, would say that exercise was a crock" but, after Prozac, "gushed on about how she loved it." "Perhaps," Sara wonders, "Prozac would help me?"[32] In "Medicated," the narrator, Sarah Downey, a depressed but now treated teacher, is on Prozac, her lover, John, on lithium (which he often forgets to take):

> I opened my canvas bag and fished out my little Sucrets tin.
> "Prozac," he announced, identifying the pills immediately.
> "You've taken them?"
> He chuckled, then he frowned. "I've taken everything," he said.[33]

Finally, Blackbridge's novel *Prozac Highway* is narrated by Jam, a middle-aged lesbian performance artist and erstwhile cleaning woman. Jam's "depression" worsens throughout the novel, to the point where she feels that she has no other alternative but to take Prozac.

In each of the four texts, Prozac functions as a facilitator for, and then as a site of, protest. Each of the women narrators or protagonists employs the promise of biological ahistoricity to break from very particular, communal pasts: the past as constructed by prior conventions of the woman's mental-illness narrative and the past of a psychoanalytic paradigm that was even more confining. The women within these Prozac narratives would seem anything but stuck behind wallpaper or constrained by a civilization built by the fearful sons of psychoneurotogenic mothers. Rather, they are engaged in the active creation of the terms of their illness and the active search for their own happiness. Each voices dissatisfaction with psychotherapy or psychoanalysis and seeks Prozac in the hope of becoming productively hyperthymic, optimistic, decisive, and quick of thought in a culture that marks those who are not as pathological. To varying degrees, all experience euphoric initial responses to the drug—or even to the act of receiving a prescription. The result is a productive new insight or understanding. In time, however, the women discover a new, chemical form of oppression in the space between cultural expectation and drug effect. Each then suffers a fall from grace when Prozac stops working or works differently than expected. Ultimately, the characters find the stability of a lasting resolution—a form of awareness that claims to reject Prozac through the discovery of a genuine self free from the constraints of language or of institution.

The eventual critique of Prozac as a specifically gendered form of oppression co-opts the biological revolution and uses it against biology itself, inasmuch as these narratives reject many of the assumptions that I have traced through this book regarding the interconnectedness of psychotropic medications and heterosexual gender norms. Further, this stance serves to differentiate these narratives from other, high-profile members of the Prozac literary family. Kramer's now-passé *Listening to Prozac,* Peter and Ginger Breggin's *Talking Back to Prozac,* Wurtzel's *Prozac Nation,* and Glenmullen's *Prozac Backlash* are just a few of the more prominent examples of texts that assume Prozac to be an agent that restores heterosexual normativity and stability. These best-selling case studies offer notions of closure—once cured, the women return to the men in their lives—that suggest a direct continuity with the themes seen in *Newsweek* in the 1950s and thereafter perpetuated in pharmaceutical advertisements.[34] For instance, the "marital dissatisfaction" experienced by Kramer's patient "Julia" magically disappears after treatment with Prozac, while Wurtzel comes to appreciate "real love" only after she takes medication.[35] Most problematic is Glenmullen's book, which gives the impression that his patients have seen too many Prozac ads. His patient Ann, for example, begins treatment after her boyfriend breaks up with her and, as we saw in chapter 1, achieves almost immediate results after he puts her on Zoloft: "We got back together a few months later. We've been married for two years now, quite happily."[36]

Poised in opposition are works that read against the notion that wonder drugs wondrously produce hypernormativity, that cultural stability is intimately wed to heterosexist norms, and that threats to the nuclear establishment are pathologized as such. For example, Slater's narrator—a single woman living in a platonic relationship with a man—never once mentions her private life.[37] Among our other protagonists, Sara of "Shrinks" seeks a form of treatment that will empower her to leave a long-term relationship and return to graduate school, Sarah of "Medicated" is a young widow who dates around, and Jam of *Prozac Highway* employs medication in the name of a lesbian, cybersex seduction, with nary a patriarch in sight. Certainly, each of these characters adheres strictly to the well-worn codification of mental illness as white, middle class, and female.[38] But, despite their homogeneity on this score, they all suggest that roles and relationships might have changed in the era of Prozac. They also explore ways in which Prozac can be employed concomitantly as an agent that reifies the hypernormal mainstream and as an agent of rebellion against that mainstream.[39]

In what follows, I briefly trace similarities in narrative form in these works, read through the three-phase law of the wonder drug. I examine how each personalizes the dynamics of Prozac in the name of protest and then conclude with a discussion of the ways in which such protests are called into question, if not undone, by the anything-but-postmodern, and often-psychoanalytic, trope of Prozac as it functions within each narrative.

PHASE I: THE FAILURE OF THE PAST

Freud's ideas profoundly changed man's conception of his self.
—Frank Alexander and Sheldon Selesnick, *The History of Psychiatry*

The *Lambda Book Report* calls *Prozac Highway* "post-modern storytelling at its best."[40] Here, the descriptor *postmodern,* affixed to Prozac as if by force of alliteration, is intended to connote the book's frequent disregard for temporality. The book's ongoing account of Jam's descent into depression unfolds almost entirely in the disembodied present tense, as if in the real time of the Internet chatroom winding through the novel. Many of the characters never appear in person but, instead, are known only through the names that they use when logging on to the listserv "ThisIsCrazy": "From:Junior to:ThisIsCrazy . . . Is anyone awake out there? . . . from:Terry to:ThisIsCrazy . . . Junior, of course I'm awake. Do you think if we stood at opposite ends of the earth and screamed anyone would hear?"[41]

Over the course of the novel, the members of the listserv offer Jam, and numerous other members "in crisis," a level of empathy and support unmatched by characters in the "meatworld." However, the connection among cybercharacters is disrupted by the embodied friends and former lovers who repeatedly come to the door of Jam's apartment, forcing her away from the intimacy of the Internet. Similarly, the text is disrupted at various points by random vignettes from Jam's past that serve to demonstrate the futility of Jam's prior, human relationships (in contradistinction to the far more satisfying relationship that she has with her computer). In one vignette she is abused by a lover; in another she lives unhappily in a commune. The most significant of these episodes, however, is that recounting her failed attempt at psychotherapy twenty years earlier: "The psychologist Jam was assigned to was young and handsome and very straight. . . . Neither of them understood anything about the other. John thought he was an attractive and successful young man, the obvious object of transference from his female clients, and

Jam thought he was boring. John thought Jam was a disturbed youth with a dead-end life, and Jam thought she was miserable but cool. But because she was going crazy and had come to John for help, John's version ruled."[42]

A "closet bisexual with a series of failed teenage relationships behind her," Jam is in the process of discovering her identity as a lesbian. Yet, in treatment, she transforms herself into John's vision of normative femininity, neatly dressed and on her way to "make something of herself": "John was pleased she had finally decided to take his advice. He . . . coached her on job-finding. 'You can't wear running shoes to an interview,' he'd tell her. . . . She started taking notes in their sessions, bringing her Sally-Anne outfits to him for approval." Even though Jam eventually wears the "Sally-Anne outfits," her condition does not improve in psychotherapy; rather, her mood worsens considerably. Beneath the happy facade that she presents to John, she becomes increasingly despondent and depressed and soon begins cutting her arms and legs with a razor blade, all the while hearing a self-critical voice that reminds her to *"hate myself, hate myself."*[43]

Antitherapeutic encounters with psychotherapy are described in the other texts as well. In "Shrinks," Sarah suffers through a life of being misunderstood by her "thirty shrinks": "She was not yet thirty years old, so it averaged out to more than one a year." Even her "feminist shrink" is wholly ineffective, ultimately working to exacerbate the very symptoms that she seeks to treat ("she'd been in psychoanalysis so long that she learned to magnify every fear instead of letting it pass").[44] And, in "Black Swans," Slater directly addresses the connection between psychotherapy, language, and women's oppression by recalling her behavioral treatment with Dr. Lipman, the first of several therapists: "He was older, maybe fifty, and pudgy, and had tufts of hair in all the wrong places. . . . I had a bad feeling about him. . . . Maybe he could help me. . . . He seemed so sure of himself that for a moment I was back in language again, only this time it was his language, his words forming me." The treatment is unsuccessful. As she leaves Dr. Lipman's office, which is located in McLean Hospital near Boston, Slater observes: "I saw a shadow in the window. Drawn to it for a reason I could not articulate, I stepped closer and closer still. The shadow resolved itself into lines—two dark brows, a nose. A girl, pressed against glass on a top floor ward. Her hands were fisted on either side of her face, her curls in a ratty tangle. Her mouth was open, and though I could not hear her, I saw the red splash of her scream."[45]

The location of these scenes in the past tense works to critique the narrative problematics of psychotherapy and psychoanalysis in the texts. In each narrative, psychotherapy focuses on a distinctly nonpostmodern temporality, a temporality that leads back to all the wrong places. A dialectic of early-life relationships and cultural models, as in the assumption of transference or the assumed power imbalance between Dr. Lipman and Slater, here relies on a very specific idea of illness and health. Such treatment, often as straight as the character John, seeks to fit women into a rigid structure of the normal—a normal inherent in expectations, expected in cures, and embedded in language. When difference presents itself, as it does in the character of Jam, it is often met with silent pressure to conform to the law of the doctor. In other words, psychoanalysis and psychotherapy are presented as central to a system of diagnosis and treatment in which psychiatric normality is coincident with heteronormative identities.

Such criticism aligns these narratives with contemporary feminist and queer critiques of psychoanalysis. Carolyn Stack, to recall my discussion in chapter 1, employs what she describes as "postmodernist ideas" to argue that, "as long as psychoanalysis promulgates the concept of 'penis envy,' as long as we use this image no matter how we understand its symbolic meaning, we reify the phallocentric narrative that men have/are the desired object that women lack. This heterosexist trope of desire rambles through our personal lives, our work with patients, and our professional relations, reinforcing and reenacting itself each time it shows up."[46] In each text, similar critiques of "heterosexist trope[s] of desire" are used to present psychotherapy and psychoanalysis as treatments that take away the possibility of protest.[47] In each, a woman's agency in a psychotherapeutic dyad is effaced by the language of structures and the structure of institutions. Slater thus describes Dr. Lipman's colonizing "words forming me" and McLean Hospital as silencing screams audible only to those on the same frequency. Slater's observations call to mind the silent and creeping women in "The Yellow Wall-Paper" who are similarly abject and obscene—"there are so many of these creeping women, and they creep so fast."[48]

Yet, despite their critical stance toward the assumptions and treatments of psychoanalysis, the protagonists are unable to break free of the power of its normativizing constraints. The psychoanalytic (and temporally premedicated) expectations and institutions exert control, even though their repressive functions are recognized by the protagonists.[49] Jam comes to consider herself "crazy," tries to please her therapist, and for a time takes his notion of progress as her own. Over years of therapy, Sarah continually struggles to "know exactly what she felt, or was supposed to feel."[50] And Slater momentarily self-identifies as Dr. Lipman's patient. The implication is that the power of psychoanalytic constraints extends to the level of interpellation. Patients are then left with the option of marking themselves normally by wearing the "Sally-Anne outfits," pathologically by cutting themselves on the arm, or schizophrenically by doing both at once.

THE DISCOVERY OF PROZAC

This resistance to biological explanation stems in part from the permanence of personality; we tend to search for causes only when something about a person has unexpectedly changed. But it also shows how unaccustomed we are to understanding behavior in terms of altered brain function. —Larry J. Siever, *The New View of Self*

The initial therapeutic response to an ssRI antidepressant is often made manifest by a brief period of near euphoria. Long-standing symptoms disappear somewhere between the third and the sixth weeks of treatment, and feelings of being energized, unburdened, and free are reported. During this serotonin boost, synapses are flooded with a surplus of neurotransmitter and respond with an often-dramatic (if not entirely understood) alleviation of mood and affect, as if a mirror-like fog has suddenly lifted.

Literary Prozac appears to work by much the same mechanism of action. In the story "Medicated," for example, Sarah experiences depressed mood, anhedonia, insomnia, and other *DSM-IV*-inflected symptoms following the murder of her husband (two years before she starts taking Prozac). After psychotherapy has proved ineffective, she decides to visit a physician very similar to the kind that Slater calls "the Prozac Doctor" and Jam describes as "the pills shrink" (as opposed to a "listening type shrink").[51] Put on medication, Sarah notices little change at first. However, after "a few weeks," the "antidepressants . . . began to work so well—lifting the gloom like a dentist's x-ray vest off my shoulders—that I almost felt depressed all over again": "How could this be, I asked myself. Was my despair such a trivial thing that a few well-chosen chemicals could dispel it? . . . I would occasionally miss one of my therapy sessions with Dr. Hagler, but he always made sure to keep the bottle of Prozac full to the brim."[52]

In short order, long-held symptoms and beliefs begin to fall away. Sarah, who had avoided the site of her husband's murder, spontaneously visits the scene of the crime several months after starting Prozac. She describes the visit with very little attention to affect and very little of the insight-speak that accompanied her more analytically based actualizations. By contrast, the language of the Prozac cure sounds as follows: "One morning, about two years after my husband's death, I entered the Wawa market—the very same one. I purchased a loaf of white bread and a quart of milk and a Kit-Kat bar. Then I left. I had breathed normally the whole time. The next fall, I went back to school."[53]

Sarah's empowered "I" is a subjectivity realized by other Prozac-treated characters as well. Sara's mother in "Shrinks," once a depressed woman who wore only gray, dresses in bright chiffon and opens a catering business. And Slater, posttreatment, describes herself as a living embodiment of Kramer's hyperthermic, "happening kind of person":

> Most things, I think, diminish over time, rock and mountain, glacier and bone. But this wasn't the nature of Prozac, or of me on Prozac. One day I was ill, cramped with fears, and the next day the ghosts were gone. . . . For I had swallowed a pill designed through technology, and in doing so, I was discovering myself embedded in an animal world. I was a purely chemical being, mood and personality sweeping through serotonin. We are all taught to believe it's true, but how strange to feel that supposed truth bubbling right into your own tweaked brainpan. Who was I, all skin and worm, all herd? . . . In dreams, beasts roamed the rafters of my bones, and my bones were twined with wire, teeth tiny silicon chips.[54]

This construction of Prozac as a "bubbling" truth, or a sudden feeling of release, is a consciously sculpted image in other contexts. Prozac advertisements, for example, are often framed entirely within the moment of encounter. Language is often worded in the here and now—"Prozac: It Delivers the Therapeutic Triad"—while images depict patients whose worries have long since ablated.[55] The message is that one need not be concerned with a temporal sense of narrative in order to attain Prozac's type of cure. Within the texts, this presentism also functions as a political tool. Here, an awareness focusing on the immediate does not merely imply a good marketing strategy, couched in the implicit critique of talk therapies. Rather, the narratives suggest ways in which biology introduces new possibilities of autobiography. In each text, the Prozac moments are set in direct counterpoint to psychotherapeutic normativity. Prozac's entry into the plot signifies the promise—or at least the possibility—of a selfhood free of the gendered weight of the psychoanalytic paradigm, as if by the removal of the "x-ray vest" of patriarchy. Biology replaces a language connected to a man's long-suffering neurosis and its discontents—John's expectations or Dr. Lipman's colonizing speech—with a language based on the "neutral" precision of science. Split selves become entirely known selves when read through the logic of the genome. Meanwhile, slips of the tongue and other shards of the underworld are exposed as wholly rational phenomena, and dreams become no more than the interaction of neural chemicals, identifiable and alterable.

Take, for example, Slater's refutation of the notion of the unconscious. A psychoanalytic model assumed the psyche gendered by the problematic divide of conscious (father, superego, precision, science, civilization) and unconscious (mother, desire, repression, nature, leisure) and saw the need for treatment when the latter realm threatened to return as symptoms, rupturing the progress narrative of the former. Yet, in Slater's narrative, the ingestion of a pill leads to a discovery of a self within a larger, reciprocal category of animal or bone. Here, the individual and individually gendered subject—previously known as the castrating, momist mother or the jealous, if otherwise compliant, daughter—is subsumed within larger, homogeneous categories *kingdom, phylum,* or *silicon chip.* As Michael Stone puts it, "As the century draws to a close, the transition from focus on the individual psychology to the chemistry and physics of the soul is in full swing."[56]

Slater's text implies that this shift from individual to communal categories empowers women by providing a language with which to describe their depression and anxiety and, subsequently, themselves. The possibility of such agency, chemically and physically attained, might itself be a form of liberation. As such, Prozac provides freedom from the individual past—the past of Sarah's husband, for example, or of his murder. More important, Prozac also provides freedom from the larger, institutional past (thus disavowing the murder's connection to a primal cultural taboo). By embedding human experience in newly formed categories, Prozac discursively renders obsolete the fundamental binaries of psychoanalytic normativity: mother and father; absence and phallus. As Jam explains, "Most psychiatrists had moved into the prescription writing business, leaving Oedipus and his buddies behind."[57] Without Oedipus these women are no longer constrained—if only briefly.

Most important, however, Prozac provides the freedom to work. Sara's mother opens a business, and Sara herself considers a return to school. Sarah becomes a teacher. And Slater can suddenly go anywhere, "do anything."[58] Depression is, of course, a disease marked by unproductivity. Poor concentration, low energy, and shattered self-esteem are but a few of the symptoms that render work, and life, exceedingly difficult. In the narratives, however, the women's return to work means more than the alleviation of symptoms. To be sure, the symptoms do improve for each during phase 1. But, in a larger sense, the symptoms themselves are deemed obsolete by a culture that no longer confines a woman to the home and provides tranquilizers when the anxiety becomes too much to bear. Hyperthymic, a woman can now produce. And, conscious, a woman can now compete. True to Klerman's vision, in other words, Prozac implies the promise of new categories and provides a discursive community of men and women, unified by the commonality of serotonin in a way that renders the binary of masculine and feminine a remnant of the past.

PHASE 2: CRISIS

Perhaps we all wage a lifelong struggle against depression, even though those of us who are blessed with happy childhoods, peppy serotonin systems, and stable adult lives may never feel the effects of the growing dysfunction in their neural connections.—Peter Kramer, *Listening To Prozac*

We're all too stressed out. . . . [P]erhaps if we had a culture that encouraged us in contemplative practices we wouldn't need Prozac.—Michael Murphy, a founder of the Esalen Institute, quoted in Bob Morris, "Divine Reinvention"

Depression was once known in psychiatric circles as the gap between expectation and fulfillment or between "what a person thinks he is going to get and what he actually does get."[59] The logic seems to makes sense. We often begin life with high expectations and lofty goals. For a time, all of our needs are met, if not completely satisfied. But, inevitably, as Thomas Kuhn well realized, the promise of a new paradigm soon becomes tempered by the imperfections in the design or the imperfections in the system within which the design functions. Either way, the result is a fall from grace.

Such is the case with Prozac. The initial sense of euphoria is often replaced by a sinking sense of familiarity, an awareness of return. Perhaps what is called *tolerance* develops. Or perhaps the drug simply stops working. Or possibly our minds remain adept at creating new neural pathways, rerouting and re-creating familiar routes to despair. And, when an initial response turns "treatment resistant," "augmentation"—with lithium, or thyroid hormone, or some other chemical booster—is then required.[60]

The cures presented in each narrative are nothing if not resistant. The path of Jam's Prozac highway, a directive that covers the entirety of the novel, ends with the contention that Prozac is doing "nothing" and that she still suffers from depression as a result.[61] Sara's high expectations are deflated by the realization that the initial euphoria is only "temporary,"[62] while the short-lived sense of security experienced by Sarah is shattered by a rock through her bedroom window. And Slater suffers the most pronounced fall from grace when her obsessional and depressive symptoms return without warning, rendering her unable to complete her research: "I ran inside. I was far from phone or friend. Maybe I was reminded of some pre-verbal terror: the surgeon's knife, the violet umbilical cord. Or maybe the mountain altitudes had thrown my chemistry off. I don't really know why, or how. But as though I'd never swallowed a Prozac pill, my mind seized and clamped and the obsessions were back . . . and something inside of me screamed *back again back again,* and the grief was very large."[63] In each case, the realization is not merely that Prozac did not live up to its promise but that that promise implied a normalizing disciplinary matrix that is itself a form of regulation and control. Each woman comes to posit biological treatments as creating their own structural constraints, flattening out the individual voice through an entirely communal process of group psychology. Here, individual writing, speaking, or research is subsumed into collective, and collectively gendered, categories, while serenity is ruptured by a rock or a knife. "*Back again back again,*" a novel form of treatment that pledged to alter only chemistry is suddenly indistinguishable from an old form of preverbal terror.

When this effect is realized, as phase 2 prepares to give way to phase 3, each narrator then fights to find a self beyond Prozac, an inner strength unbroken and uncontrolled by the short-lived, chemical seduction. By the conclusion of each text, the characters are importantly unified in the reclamation of the self as an individual and in defiance of the collective assumptions of biology and genetics. This occurs as each character claims to discover a unique identity and a unique subjectivity whose essential forms of individual expression exceed the biological notion of "chemical being."[64] Ultimately, each discovers a personal sense of productivity that claims to be free of hyperthymic cultural expectation.

In "Black Swans," Slater describes her relapse as follows: "Here's what they don't tell you about Prozac. The drug, for many obsessives who take it, is known to have wonderfully powerful effects in the first few months . . . but then peaks at about six months and loses some of its oomph. 'Someday, we'll develop a more robust pill,' Dr. Stanley said." Initially, the narrative voice becomes despondent—"my eyes hurt from crying." But then, almost as quickly, a newly agentic "I" takes control: "I woke late one night, hands fisted. It took me an hour to get out of bed, so many numbers I had to do but I was determined. . . . I rounded the pasture, walked up a hill. And then, before me, spreading out in a moonglow, a lake. . . . [M]y mind became silent. . . . [E]ven in chattering illness I had been quieted for a bit; doors in me had opened; elegance had entered. This thought calmed me. I was not completely claimed by illness, not a prisoner of Prozac."[65]

In "Shrinks," Sara's abreaction yields a similar sense of empowerment after an emotional relapse. Throughout the story, Sara wonders whether she "should" take Prozac. When she finally receives a prescription, she describes a sense of deflation almost identical to Slater's: "She waived the piece of paper with the prescription on it. . . . Suddenly her disappointment was tremendous, unbearable. 'They never make it anything you can read,' she said again, feeling her eyes get teary. 'So you can't even understand what's going on inside you when you take it.'" Yet, immediately thereafter, Sara describes a reflective and willful epiphany, a moment of self-actualization that allows her both to reach out to her boyfriend for the first time and, more important, to realize previously unexplored parts of herself: "It was then she decided to ask his [Andy's] advice. It would be the first time she had ever done so. . . . 'Andy, should I? Is it worth it?' she said, her voice sounding oddly tender. It seemed to her that she was asking some larger question than whether she should take the pill."[66]

Finally, the plots of "Medicated" and *Prozac Highway* both end with the disappointment of failed sexual relationships that explicitly stand in for medication relationships. Sarah's tryst with John, in which the lovers are connected by the "brotherhood of the scarlet letter M, this time, for medicated," ends in a painful rejection that allows Sarah to discover her own voice. John rejects medication and, in the process, rejects Sarah. Yet, as a result, Sarah speaks her own name for the first time—in the story's concluding sentence. Meanwhile, Jam's cyberspace romance involves a seduction in which sex and psychopharmacology are indistinguishable from each other—"I'm sitting here with my shirt up, you staring, fingers flicking my nipples, the other hand, my hand, trying to type some conversation about psych drugs." Here as well, the relationship fails. Jam's lover "Fruitbat" is consumed by another medication, and Jam's own affair with Prozac ends in disaster. The result at the end of the book, much like the voice looking over the lake in "Black Swans," is a sudden awareness of nature—"I'll even water the lupines. Maybe"—and the unspoken assumption that Jam then finds the resolve to finish writing her short story.[67]

PHASE 3: RESOLUTION AND THE NEW SELF

But this shrink had him on Prozac, too. Got him horny. Let me tell you. Five times a day! I said "Walter, I'm not made of steel! You may be Superman but I'm a forty-six year old woman with a hysterectomy last year! Give me a break!"—Thom Jones, "Superman, My Son"

I would like to suggest that the "I" who emerges from these literary surges and reuptakes, or the voice that evolves at the end of narratives of ingestion and disenchantment, is a feminist Prozac self. Through experience, and through the recognition of a specific history, she has learned the difference between passive and active forms of agency and has come to realize that, although psychotropic medications are potentially liberating, they threaten to bring about the former. Ultimately, each character understands that, while beneficial, Prozac has come to function as an extension of a patriarchal "they": "Here's what they don't tell you"; "They never make it anything you can read." While medications help alleviate symptoms, they also threaten to objectify their subjects by consumption.

It is exceedingly important to note, however, that Prozac also functions as a key component in the process of enlightenment—a component that is in no way rejected at the conclusion of the narratives. To be sure, each narrator discovers a new sense of self. But, in each case, this self is a self still *on* medication. Although not entirely dependent on Prozac, Slater continues taking it and "lives life in those brief stretches" of actualization.[68] Sara keeps tight hold of her prescription. Jam never does throw away her Prozac bottle and remains "on 20 mills."[69] And Sarah is, unlike John, medicated to the end. In each case, the narrators claim awareness beyond medication. But the texts reveal that the notion of outside is still wholly inside since the mind that finds reality beyond Prozac is also a mind still under the influence of its serotonin-boosting effects. Phase 3, to recall, is marked, not by disillusionment and discontinuation, but by a lasting, if wounded, resolution.

The sense of an ending that rejects the prison of Prozac while remaining respectful of the medication's real effects connects these four literary works to contemporary feminist critiques of psychotropic medication. Even highly vocal adversaries of psychopharmacology are advocates of much less rather than none at all. For example, Zita's critique of hyperthymia is tempered by the contention that a "natural body," purified of chemical and cultural contaminations, "may not be the best [option] for a particular woman suffering from dysthymia or other emotional complications."[70] Meanwhile, Judith Kegan Gardiner, whose influential essay "Can Ms. Prozac Talk Back?" set the tone for latter critiques, argues, "I don't think feminists should agree to 'just say no.' . . . [W]omen need to understand the consequences of our choices fully, remaining wary of the drug industry . . . but also of the automatic dismissal of biochemical reactions as well as medications."[71] In other words, much like the women narrators of the works discussed in this chapter, women in contemporary society should be able to accept the benefits of Prozac but remain conscious of its potentially colonizing, potentially normalizing effects.

Such measured critique can mean many things. As I mention above, it is important not to overlook the fact that Prozac does work, often safely and efficiently, in alleviating pain and suffering. The ease of prescription and the minimal risk of untoward effects have meant that more persons, and more women than men, are successfully treated for diseases long underdiagnosed and undertreated in the United States. As a result, a condition for which treatment was once exclusive and costly has become a disease whose cure, when effective, is all the more egalitarian and safe.

However, in the context of a discussion of gender and the narration of identity, I suggest that the distinction of both taking Prozac and finding a self outside Prozac is a position that needs to be considered for two reasons. First, this medicated-yet-liberated ending marks the sharpest point of differentiation from earlier generations of women's mental-illness narratives, if not from earlier feminist critiques of psychiatry, that to varying degrees promoted overthrow as a means of emancipation. "The Yellow Wall-Paper," for example, concludes with the proclamation "I've pulled off most of the paper, so you can't put me back!"[72] In *Sexual Politics,* Kate Millett calls for nothing short of a revolution against the Freudian counterrevolution: "There is no way out of such a dilemma but to rebel and be broken, stigmatized and cured. Until the radical spirit revives to free us, we remain imprisoned in the vast, gray stockades of the sexual reaction."[73] Biological psychiatry is not, however, greeted with the same political stance as Millett's attack on biological determinism is. In the Prozac narrative, liberation is attained from within, while the structure itself—a now more benign, more egalitarian pattern of wallpaper—is left wholly intact.

Second, the idea of being "on" Prozac but at the same time remaining "aware" of the self beyond Prozac ultimately amounts to the same subject position posited by biological psychiatry and specifically by its rebellious claims of victory over psychoanalysis.[74] Consider Slater's argument, for example. At the end of "Black Swans" she literally wills herself into a cure: "I had to do. I was determined." As a result, she claims to be no longer a "prisoner of Prozac."[75] But this notion of victory is itself also an acceptance of the Prozac promise rather than the discovery of a reality beyond it. All is conscious in this consciousness, and the very possibility of an unconscious self, or a divided self, or especially a castrated and so gendered self, is, thus, rendered impossible. I mean to say that the self that can take conscious control of the unseen or will herself to speak, or to act, or to exercise, or to break free of stockades, or to assume the role of master of her own home, is the very self posited by biology and promoted by Prozac. Here, the Cartesian subject reemerges, as if the Enlightenment's last laugh on modernism. And here, through an act of will and the timeless gumption of mankind, psychoanalysis is defeated once and for all. Thus is the protest against Prozac also an enactment of the Prozac project, and thus does a narrative of replacement also become a narrative of return.[76]

The Return of the Repressed

The problem with the Oedipal model, once again, was that it posited a clearly troubling binary of having and wanting in the constitution of a gendered world. Boys, in individual and in communally essential evolution, had. Theirs was an awareness of the power of protuberance and, with it, the social sanctions of reason and evolution. Girls, meanwhile, lacked. Theirs was the realization of absence, of space unfilled. This division led to marked differences in development. When boys became men, they did so always and already aware of the terrifying possibility of dismemberment. Since the fear of castration, or of being turned into a girl, was one of the most powerful forces in male psychical development, it served as a "forceful . . . motive towards forming the superego." For girls, meanwhile, an awareness of absence, of space unfulfilled, meant that they had less to lose. They accepted castration as "an established fact": as girls saw themselves as already castrated, they thus had relatively less impetus to form a strong superego. This key difference—between a superego formed against the threat of castration and a superego formed by a process of laissez-faire—led to differences in moral character between the sexes. As Freud wrote, "I cannot escape the notion . . . that for women the level of what is ethically normal is different from what it is in men. Their super-ego is never so inexorable, so impersonal, so independent of its emotional origins as we require in men. . . . [Women] show less sense of justice than men, that they are less ready to submit to the greater necessities of life, that they are more often influenced in their judgments by feelings of affection or hostility."[77] When extended over space and time, this imbalance became a metonym for the binaried nature of mankind. "Civilization," formed in the upper, conscious domain of the dichotomy, was the realm of science, of reason, and of order.[78] Here, men, with their developed superegos, were the enforcers of rules and the makers of institutions. Women, however, were by necessity relegated below, to the chthonic (and, thus, always threatening) realm of emotionality and indecision known as *the unconscious.* Their weak superegos "soon come in opposition to civilization and display their retarding and restraining influence," thus threatening the generativity of the upper domain with the constant threat of the symptom.[79] These two parts then fused as a larger whole, as father and mother, culture and nature, androgen and estrogen. And thus, with a top and a bottom locked together as if in a psychical missionary position, did civilization progress.

In the light of such assumptions, the allure of biology is easy to see. To be sure, it offers a method of treatment that is as cost-effective as it is user-friendly. But, on a deeper level, it also promises to these texts what it promises to American psychiatry. The idea that the unconscious can be made conscious—and, thus, that all is in fact conscious—carries the implicit (and wholly materialist) ablation of a binary built on seemingly outdated gender norms. If all is conscious, then men and women live in the same domain and work on the same level playing field. Prozac guarantees that a new technology will cure symptoms with a minimum of side effects and, additionally, that both symptoms and cures remain at a remove from a "real" self: the biological structure that defines both symptom and cure also defines a self independent of social constructions, cultural archetypes, and originary myths. PET scans know nothing of castration. Serotonin, an all-egalitarian compound, functions largely the same in women and in men, in African Americans and in Native Americans; psychotropic medications perform the same functions in heterosexuals, in gay butch bottoms, and in monks.

Yet the Prozac narratives expose the fallacy of this act of ablation and warn of the stakes of this communal disavowal. In "Black Swans," as one remarkable example, Slater becomes a "happening" person while taking Prozac: "Every noon I took my pill. . . . Mornings now, I got up early to jog, showered efficiently, then strode off to the library. I was able to go back to work." Protected by the medication, she applies for and receives a grant to conduct research in Appalachia. On arriving in the "rippling mountains of poverty," she encounters the "mountain women":

> In the oven I saw a roasted bird covered with flies. In the bathroom, a fat girl stooped over herself, without bothering to shut the door, and pulled a red rag from between her legs.
>
> Her name was Kim, and her sister's name was Bridget, and their mother and father were Kat and Lonny. All the females were huge and doughy.[80]

These mountain women form the terrifying unconscious of Slater's productive self. Her voice fills with distance and disgust as she describes their complacency, their unexercised habitus, their squalor. Yet the space that separates her from them is not merely one of class or living standard.[81] Rather, and more important, Slater is separated from these women by gender. They are the blood-marked femininity, the dysphoric objects of her study. They are the long-forgotten past. And she, come down from the overworld but still treated, protected, and ultimately normalized by Prozac, is their tempered voice of reason.

In these treated, hyperthymic moments in the texts, Prozac provides the women protagonists with a man's strong superego. The literary effect of Prozac is, not only that women who take it become hyperthymic, but that hyperthymia, as it is described, constitutes a point of development along a suddenly problematic, exceedingly psychoanalytic continuum. In each text, the ingestion of Prozac allows a woman to change the course of her Oedipal trajectory, if only for a brief, fleeting moment. Here, a narrative of defeat becomes a narrative of privilege, and a life of envy becomes one of rational generativity. On Prozac, the pallid Slater is able to work, to jog, and to separate momentarily from the abjection that is her birthright. The Sarah of "Medicated" teaches, while the Sara of "Shrinks," now moral, is ready to return to graduate school. Even *Prozac Highway*, the text least likely of the four to reenact a heteronormative structure, presents Jam's Prozac encounter in a language that re-creates a division between making and bearing. Although Jam argues that Prozac does "nothing," the plot is interrupted seven days into treatment by a scene from its own unconscious, where Prozac assumes an active—indeed, an erotically active—position. The book's only penetration is described as if in a dream or slip of the tongue since, in the conscious world, Jam and Fruitbat never actually meet. Jam writes: "And then they're somewhere else in bed and Fruitbat is lying on top of Jam. Maybe she has a dildo on, sure, a dildo, slow easy strokes deep into Jam's cunt and Jam gives everything."[82] Fruitbat is Prozac, and, immediately thereafter, Jam begins work on her "virtual performance." Consumed and penetrated, these women assume ownership of that phallus constructed in pharmaceutical advertisements, that superego denied them by Freud, if not by their own hypothermic body temperature. Each, in other words, becomes civilized. Biology may have convincingly argued that the Oedipus complex is the result of hormones and peptides, framed and finally understood as an "inexorable (because they are useful!) part of human society."[83] But, in spite of the evidence of prenatal androgens seen and demonstrated, the notions of useful progress and productivity, of illness and health, remain contained within familiar and familiarly divided categories, separated in a textual dichotomy between having and wanting to have. Re-creating gender as a relational concept, the Prozac that emasculates the man in chapter 2 then returns, as it were, to empower the woman.

A recognition of the psychoanalytic function of Prozac allows us to understand more fully what takes place when phase 1's euphoria becomes phase 2's crisis, within the suddenly Oedipal law of the wonder drug structuring each narrative.[84] As Prozac stops working and is replaced by a momentary but terrifying fall from grace, the characters react in almost similar fashion. Slater, for example, cries and then rediscovers the beauty of nature. In the process, she becomes less productive—"I must pause many times as I write this"—because the symptoms of depression and obsessive-compulsive disorder have "returned."[85] Meanwhile, Sara, a character marked by her toughness, cries and becomes tender for the only time in the story, and Jam suddenly thinks about watering her plants. When Prozac stops working, each woman's masquerade is uncovered, as if by emotional symptoms returning from the newly formed yet familiarly coded unconscious.[86]

To be sure, these four works are in many ways victorious in their individual and communal acts of resistance against the form. Characters demonstrating what might be considered alternative interpretations of Prozac—as in nonnuclear or nonheterosexual—become effectively empowered as each narrative develops. The result is a new, more agentic writing of the female mental-illness narrative. However, within this victory, this revision and re-creation, lies a troubling act of erasure. For protest is, ultimately, undone by the origins that Prozac, and the biological discourse for which it stands, deems inaccessible. The language of the chemical imbalance co-opted by these narratives serves as an effective tool with which to break from the past. But, in so breaking, these narratives accept—and, in accepting, reenact—some of the more troubling assumptions of psychiatry (psychoanalysis and psychopharmacology both).

The ahistorical, atemporal promise of Prozac is, thus, a false promise indeed. Freud may not have been correct about the biology, or the destiny, of contemporary civilization. But his insight that narrative form is itself gendered—in a structure that allows either a telling or a reading of the phenomenon of a wonder drug, depending on one's position in the transference/countertransference, phallus/absence dialectic—holds remarkably to the point. The notion that the discourse of biology breaks down the psychic binary, disproving the unconscious once and for all, works, instead, to efface the ways in which the assumptions of the unconscious are also structured, like a language, into biology's very language.

Prozac represents more than a rejection of psychoanalysis. Cloaked in the novelty of the neurotransmitter, it also represents a continuation of a conversation in which postmodern history is but the most recent contribution. In spite of social change, women nonetheless represent the underside of this narrative of progress. Theirs is the emotionality from which civilization needs to be protected, the nature that always threatens to rupture the tranquility of culture. Prozac may well have offered a different pharmacokinetics, a new volume of distribution. But the mechanism of action remains unchanged. Prozac not only works to break down a binary but also serves as discursive assurance that the binary remains intact. The Prozac of liberation is also, and ironically, the Prozac of the return of the repressed. The speech may protest against the binary. But the protest is in constant peril of censorship by a language that both maintains the system and denies access to the origin of the problem ("parenting being behavior that is fundamental to survival of the species," to recall Nada Stotland, but at the same time "very complex").[87] Metabolized and protein bound, progress continues.

Again, my critique is in no way meant to undermine women writing, or women in the role of protagonists, or men writing as women, in protest against the cultural assumptions signified by Prozac. Rather, it is to argue that such protests, and specifically the narrative conventions often structuring their discourse, must be considered within the larger historical and cultural forms in which they function—forms that are often codified in predictable ways, if not expressed in the cultural construction of dreams and slips of the tongue. Here, the very notion of a practical self, or a visually unified self, or a biologically productive self, seems always and already to depend on the requisite presence, in some remote region of the mind unaffected by Prozac, of mountain women and black swans or of lupines that need to be watered. Without this awareness, such protests, and the notions of selfhood that they posit, risk stealthily perpetuating the forms of oppression that they seek to defy. Yet the problem ultimately lies, not within these or other acts of resistance, but within a language and a meaning system that seeks to envelop even voices of protest within a larger conversation, always listening and talking back in the name of reification.

Chapter Six

CONCLUSION

$\mathcal{P}$erhaps the problem with psychoanalysis was its claim to the unseen. Its treatments were intimate and private, its methods resistant to exposure, its knowledge hidden within the bodies of men who looked like blank screens while at the same time remaining outside their patients' purview. As master of all that was and of all that was not, psychoanalysis staked its claim to power and knowledge on its ability to read for ruptures in the text, points of doubling back, while discovering remnants of the past that lived imperceptibly in the present. The invisibility that psychoanalysis formulated in its theory and institutionalized in its practice then became its means of discovering something hidden, and often embarrassing, about the rest of us. Even our most thoughtless moments could not escape interpretation. "The repetition of the same thing will perhaps not appeal to everyone as a source of uncanny feeling," Freud wrote in "The Uncanny." But, "from what I have observed, the phenomenon does undoubtedly, subject to certain conditions and combined with certain circumstances, arouse an uncanny feeling, which, furthermore, recalls the sense of helplessness experienced in some dream states."[1] The repetition of the same thing was, in other words, given experiential meaning only when the repetition was perceived—and, more important, identified—as such. Subject to certain conditions, a recognition then formed along neglected neural networks, firing rusted axons and jumping desiccated synapses on a path back to a point of traumatic encryption whose relevance could be made transparent, and then only partially so, only by the conditions and circumstances set forth by psychoanalysis.

Frustrated with secrecy, and uncomfortable with a process that kept its patrons and its critics similarly in the dark, the biological revolution pulled down the psychoanalytic apparition. And, when the masses came streaming in, it became disappointingly clear that what had looked from the outside like a foreboding palace was simply a place that they already knew and had strangely been to many times before. Left to its own devices for too long, psychoanalysis had merely constructed boundaries around the obvious and the requisite: a husband's need for his wife, for example, or the ways in which a son learns to love his mother. Biology exposed the fallacy of mystery and the immorality of the intimacy of the unique. *Latent,* it claimed, was nothing more than another level of *manifest.* Renaming the *mind* the *brain,* biology lay bare the reality that there was no special relation beyond the perception of one. Scopophilics, hysterics, masochists, psychoanalysts, and the many other fetishists of nostalgia would, instead, have to learn that their quirks carried little validity in a world ruled increasingly by outcomes and biological substrates. The fMRI saw beneath their perceptions and perversions, and their perceptions and perversions did not, in any case, matter because they all had the same health plan.

Why, then, did a discourse demanding to expose and demystify a specific notion of gender come to perpetuate the gender categories that it claimed to render irrelevant? As biology saw it, psychoanalysis had constructed an intricate labyrinth to cover over the teleologies in its midst, a process that ultimately blinded psychoanalysis to its own observer biases. Yet, in its enactment (or, perhaps, in the process whereby ideas and discoveries, like love relationships, often frustratingly re-create similarity from the promise of difference), biology's insistence on specialized techniques, its embrace of the so-called real in its push to legitimacy and respectability, effaced its own predetermined assumptions about reproduction and progress. Left to its own devices and its own compulsions, biology then constructed boundaries around the obvious and the requisite. Mothers were defined in opposition to fathers and were diagnosed, ultimately, by their attention to their sons. "Data from animal studies suggest that maternal smoking during pregnancy leads to reduced serotonin uptake and alterations in the dopaminer-gic neurons in the fetal brain," Rasanen, Hakko, Isohanni, et al. wrote in 1999 in "Maternal Smoking during Pregnancy," announcing momism's bio-logical return to the scientific press (as much as it had ever left). "Because of the low rate of criminal offenses among women, the present analyses are restricted to men ($N = 5,636$). Compared to the sons of mothers who did not smoke, the sons of mothers who smoked during pregnancy had more than a twofold risk of having committed a violent crime or having repeat-edly committed crimes, even when other biopsychosocial risk factors were controlled."[2] Doubly blind to a fault, the authors failed to see the irony in the situation.

Over the course of this project, I have suggested several primary reasons for the sense of déjà vu that hovers over articles such as "Maternal Smoking during Pregnancy" where the control of biopsychosocial factors does not seem to negate the many larger biopsychosocial determinants of outcome. History, development, economics, stereotypes, metaphor, mores, politics, and expectations are but a few of the conditions that combined with circum-stances to create a doubling back in the text of American psychiatry over the past half century. My resistance to selecting more carefully from this list, however, is due to the fact that what interests me still about the poten-tial connections between Freud and Prozac, or between two theories that blamed the biopsychosocial "mother" for the ills of men in spite of protests to the contrary, lies in the repetition of process as much as the process of repetition. Unlike Freud's description of the uncanny, the "repetition of the same thing" was not in this case the repetition of the same "thing." Rather, the uncanny similarity between psychoanalysis and biology was the act of repetition itself, inasmuch as repetition implied recurrence without insight over time.

On this score, I have argued, psychiatry went backward, reading its own progress through reverse transcriptase. What psychoanalysis knew well, in spite of the many gaps in its awareness, was that the symptoms of the patient were given particular meaning when mediated through the symptoms of the doctor. In spite of (or because of) its claim to the unseen, psychoanalysis provided a theory of the observer and a conceptual system in which observa-tion was inseparable from projection. People, doctors, and patients alike saw themselves in each other and only then made sense of their place in the world.

"Without any special reflection we impute to everyone else our own consti- tution, and therefore our own consciousness," Freud wrote in "The Uncon- scious," "and this identification is a necessary condition of understanding in us."[3] Observer bias was, in other words, of us and was an essential compo- nent of our discoveries, omissions, and therapeutic collaborations.

Biology overlooked this point in its rush to create a system in which pro- jection was uncoupled from actualization or social responsibility. In its ob- session with the fMRI, biology forgot that the relationships between doc- tors and patients, or between neuroscientists and electron microscopes, were based on dialectics of selves and others and the intersubjective imputation and recognition of constitution and consciousness. To be sure, this approach allowed psychiatry to treat imbalances of peptides that had previously been misidentified as imbalances of persons. But, in so doing, its passionate efforts to open up the mystery surrounding the patient, to discover her reduced serotonin uptake and altered dopaminergic neurons, left psychiatry without a viable theory of the psychiatrist. Biology then became even more guilty than psychoanalysis was of claiming dominion over the unseen, only, in this case, the emptiness was in part a self-reflection. The disappearance of the father, in other words, opened up a space for the reemergence of the mother, whose actions seemed oddly familiar but just could not be placed.

The challenge for psychiatry, as it struggles with the implications of what it was and what it will become, is to develop a theory of itself and of its own complex constitution. Psychiatry needs to expose its own synapses and den- drites with the same vigor with which it has exposed those of its patients and, in so doing, develop a perspective—indeed, a biological perspective—on the ways in which its perceptions and projections shape its own interactions. Psychiatry must also become more aware of its own, uniquely biased specta- tor positions, in relation to those who look to it for conversations as much as for encapsulated solutions. And psychiatry must better realize the implica- tions—indeed, the gender implications—of its diagnoses, its prescriptions, and its many other, erotically charged encounters and exchanges.

Without a more honest definition of itself, psychiatry will continue to be defined by everyone else. Even now, health plans structure its interactions, pharmaceutical companies dictate its practices, and funding agencies decide its long-term viability and security. In each case, the implication is that the profession is shaped from the outside because the inside has nothing to offer.

In time, and with continued layers of effacement, psychiatry then loses the capacity to understand how its unique perspective of the biological gives it something important to say about the social, the interpersonal, and the environmental. And it relinquishes its ability to address the central and centrally productive problematic of its existence: how a narrative of progress can at the same time be a narrative of return.

$\mathcal{Notes}$

ONE *Introduction*

1 To quote Bertram Brown, the former director of the National Institute of Mental Health, in the 1950s "it was nearly impossible for a nonpsychoanalyst to become chairman of a department or professor of psychiatry" ("The Life of Psychiatry," 492).

2 World War II was a key point in the history of American psychoanalysis. The war allowed for the first demonstrated "success" in the treatment of neurotic symptoms in noninstitutional settings: supportive psychotherapy, combined with rest and food, allowed over 60 percent of frontline "neuropsychiatric casualties" to return to combat duty within two to five days. Over the course of the war, the numbers of physicians assigned to the neuropsychiatric corps jumped from thirty-five in 1941 to twenty-four hundred in 1946. This success provoked the institutionalization of the practice of psychiatry in the postwar period and the spread of psychotherapy and psychoanalysis into broader clinical settings. In large part as a result, psychoanalysts rose to assume leadership positions in American psychiatry, also paving the way for the psychoanalyst William C. Menninger to become in 1946 the first psychiatrist elevated to the rank of brigadier general. See Grob, "The Origins of *DSM I*," 427.

3 Psychoanalytic concepts were requisite components of the training of all psychiatrists. By 1955, eighty-seven of the ninety-three American psychiatric training programs taught psychodynamic concepts to their residents. These residents,

meanwhile, spent up to three thousand hours over the course of their three-year training periods practicing long-term, psychodynamic psychotherapy. See Wallerstein, "The Future of Psychotherapy."

4 On the term *objectifiable*, see n. 8, chap. 4, below.

5 Wexler, "Cerebral Laterality and Psychiatry," 279. See also Hobson and McCarley, "The Brain as a Dream State Generator"; Guze, "The Clinical Diagnosis of Hysteria."

6 Lasagna, "The Role of Benzodiazepines"; Ludwig and Othmer, "The Medical Basis of Psychiatry"; Greden and Casariego, "Controversies in Psychiatric Education"; Klerman, "The Advances of *DSM-III*."

   Although *psychotropic* initially implied "antipsychotic" medication, use of the term has expanded over the past 50 years to connote all types of prescription psychoactive medication (see, e.g., Burt, Suri, Altshuler, et al., "The Use of Psychotropic Medications during Breast-Feeding"). My use of the term implies this latter definition.

7 Stone, *Healing the Mind*.

8 See Tasman, Riba, and Silk, *The Doctor-Patient Relationship in Pharmacotherapy*. Combination therapy implies the joining of two treatments assumed to work on entirely different axes; one treatment for the brain, the other for the soul.

9 Healy, *The Antidepressant Era*.

10 As just one of many examples, the psychiatrist Gerald Klerman describes the success of "biological, objectifiable psychiatry" as a "victory for science" ("The Advances of *DSM-III*," 539). See also Grob, "The Origins of *DSM I*," and "Psychiatry and Social Activism."

11 See, e.g., Rosenbaum, "Behavioral Inhibition in Children."

12 Nopoulos and Andreasen, "Gender Differences in Neuroimaging," 2.

13 Kuhn, *The Structure of Scientific Revolutions*, 6.

14 Rogler, "Making Sense of Historical Changes," 10.

15 Stone, *Healing the Mind*, 320–25. See also Ayd, "The Early History of Modern Psychopharmacology."

16 McHugh, "The Death of Freud," 36. See also McHugh and Slavney, *The Perspectives of Psychiatry*.

17 Valenstein, *Blaming the Brain*, 1.

18 Shorter, *A History of Psychiatry*, vii. While I cannot resist pointing out here that Shorter himself is making a Marxist move by claiming to expose ideology with liberatory reason, I leave an extended discussion of this point until later.

19 For example, the theme of the 2001 annual meeting of the American Psychiatric Association was "Mind Meets Brain: Integrating Psychiatry, Psychoanalysis, Neuroscience." Scholarly efforts at integration have also come from the analytic community. See Watt, "The Dialogue between Psychoanalysis and Neuroscience."

20 Cooley, "The New Nerve Pills and Your Health," 71; *Archives of General Psychiatry* 22 (April 1970): 290–91; Kramer, *Listening to Prozac,* 10–12.

21 Stack, "Psychoanalysis Meets Queer Theory," 77, 72, 73, 74.

22 Both these points are more fully discussed in contemporary psychoanalytic writing that grapples with the role of medications in the psychoanalytic process. For an excellent example, see Gabbard and Bartlett, "Selective Serotonin Reuptake Inhibitors."

23 Stack, "Psychoanalysis Meets Queer Theory," 71, 72.

24 See, among other sources, Freud, "Some Psychical Consequences of the Anatomical Distinction between the Sexes," 248.

25 Glenmullen, *Prozac Backlash,* 20, 7–8, 29. Maura's soft features form a sharp contrast to the hard science of serotonin blockade and neuroreceptors that act on these women as they lean back in Glenmullen's chair. In these and other descriptions, Glenmullen's deconstruction of Prozac also reconstructs and perpetuates stereotypes about women on wonder drugs for the past half century.

26 Slater, "Black Swans," 160.

27 At the writing of this text, e.g., the *DSM* does not account for cultural "variables" in its five axes of illness.

28 Leibenluft, foreword to *Gender Differences in Mood and Anxiety Disorders,* xv. See also Zlotnick et al., "Gender, Type of Treatment." Here, again, we find the assumption that psychiatry has been revolutionized by a gaze that shifted from life events to biological brain structures.

29 For instance, Luhrman's study of psychiatric training, *Of Two Minds,* offers an important critique of the construction of power and knowledge in American psychiatry. At the same time, her insistence on "two minds" (220)—therapy vs. medication—ultimately works to reify the very same binary insisted on by Shorter.

30 Corrodi et al., "The Effect of Some Psychoactive Drugs," 363.

31 See "Pills vs. Worry," 68.

32 Hale, *Rise and Crisis of Psychoanalysis;* Buhle, *Feminism and Its Discontents;* Zita, *Body Talk.*

33 Hale, *Rise and Crisis of Psychoanalysis,* 276.

34 See, e.g., Buhle, *Feminism and Its Discontents,* 280–318; Cuordileone, " 'Politics in an Age of Anxiety.' "

35 Berger, "The Pharmacological Properties of Miltown," 415.

36 "How Tranquilizers Work," 47; Cooley, "The New Nerve Pills and Your Health," 74; "Pills for the Mind," 63.

37 Millett quoted in "Who's Come a Long Way Baby?" 16; Johnson, *Lesbian Nation,* 166.

38 Kramer, *Listening to Prozac,* 16–17.

39 Slater, "Black Swans," 156.

40 Stotland, "Gender, What's the Difference?" 813.

41 Danquah, *Willow Weep for Me,* 256, 258–59, 266.

42 Ibid., 200–224, 256–58. See also Angier, "Grumpy, Fearful Neurotics." An unexpected development further links *Willow Weep for Me* with the "Prozac narratives" that I describe in chapter 5. The book concludes with a series of questions for and answers by the author, followed by the explanation that "Meri Nana-Ama Danquah was interviewed by Dr. Freda C. Lewis-Hall, Director of the Lilly Center for Women's Health" (Danquah, *Willow Weep for Me,* 11 unfoliated pages following p. 272). Created and funded by Eli Lilly, this same center has recently been at the forefront of Lilly's successful efforts to win FDA approval for Prozac as a treatment for premenstrual dysphoric disorder.

43 Ayd's narrative, e.g., describes the "pioneers of biological psychiatry" who began their innovative work in the abject cellars of the field, far beneath the ivory tower of psychoanalysis ("The Early History of Modern Psychopharmacology," 71). Stone observes that the confluence between the "demonstrated success" of biological methods in the 1970s and the growing discontent concerning the "lack of data supporting psychoanalytic postulates" led to the widespread belief that mental illness, personality, and even object choice are "primarily constitutional rather than psychodynamic in nature" (*Healing the Mind,* 321). And, in spite of his many important critiques of biological research methods, Valenstein devotes chapter 2 of *Blaming the Brain* to a surprisingly straightforward telling of the "Discoveries of Psychotherapeutic Drugs" (9–58).

44 Healy, *Antidepressant Era,* 179.

45 Shorter, "From Freud to Prozac," 291. The argument that wonder drugs create their own markets in the name of economic gain and professional advancement, thereby defining both the need for the drug and the illness for which the drug is indicated, finds resonance in other related literatures as well. Peter and Ginger Breggin's *Talking Back to Prozac* and *Talking Back to Ritalin* are high-profile members of a flourishing post-Szasian, post-Laingian genre of what might be called *public empowerment through informed, if already interpolated, repartee.* ("Every child needs a hero," fellow whistle-blower Jeffrey Masson writes on the back cover of the Breggins' *Talking Back to Ritalin,* "a champion who will speak truth to power. That hero is Peter Breggin.") *Talking Back to Ritalin,* e.g., is a book marketed for physicians and patients with the claim that "there are dozens of books on the market which take a more positive view on these medications but this is the only book that examines their mechanism of action and their adverse effects in depth and detail" (x)—ironically a claim very similar to Valenstein's earlier in that same year. The Breggins compile and quantify "the actual evidence" about Ritalin, an impressive twenty-page bibliography of scientific articles, in support of the contention that Ritalin both causes and treats attention deficit hyperactivity disorder: "Ritalin and amphetamines are stimulants. As such they can produce the very symptoms they are supposed to control" (7). The common point here is that agency resides at the

top of the system, drug companies, in concert with physicians, researchers, and even the drugs themselves, creating economies of need and want that did not previously exist. A similar point, in a markedly different formulation, connects these histories and public-service books to important feminist critiques of psychopharmacology. For example, see the discussion of "diagnostic bracket creep" in Zita, *Body Talk,* 61–84.

46 For example, scientific knowledge is assumed to be refigured and reinterpreted in popular culture in much the same way in Greg Meyers's *Writing Biology.* Meyers argues that popularizing articles adhere to a sequential "narrative of nature," in which "narratives of science" are "translated into the syntax and vocabulary emphasizing the externality of nature to scientific practices," thereby making science more palatable for popular consumption (141–42).

47 Healy, *The Antidepressant Era,* 5. Yet Healy's examination focuses almost entirely on "the rise of biological language in psychiatry," as traced through reports of "watershed studies," "data," and "pharmaceutical company reports." Only at the very end does "popular culture" receive an exceedingly brief role—in the form of Peter Kramer's *Listening to Prozac.* The actual "language," however, is never examined at all. Rather, it is assumed to be a derivative of the syntax generated by what Healy calls "stories of discovery." Healy, *The Antidepressant Era,* 143, 169.

48 See Stolberg, "Clinical Guides Often Hide Ties."

49 Smith, *Small Comfort,* 4–5.

50 For one example, see Hudson and Pope, "Affective Spectrum Disorder."

51 This structure then mediates the ways in which each author assumes "gender" interactions to take place only at the end point of a progression of knowledge from science to culture. The possibility that science might be involved in the relations of women and men is not imbricated within but rather results from scientific penetration. (This is a generous reading—since few of these works focus on gender at all. Not one of these works addresses controversies concerning the overprescription of psychotropic drugs to women or the protests of the women's movement specifically against the institution of psychiatry. Ayd, e.g., seems to inhabit a world in which the generalizability of clinical trials blocks access to the implications of his "discoveries" for gender as well as for race, class, and other variables constructed as outside the pharmaceutical purview.) For example, Valenstein separates his scientific evidence from a realm where popular culture shapes women's agency. Here, knowledge is created in a lab, while controversies concerning feminist protests and gender-imbalanced prescription rates take place on another continent (*Blaming the Brain,* 56). Healy directly addresses the possibility that "there was a particular concern about the use of tranquilizers by women, which was interpreted as a clear effort by some to suppress women." Without analysis, these concerns are dismissed as old wives' tales, in line with "pharmacological Calvinism," a prevailing cultural belief system in which "drug use is held to be bad and potentially even

dangerous if it makes you feel good. A drug that makes the subject feel good is either somehow morally wrong, or is going to be paid for with dependence, disease" (*The Antidepressant Era*, 227, 228).

52 Parry, Cooperstock, Manheimer, and many other quantitative and qualitative researchers cited in the chapters that follow present evidence that antidepressants, anxiolytics, and other medications have been supplied to women at rates as much as 75 percent higher than those for men. See chapter 4 below; or Manheimer et al., "Psychotherapeutic Drugs."

53 Buhle's work on the 1950s, e.g., provides a context for my argument that the discourse of medications became imbricated into the tensions of momism (see her *Feminism and Its Discontents*), while Zita importantly defines the expectations of women on Prozac as a 1990s phenomenon (see her *Body Talk*).

54 Keller, *Reflections on Gender and Science*, 17.

55 I thus also mean to reference the conservative psychoanalytic thought that rose to prominence in the 1950s and 1960s as a direct result of these theories. In rejection of Alfred Adler ("masculine protest"), Karen Horney ("the dread of woman"), and other theorists who employed psychoanalysis in the project of deconstructing coherent gender roles (and specifically a coherent masculinity), Reik, Bieber, Jung (and later Robert Stoller and Allan Schore) steered psychoanalysis down the path of gender orthodoxy by directly linking mental health with conventional heterosexuality, marriage, and essentialized notions of motherhood. Bieber's work in 1962, e.g., posited heterosexuality as an unproblematic, "natural" path of human development and feminism, homosexuality, and other deviances from the norm as "pathological" (Bieber et al., *Homosexuality*; see also Reik, *Of Love and Lust*).

56 Freud, *An Autobiographical Study*, 37.

57 Freud, "Some Psychical Consequences of the Anatomical Distinction between the Sexes," 248.

58 Freud, *Civilization and Its Discontents*, 123–46.

59 I elaborate on this point in chapters 2 and 3. See also Minsky, *Psychoanalysis and Gender*, 43.

60 Foucault, *The History of Sexuality*, vol. 1, *An Introduction*.

61 Lewis, "Psychiatry and Postmodern Theory."

62 See Butler, *Gender Trouble*, 141.

63 Again, part of my point is that the Freudian concepts on which I call were taken up both by American popular culture in the 1950s and "orthodox" voices in psychoanalysis itself (e.g., Reik) in the common project of restoring a specifically gendered social order.

64 Žižek, *The Plague of Fantasies*, 45–86. My definition of the "traditional" function of psychotropic drugs is implied in the reading of Prozac in Stack's "Psychoanalysis Meets Queer Theory": psychopharmaceuticals that work to divide man from woman, top from bottom, and other "heterosexist" binaries in a manner that

allows me to make a connection to Freudian notions of conscious and unconscious.

65 Freud, "Some Psychical Consequences of the Anatomical Distinction between the Sexes," 248.

66 This term is co-opted from Žižek (*The Plague of Fantasies,* 45–86) yet modified slightly in order to point out Žižek's playfully operative disavowal of the psychological function of narrative history.

67 Although such a conceptualization is beyond the scope of my analysis, one can also think of medications in Foucaultian terms for the regulation of behavior and the diminishment of excitation, both requisite for "stability." This latter definition implies a late-nineteenth- rather than a late-twentieth-century notion of sexuality. And, more to the point I am trying to make, this notion of sexuality is clearly more Freudian than it is progressively biological. Freud's "pleasure principle," as just one example, did not provide pleasure, but instead modulated it so that the educated individual would not become overstimulated. Yet this seemingly outdated sexuality is, I argue, the very sexuality that psychotropic medications come to perform.

68 As Zona complains about the newfound potency of her husband, Walter, in Thom Jones's story "Superman, My Son," "But this shrink had him on Prozac, too. Got him horny. Let me tell you. Five times a day! I said 'Walter, I'm not made of steel! You may be Superman but I'm a forty-six year old woman with a hysterectomy last year! Give me a break!" (33).

69 Stack, "Psychoanalysis Meets Queer Theory," 77.

70 See, e.g., Collins, *Black Feminist Thought,* 222–25; Omunuwa, "Health Disparities in Black Women."

71 Until recently, psychiatric definitions of *race* implied "nonwhite." To the present day, these discussions often appear limited to the discourse of schizophrenia. See Lewine and Caudle, "Racial Effects on Neuropsychological Functioning in Schizophrenia"; "Schizophrenia Linked to Racism." For a highly misguided illustration, see also Satel, *How Political Correctness Is Corrupting Medicine.*

72 Piderhughes, "Understanding Black Power"; Lipscomb, "Drug Use in a Black Ghetto."

73 See Healy, *The Antidepressant Era.*

TWO *The Name of the Father, the Place of the Medication*

1 Stotland, "Gender, What's the Difference?" 813.

2 "Why is it that the same gene can have different effects depending on whether it comes from the male or the female parent? How do differences in hormones interact with differences in rearing and circumstances to cause differences in behavior both simple and complex (parenting being behavior that is fundamental to sur-

vival of the species but very complex)?" (ibid., 813). The complexity of hormones, genetics, and environment is, in other words, understood through the assumption that the "fundamental" survival of "the species" depends on the interaction of a male and a female parent, described in the singular, who together make up the binary of "parenting." This point becomes relevant for my later reading of psychiatric binaries.

3   Similarly, the "Images in Neuroscience" column in the June 1999 issue asks viewers to observe an MRI-produced "optical imaging of neuronal activity: an image of the surface and vasculature of a 9-mm-by-6-mm portion of primate visual cortex" (815). Yet, past the MRI, no reference is made to the optical imagers.

4   "Advantage confirmed," a bright five-page advertisement for the antidepressant Wellbutrin proclaims on its first page, above a young man and woman who smile as they stand arm in arm. Enlarged on the second and third pages, the couple tighten their hold on each other and fall supine, beneath bright, power-point text explaining that Wellbutrin has "significantly less sexual dysfunction than Zoloft, with comparable efficacy." I examine these advertisements in closer detail in chapter 4.

5   See, e.g., Hackett, "The Psychiatrist." In subsequent chapters, I argue that the emphasis placed by many historians on the 1970s as the site of the biological revolution effaces the ways in which the events that took place in psychiatry during that era were predated by a larger and more explicitly gendered biological revolution in American popular culture in the 1950s. Here, however, I take the standard, 1970s narrative at face value—inasmuch as it is clearly the narrative supported by the evidence of the *AJP*—while pointing out the numerous inconsistencies in the tale as it is told.

6   Brown, "The Life of Psychiatry," 492.

7   *American Journal of Psychiatry* 156, no. 3 (March 1999): A41–A42.

8   Maciver and Redlick, "Patterns of Psychiatric Practice," 692, 694, 695, 696.

9   Psychoanalytic concepts were requisite components of the training of all psychiatrists, e.g. By 1955, eighty-seven of the ninety-three American psychiatric training programs taught psychodynamic concepts to their residents. These residents, meanwhile, spent up to three thousand hours over the course of their three-year training periods practicing long-term, psychodynamic psychotherapy. See, e.g., Wallerstein, "The Future of Psychotherapy."

10 See Rogler, "Making Sense of Historical Changes."

11 Freud, *Inhibitions, Symptoms, and Anxiety*. As I explain in chapter 3, this piece marks an important landmark in Freud's understanding of anxiety.

12 Freud, "Analysis of a Phobia in a Five-Year-Old Boy," 122.

13 See, among other sources, Freud, "Some Psychical Consequences of the Anatomical Distinction between the Sexes."

14 For a more complete discussion of neurotic disorders, see chapter 3 below.

15 As Rosalind Minsky writes, "The cultural requirement of 'masculinity' crucially depends on acceptance of symbolic castration by the father and the repression of the boy's mother, and all she represents, into the unconscious. This severing of his femininity, half of what comprised his potential self, is the enormous emotional price which must be paid for a 'masculine identity' within patriarchal cultures" (*Psychoanalysis and Gender,* 43).

16 Maciver and Redlick, "Patterns of Psychiatric Practice," 697. Such skepticism is also interesting in the light of the established use of sodium pentothal and other "somatic" therapies within psychoanalysis.

17 Kalinowsky, "Appraisal of the 'Tranquilizers,'" 294–95.

18 Bailey, "The Great Psychiatric Revolution," 390–91. The Freudian contributions to Bailey's division of feminine nature and masculine reason are addressed in chapters 3 and 5 below.

19 Hoch, "Progress in Psychiatric Therapies," 242, 243.

20 Wikler, "The Uses of Drugs in Psychiatric Research," 961, 963.

21 Schenk, "Anxiety-Depression and Pharmacotherapy," 79.

22 *American Journal of Psychiatry* 112 (1956): 7, 116 (1960): 4.

23 Walker, *Couching Resistance,* 32.

24 *American Journal of Psychiatry* 120, no. 6 (1964): 57. Here as well, the sagacious psychotherapist is identified by his foregrounded, off-centered, enlarged position and his spectacles. Both signify his specialized means of looking more deeply at, and understanding, his patient, all the more with Deprol's help.

25 Eysenck, "The Effects of Psychotherapy," 319–20. See also Eysenck, "Training in Clinical Psychology."

26 Eysenck, "The Effects of Psychotherapy," 323.

27 Hoch, "Progress in Psychiatric Therapies," 242, 243.

28 Glueck, "Psychodynamic Patterns in the Homosexual Sex Offender," 584.

29 Ibid., 585. See also Glueck, ed., *Psychiatry and the Law;* Guttmacher, "The Homosexual in Court"; Bowman and Engle, "A Psychiatric Evaluation of Laws of Homosexuality."

30 Glueck, "Psychodynamic Patterns in the Homosexual Sex Offender," 585, 586, 587.

31 Freud, "From the History of an Infantile Neurosis," 72, 104. The Wolf Man's pleasure lay in attaining a narcissistic sense of passivity. The Rat Man's neurotic crisis was set off by a misplaced pair of eyeglasses (see Freud, "Notes upon a Case of Obsessional Neurosis").

32 See my discussion of *Civilization and Its Discontents* in chapter 3.

33 In other words, the rigidity of the psychoanalytic system allows for the interpretation of a potentially disruptive category—*homosexual men*—as instead affirming its beliefs. By explaining the men's "homosexuality" and "genital diminution fears" through their absent fathers, as opposed to their economic circumstances, prison conditions, or other artifacts and resistances, the psychodynamics of the article in

effect redefine the "men" as "women," whose weak superegos and underdeveloped consciouses threaten the normal functioning of their own bodies and, I argue in chapter 3, of their bodies within civilization.

34 Glueck, "Psychodynamic Patterns in the Homosexual Sex Offender," 589; Maciver and Redlick, "Patterns of Psychiatric Practice," 692.

35 Manheimer, Davidson, Balter, et al., "Popular Attitudes and Beliefs about Tranquilizers," 1246–50.

36 Ibid., 1246, 1249, 1250.

37 Eaton and Goldstein, "Psychiatry in Crisis," 432.

38 Szasz, *The Myth of Psychotherapy,* 16–17. See also Szasz, *Ideology and Insanity,* and "Blackness and Madness"; Laing, "Transcendental Experience"; Laing and Esterson, *Sanity, Madness, and the Family.*

39 Whitman, Armao, and Dent, "Assault on the Therapist," 428.

40 Spitzer, Endicott, and Robins, "Clinical Criteria for Psychiatric Diagnosis," 1187.

41 Klerman, "The Evolution of a Scientific Nosology," 91.

42 These concerns are summarized in Leigh, "The Role of Psychiatry in Medicine."

43 Sharfstein and Clark, "Why Is Psychiatry a Low-Paid Medical Specialty?" 831.

44 McCarley, "The Psychotherapist's Search for Self-Renewal," 221, 223.

45 Brown, "The Life of Psychiatry," 492.

46 Klerman, "The Advances of *DSM-III*," 539.

47 See Wilson, "The Transformation of American Psychiatry," 399, 400.

48 *DSM-III,* 7.

49 On the term *objectification,* see n. 8, chap. 4, below.

50 Wexler, "Cerebral Laterality and Psychiatry," 279.

51 Hobson and McCarley, "The Brain as a Dream State Generator," 1335. "Formal features of the generator processes with strong implications for dream theory include periodicity and automaticity of forebrain activation, suggesting a preprogrammed neural basis for dream mentation in sleep; intense and sporadic activation of brain stem sensorimotor circuits including reticular, oculomotor, and vestibular neurons, possibly determining spatiotemporal aspects of dream imagery; and shifts in transmitter ratios, possibly accounting for dream amnesia. The authors suggest that the automatically activated forebrain synthesizes the dream by comparing information generated in specific brain stem circuits with information stored in memory" (ibid.).

52 Guze, "The Clinical Diagnosis of Hysteria," 221.

53 As Joseph Cyyle and Steven Hyman claim, "To guard against subjective biases, the strategy of the double-blind, placebo-controlled study was developed, a strategy that is now considered the gold standard to which most new medications are subjected" ("The Neuroscientific Foundations of Psychiatry," 23).

54 See, e.g., Lasagna, "The Role of Benzodiazepines."

55 Ludwig and Othmer, "The Medical Basis of Psychiatry," 1087; Greden and Casa-riego, "Controversies in Psychiatric Education," 270.

56 Hackett, "The Psychiatrist," 432. Leigh later argued that "Psychiatry shares with the rest of medicine all basic goals, assumptions, and approaches as well as many techniques. Any apparent 'differences in approach' between psychiatry and general medicine arise from a confusion between the essentials and the specialized techniques and procedures developed in psychiatry. The educational task of psychiatry—to integrate relevant knowledge and skills from the behavioral sciences with the biological sciences and to operationalize a comprehensive approach to patient care—can be accomplished by the general psychiatrist through consultation and collaborative care of patients" ("The Role of Psychiatry in Medicine," 1581–82).

57 This dynamic is also seen in the progression of images reproduced in chapter 4. A survey of the *AJP* from the years 1975–79, e.g., reveals only seven campaigns depicting psychotherapists or psychiatrists. And no psychiatrists appeared in advertisements in the journal in 1999.

58 In the mid-1950s, to recall the Deprol advertisement, the power structure of the images was simple to diagnose: it flowed down a grid as if by Le Chatlier's principle, from viewing psychiatrist, through a scopic lens, and onto the image. By the end of the 1970s, however, the visual system implied that the psychotherapists had to beg the good graces of the images.

59 Pulver, "Survey of Psychoanalytic Practice," 615, 617.

60 See, e.g., Greenblatt and Shrader, "The Clinical Choice of Sedative Hypnotics"; Lader, "Anxiolytic Drugs."

61 Klerman, "The Advances of *DSM-III*," 542.

62 Ibid., 539; Spitzer, Endicott, and Robins, "Clinical Criteria for Psychiatric Diagnosis." See also "An Interview with Frank Berger."

63 Wilson, "The Transformation of American Psychiatry," 399. Rogler repeats these claims in "Making Sense of Historical Changes," 10–14.

64 Luhrman, *Of Two Minds*, 220–21. Luhrman argues that the 1970s thus permanently altered the face of American psychiatry.

65 Sturm and Klap, "Use of Psychiatrists, Psychologists, and Master's-Level Therapists."

66 Katon, VonKorff, et al., "Adequacy and Duration of Antidepressant Treatment"; Katzelnick, Kobak, et al., "Prescribing Patterns of Antidepressant Medications."

67 Fairman, Drevets, et al., "Course of Antidepressant Treatment," 1180. Even pharmaceutical advertisements have contributed to the effacement of psychiatry: psychiatrists are simply never represented; images overwhelmingly depict patients and medications. The ads themselves began to bypass the psychiatrist altogether when they were allowed to appeal directly to the "consumer" in August 1997.

68 These advertisements, and their glaring points of conflict with psychiatry itself, will be examined in greater detail in chapter 4.

69 Kornstein, Schatzberg, et al., "Gender Differences in Treatment Response," 1445. Numerous other studies make a similar argument. See, e.g., Kornstein, "Premenstrual Syndrome"; Kornstein, Schatzberg, Yonkers, et al., "Gender Differences in Presentation of Chronic Major Depression"; Kornstein, Schatzberg, Thase, et al., "Gender Differences in Chronic Major and Double Depression"; Hamilton, Grant, and Jensvold, "Sex and the Treatment of Depressions"; and Steiner, Wheadon, and Kreider, "Antidepressant Response to Paroxetine."

70 Olfson, Marcus, and Pincus, "Trends in Office-Based Psychiatric Practice," 451, 455.

71 Tasman, Riba, and Silk, *The Doctor-Patient Relationship in Pharmacotherapy*, 3.

72 Gabbard, "Empirical Evidence and Psychotherapy," 2.

73 Shorter, "From Freud to Prozac." See also Hale, *Rise and Crisis of Psychoanalysis*, 300; Wallerstein, "The Future of Psychotherapy."

74 In the chapters that follow, I present evidence that the "complexity" of medications is the result of properties affixed to them in popular culture in the 1950s, two decades before the alleged revolution—a point that explains both the "actions" of medications in the present day and psychiatry's inability to perceive these actions.

75 Cartwright, *Screening the Body*, xi, xii.

76 Cook, "Medical Identity," 63. Although the subject is beyond the scope of my analysis, literature in science and technology studies has explored the agency of technologies and artifacts in ways directly relevant to the matter of medications. See Stone, *The War of Desire and Technology*; "Techno-Prosthetics and Exterior Presence"; Cartwright, Penley, and Treichler, eds., *The Visible Woman*; Dumit, *Picturing Personhood*.

77 This occurs through a process of modification and expectation (see Szasz, "The Case against Psychiatric Power").

78 Zita, *Body Talk*, 70.

79 To recall Sing Sing Prison, the facade of psychoanalytic coherence misrepresented the inability of psychoanalysis to safeguard society from homosexual pedophiles.

80 See Pies, *Handbook of Essential Psychopharmacology*.

81 Minsky, *Psychoanalysis and Gender*, 150.

82 Freud described hysteria as the identification with, and inability to choose between, male and female objects. Hysterical men thus vacillated "ambivalently" between poles of domination and submission. Freud, "Hysterical Phantasies and Their Relation to Bisexuality," 157–58, 165–66.

83 My references to Freud in this concluding section are in part meant to acknowledge his insight in the cases of the Wolf Man and the Rat Man that masculine vulnerability and passivity are not connected to status, income, or position in life but are, instead, components of a broad range of experiences. As such, Freud ironi-

cally provides a means for deconstructing the divide between top and bottom, man and woman, that is in many ways his legacy to psychiatry. As Peter Stallybrass and Allon White argue in *The Politics and Poetics of Transgression*, "The 'top' attempts to reject and eliminate the 'bottom' for reasons of prestige and status, only to discover that not only is it in some way frequently dependent on the low-Other, but also that the top includes that low symbolically as a primary eroticized constituent of its own fantasy life. . . . [W]hat is socially peripheral is . . . *frequently symbolically central*" (5–6; emphasis added).

84 For a further explanation of the use of the term *psychosis* that I have adopted here, see, e.g., Freud's 1911 "Case History of Schreber," an analysis of Judge Daniel Schreber's "negative Oedipus complex," read through Schreber's 1902 memoir *Journal of My Nervous Illness.*

I mean to reference the primitive narcissistic aspect of identification as an act of devouring and to conflate the ingestion of the patient with the ingestion of the doctor. I also mean to reference the pathologization by psychiatry of homosexuality through the 1970s. See Alexander and Selesnick, *The History of Psychiatry*, 356.

THREE *Anxiety, the Crisis of Psychoanalysis, and the Miltown Resolution*

1 Jagger and Richards, "Mother's Little Helper."

2 Gordon, *I'm Dancing as Fast as I Can,* back cover. "The air is so thin you can barely breathe. You've made it—and the world says you're a hero. But it was more fun at the bottom, when you started." Susann, *Valley of the Dolls,* 1.

3 Numerous retrospective studies argue that white, middle-class women between the ages of twenty-five and fifty were far more likely than the general population to be prescribed Valium by their doctors. Parry, e.g., sampled four thousand adult respondents and found that tranquilizer use was disproportionately high among women (see Parry et al., "National Patterns of Psychotherapeutic Drug Use"). Balter's National Institute of Mental Health studies examined tranquilizer utilization and concluded that women were anywhere from twice to three times as likely as men in all age groups to be prescribed these medications and to ingest them "in advance of a possibly unpleasant event" (Balter et al., "The Extent of Anti-Anxiety/Sedative Drug Use," 773). (Balter ultimately defended the use of tranquilizers in the United States.) Manheimer et al.'s study "Psychotherapeutic Drugs," from roughly the same time period, sampled one thousand randomly selected respondents and found women "more than twice as likely as men to be tranquilizer users" (449–50). And Chambers asserted that, among regular tranquilizer users in the state of New York, 70.5 percent "were female" and that these women "were more likely to be married than to be single" ("An Assessment of Drug Use in the General Population," 55, 56).

Of note, some historians have called into question both the meaning and the implications of prescribing patterns and utilization studies. Healy, e.g., expands on Balter's work to claim that, "far from there being evidence for overprescribing, a majority of physicians and patients remained concerned about the dangers of psychotropic drugs or used them rather sparingly." Healy also cites the work of Pflantz et al., according to whom "minor tranquilizer users" were "health conscious women, more likely to be employed than confined at home" (Healy, *The Antidepressant Era*, 227–28). And the pharmacologist Mickey Smith asks, "Is the question why do women take more, or why do mean take less? The assumption appears to be that less is better" (*Small Comfort*, 55).

4 Cooperstock and Lennard, "Some Social Meanings of Tranquilizer Use," 332 (see also 342–43).

5 Valenstein, *Blaming the Brain*, 56. See also Koerner, "Leo Sternbach."

6 Smith, *Small Comfort*, 4 (see also 5–9).

7 Part of the paucity of outcomes data is the result of the fact that the FDA made prescriptions mandatory for new medication only in 1951. To my knowledge, prescription rates broken down by gender did not appear until later in the decade. See Healy, *The Creation of Psychopharmacology*, 35.

8 Each title was listed in the list of "Leading U.S. Consumer Magazines" in the 1955, 1956, and 1957 *World Almanac*. For instance, in 1955, the circulation of the *Ladies' Home Journal* was 4,950,472, that of *Time* 1,860,512, that of *Cosmopolitan* 1,043,220, and that of *Newsweek* 991,452 (*World Almanac 1957*, 483).

9 See the fifth edition of *The Physicians' Reference Manual*, published in 1960 by Miltown's manufacturer, Wallace Laboratories; as well as Ayd, "The Early History of Modern Psychopharmacology." Ayd describes how, in 1950, Carter Products (of Rochester, New York, previously the manufacturers of Carter's Little Liver Pills) contacted a number of physicians to ask if they would be interested in learning about a new concept in pharmacotherapy: a drug treatment for anxiety. When most said no, Carter's promotion and development of the new medication stopped. At the time, Milltown was merely known as the name of a town in New Jersey (after which Miltown would later be named).

10 Meanwhile, Milton Berle publicly renamed himself "Miltown Berle," and the humorist S. J. Perelman's best-seller described *The Road to Miltown*.

11 "Pills vs. Worry," 69.

12 "Unsettling Facts about the Tranquilizers," 4.

13 "The Tranquilizer," 68.

14 Also in the 1950s, biological scientists announced the discovery of antidepressants, lithium, thorazine, and haloperidol. See Cade, "Lithium Salts"; Delay, Deniker, et al., "The Treatment of Excitement and Agitation States"; Divrey et al., "R 1625"; Kuhn, "The Treatment of Depressive States."

15 Gerard, "The Biological Roots of Psychiatry"; Wikler, "The Uses of Drugs in Psychiatric Research."

16 Hendley et al., "Effect of Meprobamate."

17 Kletzin and Berger, "Effect of Meprobamate," 681.

18 Frank Berger, "The Pharmacological Properties of Miltown," 413.

19 Berger, "Anxiety and the Discovery of the Tranquilizers," 117.

20 Valenstein, *Blaming the Brain*, 1.

21 Cooley, "The New Nerve Pills and Your Health," 70.

22 This influence is often correlated with the fact that, throughout the decade, psy-
    choanalysts controlled the power structure of the profession of psychiatry. See
    Gerald Grob, "The Origins of *DSM I*," 427. For a discussion of the analytic com-
    munity's resistance to the use of psychotropic medications, see Flieschman, "Will
    the Real Third Revolution Please Stand Up?"

23 See, e.g., Mari Jo Buhle, *Feminism and Its Discontents*, 280–318; Cuordileone,
    " 'Politics in an Age of Anxiety.' "

24 Rogler, "Making Sense of Historical Changes," 10.

25 The fact that the mothers pictured in these magazines were often assumed to be
    requisite components of the unconscious of men complicates Nancy Choderow's
    notion of the "reproduction" of the traits of motherhood (*Reproduction of Mother-
    ing*, 3). In popular magazines in the 1950s, motherhood was clearly reproduced for
    commercial as well as psychical consumption. Elaboration of this point is, how-
    ever, beyond the scope of this chapter.

26 This influence is often correlated with the fact that, throughout the decade, Freud-
    ian psychoanalysts controlled the power structure of the profession of psychia-
    try. For example, psychoanalysts chaired major academic departments, sat on the
    editorial boards of major journals, and held key legislative posts in the American
    Psychiatric Association. See Grob, "The Origins of *DSM I*."

27 "In this day theater, the movies, and TV have almost drowned themselves in psy-
    choanalytic plots and prose, and even Freud's official biography, far from easy
    reading, has crept into the American best-seller lists" ("The Mind," 59).

28 Hale, *Rise and Crisis of Psychoanalysis*, 276; Buhle, *Feminism and Its Discontents*, 170.

29 Gabbard and Gabbard, *Psychiatry and the Cinema*, 76, 77. The authors clearly link
    popular representation with clinical appeal. "Intrigued by successes with World
    War II casualties, young physicians had flocked into psychiatric residency train-
    ing programs in the late 1940s, the same period in which *Life* magazine and
    other transmitters of popular ideology were making psychoanalysis fashionable
    for middle Americans. By the 1950s Dr. Spock was advising mothers on the prin-
    ciples of psychoanalytically informed child rearing; psychoanalytic ideas were ap-
    propriated as cure-alls for a variety of social ills; and middle and upper middle
    class professionals looked forward to the opportunity to lie down on The Couch"
    (ibid., 75–76).

30 Cronkite quoted in Schultheiss and Schaulbert, eds., *To Illuminate Our Time*, 177.

31 *Inhibition, Symptoms, and Anxiety* marks an important landmark in Freud's

thought. Prior to this influential essay, Freud had believed anxiety to be the product of a frustrated libido.

32 Freud, *Civilization and Its Discontents,* 297 (quotation), 322 (on *instinct*).

33 In other words, this renunciation differentiates humans, and their civilized drives,
from animals guided by instinct alone.

34 Irigaray, *Speculum of the Other Woman,* 157. Culture then, to build on Irigaray's
point, is in effect self-castrated: it cuts off and disavows what was once a part of
itself. And, if this is the case, patriarchal culture can also be argued to reverse the
act of castration by returning the severed part of the self, in the act of projection
onto the woman. It may also, I mean to say, return the phallus to the woman.

35 See Rosenberg, *Divided Lives;* Evans, *Born for Liberty.*

36 See Evans, *Born for Liberty,* 247.

37 Seward, "Sex Roles in Postwar Planning," 181.

38 Many studies support these claims. See, e.g., Mintz and Kellogg, *Domestic Revolutions.* Scholars such as Rosalind Rosenberg and Sara Evans have recently contested the notion of a domestic 1950s and, specifically, the folkloric assumption
that mothers returned to the tranquillity of the home. My goal is not to debunk
these obviously problematic stereotypes but rather to understand how their existence may have set the stage for the early success of psychopharmacology.

39 Buhle, *Feminism and Its Discontents,* 193.

40 Andrews quoted in Chafe, *The American Woman,* 177.

41 As cited in Friedan, *The Feminine Mystique,* 44. Similarly, Zube's analysis of the
Ladies' Home Journal claims that postwar articles deemphasized "doing" and emphasized "being" and argues that "a major tendency of the *Journal* in the late forties
and early fifties was to portray the blessings of family and marriage, and to confirm
its stability" ("Changing Concepts of Morality," 388). Fiction in women's magazines, meanwhile, emphasized domesticity, with few if any women portrayed as
being employed (see Franzwa, "Working Women in Fact and Fiction").

42 Cited, e.g., in Evans, *Born for Liberty,* 249, 254.

43 Minsky, *Psychoanalysis and Gender,* 43.

44 See, among many other works, Horney, *The Neurotic Personality of Our Times;*
Fromm, *Escape from Freedom;* Klein, *The Feminine Character;* and Pappenheim,
The Alienation of Modern Man. For useful background, see Rose, *The Freudian
Calling.*

45 Farnham and Lunberg, *Modern Woman,* 151, 160. See also Weiner, *From Working
Girl to Working Mother,* 47.

46 See Bloom, *Dr. Spock.* See also Buhle, *Feminism and Its Discontents,* 161.

47 Wylie, *Generation of Vipers,* 1, 184, 201, 298. For a discussion of the ways in which
momism was a visual aesthetic as well, see chapter 4 below.

48 Toch and Farson, "How to Be a Good Listener," 1.

49 Ibid., 1.

50 Scheinfeld, "Motherhood Breakdowns," 16. The article goes on to explain that, "the longer couples live together, the farther they like to be when they sleep" (ibid.).

51 Safford, "Tell me Doctor," 125. The reader should note that *me* was always lower-cased and that *Doctor* was always capitalized. The column regularly appeared on the page after Harlan Miller's "There's a Man in the House."

52 Safford, *Tell me Doctor,* 50.

53 Ibid., 125.

54 Horney, *Feminine Psychology,* 74. Dyspareunia (recurrent genital pain associated with intercourse) was later classified as a psychophysiological genito-urinary disorder (see *DSM-II,* 47).

55 In "Frigidity in Women," Moore discusses Helene Deutsch's concerns about the implications of a frigidity in which "psychotic women and aggressive, masculine women experienced intense vaginal orgasm, while loving, giving, maternal, and happy women did not, even though they felt fully gratified" (571).

56 Scheinfeld, "Bigger Mamas, Bigger Babies," 6.

57 Scheinfeld, "Marriage Crises," 6.

58 "What's on Your Mind," 6.

59 "The Mind," 59, 60, 62. This conflation is an oversimplification of psychoanalytic practice that would have been apparent to anyone writing about psychoanalysis in the 1950s. Freud died in 1939, sixteen years before the *Newsweek* article appeared. Moreover, by 1955, American psychoanalysis was split into numerous factions whose major points of contention revolved around the "Freudian discoveries" taken for granted by the article, if not lauded in its attempt at cohesiveness.

60 Ibid., 59.

61 To quote Andrew Cherlin, "After nearly a decade of depression and four terrible years of war, Americans finally had prosperity as they entered the 1950s. And, except for the more limited Korean conflict, they finally had peace. Millions of men and women had been forced to postpone marrying during the hard times of the 1930s and the austerity and separation brought about by the war. It was not surprising, then, that they married in record numbers in the late 1940s and that the birth rate soon rose dramatically. What was surprising was that years after this pent-up demand for marriage and children should have been satisfied, the birth and marriage rates remained high through the decade" (*Marriage, Divorce, Remarriage,* 34).

62 Durkheim, *Suicide,* 246.

63 As well as personal crises that lead to isolation, such as divorce or the death of a spouse.

64 See, e.g., Steckel, "Financial Insecurity"; Coopersmith, *The Antecedents of Self-Esteem;* and, for an interesting if somewhat problematic approach, Langer et al., "The Effects of Anxiety and Induced Stress."

65 Suicide rates among young white men (aged fifteen to nineteen), e.g., began to rise only in the 1960s—from 4.5 per 1,000 in 1960, to 9.4 in 1970, to 15.0 in 1980, to 19.3 in 1990. See *Statistical Abstract* (1990), booklet 6, p. 17; *Statistical Abstract* (1992), booklet 6, p. 14.

66 To take just one example, Verhoff, Kulka, and Douvan's extensive time-lag research (reported in *Mental Health in America*) assessed anxiety in American adults over the twenty-year period from 1957 to 1976. The authors concluded that, over the course of that period, anxiety was at its lowest level in 1957 and theorized this year to be the nadir of the past fifty.

67 This point also holds true for the other articles I discuss in this chapter. Much like Robert Robinson's despair and the young husband's dyspareunia, *Newsweek*'s mass dysphoria is unquantified and unqualified even though it appears in a "medical information" article.

68 Also, on 24 October 1955, the world celebrated the tenth anniversary of the establishment of the United Nations, and President Eisenhower had just suffered a coronary thrombosis on a trip to Denver.

69 The biological revolution was, thus, often described as a "red brick" revolution, as opposed to the "ivory tower" of psychoanalysis. See "Pills for the Mind."

70 "The Mind," 64.

71 See Freud, *Inhibitions, Symptoms, and Anxiety,* secs. 1–3. Freud initially believed that anxiety was due to tension from frustrated sexual desire. My discussion of anxiety implies Freud's reformulations subsequent to 1925. Freud further broke down the response to a traumatic situation into "automatic anxiety" and "anxiety as a signal"—see ibid., secs. 1–3.

72 Ibid., 132. "In Freudian psychoanalysis, fear," Alexander and Selesnick summarized in the influential textbook *The History of Psychiatry* (1966), "is an alarm reaction to external danger; anxiety signalizes internal danger" (202).

73 Beginning with the 1960 census, the same barometric indicators that pointed to women's domesticity slowly but steadily began to reverse in almost direct refutation of Farnham and Lunberg's notions of maternity and femininity. Women showed, e.g., an uninterrupted ascent in involvement in the U.S. labor force. This trend has continued to the present day. Statistics on women's labor force participation show a straight linear pattern, as do those on women as a percentage of the total labor force. And, in 1950, 12 percent of married women with preschool-age children were employed outside the home. This number represents the low point in the past half century of the work history of women with children: by 1995, this figure had risen almost five times, to 65 percent. Similarly, women's education levels rose steadily beginning in the early 1960s. The 1950s represented the low point of the past seventy years for women's attainments in higher education. To take just one example, 24 percent of all B.A. degrees awarded in 1950 went to women, a figure that has risen each and every

year hence (women now earn 55 percent of bachelor's degrees). Finally, the statistics on marriage and domesticity mentioned above all represent their most extreme point in the past fifty years. The trend of earlier marriages reversed in 1960, age at first marriage rising every year without fail, from 20.3 years in 1950 to an all-time high of 24.5 in 1995. And, not surprisingly, women had fewer and fewer babies as well. The average total fertility rate (i.e., children/lifetime) fell steadily from 3.7 in 1959 to a low of 1.8 in 1975. See Weiner, *From Working Girl to Working Mother,* chaps. 3–4; Mintz and Kellogg, *Domestic Revolutions,* 178–80, 203.

74 Prioleau et al., "An Analysis of Psychotherapy versus Placebo Studies," 284. Importantly, Prioleau et al. call on the work of Hans Eysenck, whose critiques of psychoanalysis were largely ignored in the 1950s.

75 Klerman quoted in Healy, *The Antidepressant Era,* 247.

76 As noted earlier (see n. 38 above), contemporary scholars have successfully contested the assumption that, in the 1950s, mothers returned to the tranquillity of the home. However, part of my point in this chapter is that the recognition of unstable gender roles was sensed by *Newsweek* in the 1950s, through a logic based in the realization that no repression is ever complete. From a Freudian perspective, the possibility of rupture always lies beneath surfaces of tranquillity—whether domestic spheres or golden ages. There is no subject, Jacques Lacan would later realize, without the symptom, while repetition constitutes existence. Anxiety is a constantly realized threat to the civilized world because nothing repressed ever remains so. Every repression is met with resistance. The model is, at its core, hydraulic. The repressed returns, in some form, each and every time. (Or, to paraphrase Slavoj Žižek [*Enjoy Your Symptom,* 1–28] paraphrasing Lacan, the letter always arrives at its destination.)

In positing the return of the repressed, Freud assumed that, like history, life is a process of development. The patient before you tells his story in the present tense, but this story can be understood only as part of a continuum. If a patient presents in crisis, you must address the crisis. But, if a patient tells you that nothing is wrong, then you must wonder why he has come to your office. In other words, what appear to be the most stable moments in history can also be times filled with the rumblings of unrest. All that glitters is not gold, and stability is attained at a cost. Stability is, psychoanalytically speaking, never the same as true equilibrium. And thus a decade once described as a period of normalization and calm can, when read analytically, at the same time be a decade unconsciously sensing the discontent in its midst.

77 Dickel et al., "Electromyographic Studies on Meprobamate."

78 Cade, "Lithium Salts."

79 Delay, Deniker, et al., "The Treatment of Excitement and Agitation States," 267–68. Similarly, in 1958, haloperidol, a butyropenone antipsychotic that would soon

revolutionize the treatment of schizophrenia, was first synthesized, tested, and reported (in Divrey et al., "R 1625"). See also Healy, *The Creation of Psychopharmacology*.

80 See Domino, "Human Pharmacology of Tranquilizing Drugs"; Fleischman, "Will the Real Third Revolution Please Stand Up?"

81 Kuhn, "The Treatment of Depressive States"; Ayd, "A Preliminary Report on Marsilid," 84.

82 *Physicians' Reference Manual*, 2.

83 Berger, "The Pharmacological Properties of Miltown," 413.

84 See, e.g., Domino, "Human Pharmacology of Tranquilizing Drugs."

85 Marquis et al., "Behavioral Effects of Meprobamate on Normal Subjects."

86 Berger, "The Pharmacological Properties of Miltown," 413.

87 Hendley et al. "Effect of Meprobamate," 35.

88 Kletzin and Berger, "Effect of Meprobamate," 681.

89 Hellebore, or ranunculaceae, was described by Hippocrates. In *The Anatomy of Melancholy* (1621), the cleric Robert Burton described hellebore as a purger of black bile and a cure for anxiety.

90 See Altschule, *Body Physiology in Mental and Emotional Disorders*.

91 Dickel et al., "Electromyographic Studies on Meprobamate," 12.

92 Rickels et al., "An Evaluation of Tranquilizing Drugs," 413.

93 Dixon, "Meprobamate," 12, 13.

94 Pennington, "Meprobamate," 638.

95 Lincheiznich, "Meprobamate in Children."

96 Leary et al., "Tranquilizing Drugs and Stress Tolerance," 59.

97 Huebner, "Meprobamate in Canine Medicine," 488.

98 Berger, "The Tranquilizer Decade," 408.

99 Berger, "Anxiety and the Discovery of the Tranquilizers," 117 (see also 120).

100 Moreover, resident training hours spent in long-term psychotherapy showed a steady and uninterrupted decline beginning in the early 1960s (see Wallerstein, "The Future of Psychotherapy").

101 Although many in the analytic community were openly skeptical about medication treatments for emotional problems: see, e.g., Gerard, "The Biological Roots of Psychiatry"; Wikler, "The Uses of Drugs in Psychiatric Research"; Fleischman, "Will the Real Third Revolution Please Stand Up?"

102 *Physicians' Reference Manual*, 3.

103 Dixon, "Meprobamate," 12.

104 Klerman, "The Advances of *DSM-III*," 239. See also "An Interview with Frank Berger."

105 Wilson, "The Transformation of American Psychiatry," 399.

106 Rogler, "Making Sense of Historical Changes," 10.

107 "Pills vs. Worry," 69.

108 Schwalb, "Search for New 'Mental Chemicals,'" 83. An ironic point since current treatment of depression assumes the exact opposite.

109 "Truth about the Tranquilizers," 3; "New Clues about Mental Illness," 3.

110 "Pills for the Mind," 63.

111 Cooley, "The New Nerve Pills and Your Health," 71.

112 "Pills vs. Worry," 68–69. The reference to "over-the-counter" implies illicit. This was in spite of the fact that almost all prescriptions for tranquilizers were written by psychiatrists and that nonpsychoanalyst psychiatrists are cited as experts throughout the article. The implication is, the article makes clear, that peace of mind can be attained without the pain of introspection and without the need for years on a couch.

113 "How Tranquilizers Work," 47.

114 Cooley, "The New Nerve Pills and Your Health," 70. On Ayd as a pioneer in the discovery of psychoactive medications, see chapter 1.

115 Alvarez, "Live with Your Nerves and Like It," 42. Numerous other articles illustrate this point. See, e.g., Toland, "My Husband Came Home"; "Man and Wife"; "Sanity from Chemistry?"

116 "Pills for the Mind," 63.

117 As cited in Friedan, *The Feminine Mystique,* 44.

118 "Mirror in the Brain."

119 The case of Anna O. began in 1880. When Freud first became aware of it in 1882, he initially "misperceived" its significance as a case of "organic" as opposed to "unconscious" symptomatology—ironically, the very same territory recovered by Dr. Penfield. See Breuer and Freud, *Studies in Hysteria.*

120 "Mirror in the Brain."

121 "How Tranquilizers Work," 47.

122 Schwalb, "Search for New 'Mental Chemicals,'" 83.

123 Replacing theories with essential facts, Fromm's hysteria and Deutsch's neurosis with the certainty of ganglia and pallida, thus disavowed the slippage between personal and cultural pathology so central to Freud's formulation.

124 It is important to note that concomitant popular notions of biology sought to present biology as proof of sexual difference. Postwar "biologists" such as Abraham Kardiner, Edward Strecker, and Vincent Lathbury are but a few of the mid-1950s popularizers of the widespread belief that gender roles were determined by "natural differences" (see Strecker and Lathbury, *Their Mothers' Daughters,* 120–53). Kardiner, e.g., argued that preprogrammed "male pursuits" included "work outside the home" and that the female "biological role" included domestic responsibilities (*Sex and Morality,* 220)—a point later taken up by John Bowlby, among others. Men and women, Kardiner writes, were "two biologically differentiated creatures" with "diverse" social functions (231)—an assumption that would later pave the way for the protests of Kate Millett and other feminist critics of

"biology." My point here, however, is that the discourse of biological psychiatry worked in exactly the opposite way specifically because it claimed to be gender neutral and because it claimed not to be psychoanalysis. The notion of gender-based differences in brain metabolism would not appear in this particular discussion until the mid- to late 1990s and only when electrophysiology became neuroradiology. The focus of biological psychiatry on universal structures such as the thalamus, the hippocampus, and the electrical impulse thus differentiated biological psychiatry from biological determinism. In the process, biological psychiatry promised a new allegory for defining—or, more appropriately, for displacing—the awareness of the same discontent that had so troubled *Newsweek's* America. Under the psychoanalytic regime, to recall, anxiety was ostensibly a maternal event. The repression of the mother, or, rather, the repression of the desire for her, formed the unconscious. The threat of her return, or the threat that caused her repression in the first place, was what self and civilization sought at all costs to avoid. Mothers threatened to leave the home, to assume new roles and new identities. If, however, there was no unconscious, or if the unconscious was made conscious and ungendered by the electroencephalogram, then this threat was neutralized. The schizophrenogenic mother could not arise from the unseen to disrupt progress if she was first exposed as having been within civilization all along. Self and country then had little to fear from her return. The language of biology externalized and civilized the mother—rendering her structurally incapable of causing a change within—while at the same time protecting the mainstream from the awareness of a rising tide of discontent. And, if the mother was not the cause of anxiety, then it is not difficult to see how tranquilizers were effective in treatment.

125 Cooley, "The New Nerve Pills and Your Health," 71.
126 "Tranquilizers Shield Brain," 153. Here, the neural effects of the tranquilizers are validated by their effects in treating the symptoms of "neurotic mice," thereby throwing the diagnosis of neurosis (and Freud's differentiation between instincts and drives) into question.
127 For the original statement of Kuhn's position, see Kuhn, "The Structure of Scientific Revolutions."
128 A reminder of my point about remnants in the opening. Innovation and overthrow cannot help but employ the conceptual terminology of the replaced. Innovation itself, I mean to say, often employs a language always already interpolated in the old system. Once the postmodern becomes postmodern, it cannot exist without the modern. Similarly, in assuming its own hegemony, biology learns to speak by assuming a cultural role similar to that performed by psychoanalysis. As this process occurs, the notion of a paradigm shift also comes to reveal the ways in which power structures work to remain in power in unconscious ways.
129 Toland's "My Husband Came Home" is narrated by an anonymous woman; Flemming's "I Had My Husband Committed" by a Mrs. Markley.

130 Certainly, the similarity between articles about psychoanalysis and articles about tranquilizers had much to do with forces of production. As the bylines of these articles reveal, many of the same writers who wrote about psychoanalysis wrote about Miltown when it became fashionable to do so. Again, I want to suggest, however, that more was at stake than production when the signifier changed but the condensation and displacement that connected it to social restoration did not.

131 "Why People Don't Marry," 47. Articles describing the psychoanalytic condition of "marriage phobia" were all the rage in the 1950s, appearing regularly in both newsmagazines and women's magazines. For example, Dr. Friedman's research into the treatment of marriage phobia, first published (according to "Phobias about Marriage," 22) in the *Journal of Hillside Hospital,* received wide acclaim. The March 1957 *Science Digest,* e.g., published a brief story on Dr. Friedman's work entitled "Phobias about Marriage": "Dr. Friedman said that most persons with marriage phobias do not know the cause of their unwillingness or inability to marry. To outsiders these persons may have normal and valid reasons for not marrying. But actually, they 'remain unmarried due to unconscious motivating factors' which must be made conscious in the act of treatment" (22). Marriage phobia might, thus, be considered a man's autoimmune version of frigidity.

132 "Why People Don't Marry," 47.

133 "Marital Status and Living Arrangements."

134 Or, in the context of the demographic statistics mentioned earlier, a phobia that a man might show up for work to find out that Rosy the Riveter has taken his place.

135 As is, I hope, apparent, I am in no way making the claim that this is quantifiable evidence, evidence of the type that can be validated (i.e., proved to be statistically significant) through, e.g., chi-square analysis or controlled logarithmic regression. Rather, I argue that this is psychoanalytic evidence, a rupture in the facade, evidence validated by the simple fact that it exists or is at least thought to exist— although, as I argue in subsequent chapters, the linking of marriage and psychotropic medication becomes something of a transhistorical trope.

136 Schwalb, "Search for New 'Mental Chemicals,'" 86; "U.S. Women Now Mothers at Younger Age," 86.

137 "Want a Long Life? Get Married," 29.

138 I do not mean here to posit outdated psychoanalytic paradigms as universal truths. Psychoanalysis did not create the nature/culture binary, and the unconscious does not exist unless one actively looks for it—as I obviously have. Knowledge about the influence of psychoanalysis in the 1950s does, however, help explain what took place on an obscure page of the seemingly forgotten *Newsweek* magazine medicine section in 1956. Here, the embrace of a new discourse claimed to block the awareness of pressing social concerns. Existing notions of repression and return had opened the possibility of a limitless cascade, an analysis without end, at $80 an hour. The insistence on a biological substrate, however, promised an end from the

beginning, manifest in structures made visible by the surface tracing of electro-encephalography and by symptoms—muscle tension, restlessness, gastrointestinal upset—inscribed and read on the bodies of women and men. As such, Miltown represented a conscious cure for a suddenly, doubly conscious disease.

139 This is, of course, a point that psychoanalysis makes explicitly, where the return of the repressed caused neurosis. But, as *Newsweek* demonstrated on 24 December 1956, and as I argue through the remainder of this project, the neurosis remained long after Freud fell out of favor.

140 See Irigaray, *Speculum of the Other Woman,* pts. 1 and 3.

141 Braslow, *Mental Ills and Bodily Cures.*

142 Although beyond the scope of my analysis, this point also resonates with Judith Butler's notion of the *abject,* inscribed on the surface of popular culture and performed throughout the readership that it represents (see her *Bodies That Matter*). This is an interesting possibility since, like Foucault, Butler complicates the very notion of the unconscious that I take for granted in this chapter. I would readily agree that the unconscious is a social construct—as *Newsweek* well reveals, both conscious and unconscious lie on the same page. At the same time, such arguments often have a hard time explaining the need for the unconscious—or, rather, man's repetitive, compulsive need to keep creating the unconscious—in the face of always-compelling proof of its nonexistence.

143 See Freud, *Inhibitions, Symptoms, and Anxiety,* 144–50. For a contemporary discussion, see Silverman, *The Acoustic Mirror,* 88.

144 Other phase-specific defense mechanisms include sublimation, displacement, and reaction formation. Each of these is, according to Freud, an attempt to bind anxiety.

145 Repression is, unfortunately, also not globally effective. Hence, repressed feelings would later return (and, with the help of an analyst, be identified) into consciousness in the form of dreams, and jokes, and slips of the tongue. Too much repression, and this return took the form of the symptoms of psychoneurosis. The analyst's job, then, was to help the patient ease the pressure on the ego: to relax the superego's attacks on the id (as well as the destructive impulses of the death instinct, which further obstruct the free expression of the id) and, in so doing, to allow for a free expression of what lay below the anxiety, this that had been known before only by the return of the repressed.

146 *Physicians' Reference Manual,* 11.

147 Psychoanalytic anxiety was, in other words, a melancholic anxiety, an inescapable anxiety, and, most of all, a nostalgic anxiety. Subjects longed for a perfect union to which they could never return and were, instead, always reminded of a trauma that they would rather forget. Castration loomed around every corner. Women then represented what men most wanted and, at the same time, what men most feared. Worst of all, such eloquence did nothing to bind the threat. Victory—un-

like the war, unlike the invasion, unlike the bomb—was never certain. The symptom, always and already, remained. Perhaps this was much more than American popular culture ever bargained for when it embraced Freud as a golden paradigm of itself.

FOUR *The Gendered Psychodynamics of Pharmaceutical Advertising*

1 Schutzman, *The Real Thing*, 3.

2 As I imply throughout this chapter, representations of women in pharmaceutical advertisements correlate with the actual treatment of women in the medical system. Levy's "The Role and Value of Pharmaceutical Marketing" is one of many articles arguing that these advertisements serve as primary sources of information about pharmaceuticals for many physicians. Extrapolating from the membership of the American Psychiatric Association over the time period of my study (see http://www.psych.org/women/statistics.cfm [accessed 1 June 2002]), one can assume that, historically, 70 percent of the viewers of these ads have been male. However, to judge solely by the visual systems constructed by the images, one might well assume that the concerns of women psychiatrists were simply never taken into account or, more problematically, that the skill of looking like a man was a requisite component of professional training.

3 Hawkins and Aber, e.g., decry the visual portrayal of women in medical advertisements while speculating that "physicians and others who read medical journals might be influenced by overt and covert messages" to "prescribe medications to women" ("The Content of Advertisements in Medical Journals," 45). Similarly, Linn and Davis argue that "advertisements can be responsible not only for influencing physicians in their prescribing habits, but also for shaping opinions and attitudes towards women" ("Physicians' Orientation toward the Legitimacy of Drug Use," 199). In a review of studies of advertisements in medical journals, Courtney and Whipple write that "the authors all contend that such advertising reinforces doctors' prejudice against women and causes them to prescribe mood altering drugs, rather than dealing with the cause of women's problems" (*Sex Stereotype in Advertising,* 14). On those few occasions when men do appear in advertisements as patients, they are depicted as "nonemotional, rational, and stoic, exhibiting fewer symptoms of mental illness," thus conforming to what Prather and Fidell call "the cultural stereotype" ("The Content and Style of Medical Advertisements," 24).

4 On the overprescription of psychotropic medications to women, see n. 3, chap. 3, above.

5 Expanded, special-section advertising first appeared in the *AJP* in 1964; pharmaceutical ads first appeared in popular magazines in 1997.

My focus is on advertisements for medications frequently prescribed for out-

patient conditions, such as anxiety and depressive disorders. I leave out advertisements for psychotic disorders, which have historically employed different representational strategies. Each of the advertisements that I cite in this chapter
appeared in at least one other mainstream psychiatric journal (e.g., the *Psychiatric
Times* or *Psychiatric News*) as well as in various promotional publications, inserts,
and other materials supplied to doctors by pharmaceutical companies.

Although a thorough examination of the *Journal of the American Medical Association,* the *New England Journal of Medicine,* and the *Archives of Family Medicine* is
beyond the scope of my analysis, a cursory look reveals stark differences between
advertisements for psychopharmaceuticals and advertisements for other types of
medications with respect to the construction of gender relationships. Moreover,
advertisements for psychotropic medications were often altered for publication
in medical journals. For instance, compare the Valium advertisements discussed
below, in which single women appear in need of medication as a matter of course,
with the androgynous Valium ads that ran concomitantly in *MD Medical Newsmagazine* (21, no. 12 [1977]: 18).

6 Frank et al., "Characteristics of Female Psychiatrists."

7 Krupka and Vener, "Prescription Drug Advertising."

8 The term *objectifiable* became a catchphrase for attempts by Feighner, Spitzer, and
other leading psychiatrists, beginning in the 1970s, to establish a series of "objectifiable criteria" for the diagnosis of psychiatric conditions. The historian Michael
Stone thus identifies the 1970s as the period of "the flourishing of objectifiable
science" (*Healing the Mind,* 320).

9 Walker, *Couching Resistance,* 20.

10 Ibid., 20, 171–73.

11 See also Roeske, "Women in Psychiatry"; Rice and Rice, "Implications of the
Women's Liberation Movement."

12 Walker, *Couching Resistance,* 20.

13 Josephson, *From Idolatry to Advertising,* 158–59, 172 (see generally 158–72). A
somewhat similar argument is made in Bordo, "Braveheart, Babe, and the Contemporary Body."

14 DTC ads first appeared in popular magazines and on television after the FDA relaxed its regulations on the site and content of pharmaceutical ads in August 1997.
I discuss these advertisements at the conclusion of the chapter.

15 Thompson, "Sexual Bias in Drug Advertisements," 187. See also Berkwits,
"Health-Industry Advertising in Medical Journals"; Angell, "Is Academic Medi-
cine for Sale?" For a similar discussion of DTC ads, see O'Connell and Zimmerman,
"Drug Pitches Resonate with Edgy Public," A3.

16 See, e.g., Hawkins and Aber, "The Content of Advertisements in Medical Journals," 45. As Mickey Smith (*Small Comfort,* 10) notes, "Certainly the evidence indicates that women report many more symptoms of neuroses and anxiety than do

men, and that they receive many more prescriptions for minor tranquilizers." In support of his assertion that "women are uniquely vulnerable to institutional pressures toward defining their problems in medical terms," Smith cites Nathanson's "Social Roles and Health Status among Women."

17 Although Deprol was found to have psychosis-inducing properties in patients with schizophrenia, it was marketed for anxiety depression until well into the 1990s—thus outliving its more famous Wallace Laboratories progenitor, Miltown.

18 Again, in the *DSM-I* (1952), psychoneurotic disorders were defined in psychoanalytic terms: "The chief characteristic of these disorders is anxiety, which may be directly felt or expressed or which may be unconsciously and automatically controlled by the utilization of various psychological defense mechanisms (depression, conversion, displacement, etc.)" (37).

19 Garb, "Gender and Representation," 219–20.

20 Goffman, *Gender Advertisements,* 28, 37.

21 Mulvey, "Afterthoughts," 14; Propp, *Morphology of the Folktale.*

22 Numerous ads of the era similarly drew on cinematic phantasmagoria. See, e.g., the Bergman-like advertisement for Trilafon in the *American Journal of Psychiatry* 120 (1964): A3.

23 Goffman, *Gender Advertisements,* 28, 37.

24 As Sylvan Barnet helpfully claims, visual perspective is often relayed in painting through the construction of a hierarchical scale in which "a king, for instance, is depicted bigger than a slave, not because he is nearer, but because he is more important" (*A Short Guide to Writing about Art,* 37).

25 Wylie, *Generation of Vipers,* 201, 298.

26 "The myth of the Big Momma is on the upswing. When Philip Wylie crusaded some years back for misogyny, a fair-sized opposition went into action. But now everybody's in his corner. It would seem that Wylie's rantings weren't wrong: he was simply a bit too prematurely anti-Mom. The impact of the Big, Bad, Bold Momma has become part of the American way of life, and as Big Momma thus brazenly ascends the scale of things, so Big Daddy has come down" (Merriam, "The Matriarchal Myth," 332). The drawing that accompanied the article illustrated the same fears presented in the Deprol advertisement and later described by sources such as "The American Male" and Schlesinger's "The Crisis in American Masculinity": the "power" of women led to the shrinking of men. Somewhat similarly, see Rothman's discussion of the film *Psycho* (*Hitchcock,* 339).

27 Mari Jo Buhle grounds the popular appeal of momism in the resonance between popular perception and psychoanalysis. In her view, momism (and Wylie's self-described "psychoanalytic methods") rose from Freudian origins, aided by "its ability to tap into psychoanalysis as a popular discourse." The result was, as in psychotropic advertisements, an attack on motherhood that both mirrored and helped shape popular sentiment. Buhle compellingly argues that the discourse of

momism suffused psychoanalysis as well. As just one of many examples, she asserts that American ego psychologists "sought out not motherhood's beneficent, but malignant potential": "With the assistance of popularists like Wylie, psychoanalysis transformed mothers into the principle agents of children's disorders, and the maladies that plagued the nation" (Buhle, *Feminism and Its Discontents,* 127–31).

The point that Buhle overlooks, however, is that (to borrow Warren Sussman's terminology) psychoanalysis failed to dictate the politics of the consciousness of the self in American psychiatry in the latter half of the twentieth century (see Sussman, *The Transformation of American Society,* 271). Rather, psychoanalysis in the United States suffered what the historian Nathan Hale describes as a "rapid decline in the field," replaced in clinics and in training programs by a model envisioning mental illness as the result of structurally influenced disorders of brain chemistry treated by Deprol and other medications (Hale, *Rise and Crisis of Psychoanalysis,* 300). Over the coming years, biological explanations for illness and health would become the foundation for the ways in which psychiatry thought of selves, while prescriptions, not analysts' couches, framed many of the interactions between doctors and patients.

28 *Archives of General Psychiatry,* vol. 24, no. 4 (1971).

29 Friedan, *The Feminine Mystique,* 40, 51–52. Friedan attacked Freudian psychoanalysis as "an all embracing American ideology" (44) whose patriarchal structure prohibited women from questioning long-standing prejudice. As Susan Douglas writes, "The feminine mystique, elevated by Freudian theory into a scientific religion, sounded a single, overprotective, life-restricting, future-denying note for women" (*Where the Girls Are,* 124).

30 Douglas, *Where the Girls Are,* 125. In April 1963, *The Feminine Mystique* joined the best-seller list; by 1964, it had become the best-selling paperback in the country (*Publisher's Weekly,* 18 January 1965, 68, 72).

31 Parry et al., "National Patterns of Psychotherapeutic Drug Use."

32 "The New Feminists," 53.

33 "Special Report: Women in Revolt," 70.

34 "Who's Come a Long Way Baby?" 16, 17.

35 Douglas, *Where the Girls Are,* 175.

36 "Special Report: Women in Revolt," 73; Johnson, *Lesbian Nation,* 166; Koedt, *Notes from the Third Year.*

37 Millett, *Sexual Politics,* 23.

38 See, e.g., Kurland et al., "Comparative Effectiveness." See also n. 53, chap. 2, above.

39 Brown, "The Life of Psychiatry," 492.

40 Corrodi et al., "The Effect of Some Psychoactive Drugs." These actions would later be attributed to the disinhibition of the neurotransmitter GABA.

The success of Valium shaped the biological notion of anxiety, which was found to be an activation of the hypothalamic-pituitary-adrenal axis, as mediated through benzodiazepine-gammaaminobutyric receptor complexes (see Berger, "Anxiety and the Discovery of the Tranquilizers," 125). Further, lactate infusion allowed biological psychiatrists to differentiate *anxiety* and *panic*—thereby tacitly uncovering the "scientific" difference between what Freud in *Inhibitions, Symptoms, and Anxiety* misperceived as developmentally derived anxiety and fear (see Hollander, Leibowitz, et al., "Cortisol and Lactate Induced Panic").

41 "Properly used by the medical profession, it has only medicinal properties. A drug has no moral or immoral qualities. These are the monopoly of the user or abuser" (Cant, "Valiumania," 54). Valium's safe side-effect profile made it a medication prescribed by psychiatrists as well as by many other types of medical practitioners. With the success of psychopharmacology—as measured by improving efficacy and decreasing side effects—these medications became medical rather than psychiatric treatments. Although I do not address the issue here, the replacement of psychoanalysis by biology must also be understood in the context of the replacement of psychiatry by psychology, internal medicine, family medicine, and other specialties.

42 This title was later claimed by Prozac.

43 Chambers, "An Assessment of Drug Use in the General Population."

44 *Archives of General Psychiatry* 22 (April 1970): 290–91.

45 *Archives of General Psychiatry* 22 (June 1970): 481–82.

46 Histrionic personality disorder, the modern-day descendant of hysteria, is conceptualized in a psychoanalytic paradigm as a remnant of Oedipal development. Patients (overwhelmingly women) are thought to be in a bind between always seeking to re-create the father-daughter relationship and always finding men who fall short of their own, internalized, fatherly expectations. See Phillips and Gunderson, "Personality Disorders," 528.

47 As Dora explains in Freud's most famous case history, "Men are so detestable that I would rather not marry" (Freud, "Fragment and Analysis of a Case of Hysteria," 98).

48 See Chesler, *Women and Madness,* 182–205, 262–68.

49 Wong et al., "A Selective Inhibitor of Serotonin Uptake," 471.

50 "Listening to Eli Lilly," B1.

51 "The Promise of Prozac," 38.

52 Toufexis, "The Personality Pill," 53.

53 Stotland, "Gender, What's the Difference?" See also Stotland, "Gender-Based Biology"; Seeman, "Psychopathology in Women and Men"; Kessler, McGonagle, et al., "Sex and Depression in the National Comorbidity Survey"; Weissman, Bland, et al., "Sex Differences in Rates of Depression"; Regier, Boyd, et al., "One-Month Prevalence of Mental Disorders."

54 Kornstein, Schatzberg, et al., "Gender Differences in Treatment Response." Korn-

stein, Schatzberg, et al. argue that biological differences between women and men actually determine responses to antidepressant medications—and, by extension, that antidepressant medications work to validate and reify biological categories of gender and their differences. In a comparison of 235 men and 400 women with chronic major depression or double depression (major depression superimposed on dysthymia), "women were significantly more likely to show a favorable response to sertraline than to imipramine, and men were significantly more likely to show a favorable response to imipramine than to sertraline. Gender and type of medication were also significantly related to dropout rates; women who were taking imipramine and men who were taking sertraline were more likely to withdraw from the study." They concluded: "The differing response rates between the drug classes in women was [sic] observed primarily in premenopausal women. Thus, female sex hormones may enhance response to ssris or inhibit response to tricyclics. Both gender and menopausal status should be considered when choosing an appropriate antidepressant for a depressed patient" (1445). See also Goodwin et al., "Prescription of Psychotropic Medications"; Mamdani et al., "Use of Antidepressants"; Fairman, Drevets, et al., "Course of Antidepressant Treatment."

55 Wallis, "Onward Women!" 84.

56 Too, the portrayal of women in pharmaceutical advertisements had come under scrutiny, in large part owing to feminist protests emerging from the social and medical sciences in the 1980s. In a vast literature, numerous scholars derided portrayals of women based on passive stereotypes such as "housewives, mothers, sex objects, ethereal, naked or caricatured persons," to cite the critics Joellen Hawkins and Cynthia Aber ("The Content of Advertisements in Medical Journals," 56).

57 De Titta and Robinowitz, "The Future of Psychiatry," 853. See also Frank et al., "Characteristics of Female Psychiatrists."

58 Kramer, *Listening to Prozac,* 16–17. See also Zita, *Body Talk,* 61–84. I discuss these works in detail in chapter 5 below.

59 One could say that the base lagged far behind (or perhaps called into question) the illusion of change in the superstructure.

60 This is the same dominant side occupied by the physician in the 1960s—as opposed to the weaker, sinister side on which wedding rings are worn in Western culture.

61 All campaigns appear in both the *AJP* and the *Archives.* See also figure 7.

62 Edward Shorter argues that, along with physicians, drug companies "create their own markets" by ever expanding the indications for prescription drugs ("From Freud to Prozac," 291). The point is not only Shorter's, however. David Healy makes a similar claim in *The Antidepressant Era* when he discusses pharmaceutical "market formation" (179), and Jacqueline Zita describes "diagnostic bracket creep," an ever-expanding set of indications for an ever-widening series of psychiatric illnesses (*Body Talk,* 61–84). All three assume that, in concert with physicians,

researchers, and even the drugs themselves, drug companies create economies of need and want where such economies did not previously exist.

Often overlooked by the "new markets" argument, however, is the point that emerges from the advertisements: when gender is the currency of expansion, drugs and drug companies are also adept at perpetuating markets long in existence. Representations of women constitute one such preexisting market, insofar as the themes, aesthetics, and strategies seen in the ads functioned in popular culture long before they appeared in promotions for pharmaceuticals. At the same time, pharmaceutical advertisements also build on the communal understanding of how women's problems threaten the well-being of men, and they thereby perpetuate a mode of sense making in which, to recall *Science Digest*'s "Want a Long Life? Get Married," "the death rate for the married man is only about half that for the single. The difference is not so marked among females, and it is only recently that married women have had a lower mortality than the unmarried" (28–29).

63   Shorter, *A History of Psychiatry,* vii.

64   Chesler, *Women and Madness,* 21–22.

65   Or, as Kaja Silverman argues, "What an image of woman is of is masculinity's lack." In Silverman's analysis of representations of women, as cinema works "through its endless narrativization of the castration crisis, it transfers to the female subject the losses which afflict the male subject. It also arms him against the possible return of these losses by orchestrating a range of defensive operations to be used against the woman, from disavowal and fetishism to voyeurism and sadism. In this way the trauma which would otherwise capsize the male viewer is both elicited and contained" (*The Acoustic Mirror,* 15).

FIVE *Prozac and the Pharmacokinetics of Narrative Form*

1   Wurtzel, *Prozac Nation,* 329.

2   The flow of events went something like this: Prozac, the first and most certainly the best named (combining the *pro-* of *proficient* and the *-zac* of *attack*) of the selective serotonin reuptake inhibitors (SSRIs), generated works of fiction and nonfiction (and often both at once) extolling the virtues of listening and talking back to the drug, of thinking of Prozac as a metaphor as big as a nation or as personal as a diary. These works in turn gave rise to numerous scholarly and popular arguments that Prozac-based expression reflects a moment of alienation (Elliott, "Pursued by Happiness"), or an American desire for enhancement and improvement (Parens, "Is Better Always Good?"), or a recognition of the material fluidity of personality (Concar, "Design Your Own Personality"), or a fixation with drugs and pharmaceuticals (Gardiner, "Can Ms. Prozac Talk Back?").

3   Zita, *Body Talk,* 63.

4   Shorter, "From Freud to Prozac," 289.

5　Schilb, "Autobiography after Prozac," 202–3.

6　Smith, *Small Comfort*, 4–5.

7　Marks, *The Benzodiazepines*. Prozac set the graph on different coordinates entirely. Chemically designed and synthesized in an Eli Lilly laboratory in the mid-1970s, and approved by the FDA in December 1987, Prozac spurred a popular frenzy (Smith's phase 1) that gave new meaning to long-held notions of the economics of consumer demand and physician supply. Prozac was easy to prescribe, showed a "flat dose-response curve" (meaning that there is usually no advantage to increasing the dose above that which is the effective minimum [Janicak, *Handbook of Psychopharmacotherapy*, 101]), and was rarely lethal in an overdose. Moreover, Prozac was argued to be a "clean drug," exerting its effects on a highly specific aspect of neurochemical transmission. As such, Prozac was thought to be effective against much more than mere depression. Prozac treated what researchers at McLean Hospital, writing in the *American Journal of Psychiatry*, called *affective spectrum disorder*—a series of symptoms including anxiety, panic, and downtrodden mood that signaled what was, according to the McLean researchers, "one of the most widespread diseases of mankind" (Hudson and Pope, "Affective Spectrum Disorder," 558). Patient requests soared as word spread about this amazing efficacy, this widespread indication. "Prozac is much more than a fad," *Time* magazine explained; "it is a medical breakthrough" (Toufexis, "The Personality Pill," 53). "Prozac," *Newsweek* added, "is a breakthrough antidepressant that is easier to prescribe and has fewer side effects. And that makes patients—and doctors—happy" ("The Promise of Prozac," 39). As discussed in chapter 4, within a few years of its release Prozac become the drug most prescribed by psychiatrists in the United States and the second-best-selling drug in the world (Shorter, "From Freud to Prozac," 324).

8　Slater, "Black Swans," 155.

9　Blackbridge, *Prozac Highway*, 132.

10　"Psychotherapy and psychoanalysis consume ever larger amounts of the health budget, with little evidence that they work for anything in particular" (Klerman, "The Evolution of a Scientific Nosology," 91).

11　"Depression, like mourning, hides an aggression against the lost object and thereby reveals the ambivalence on the part of the afflicted with respect to the object of his mourning" (Freud, "Mourning and Melancholia," 239–40). Of course, great differences exist within psychoanalytic practice about the importance of uncovering and realizing this past. At the same time, conceptual acknowledgment and awareness of a past represent a basic point that connects models and concepts as disparate as Freud's *transference,* which "gives us new impressions or reprints" and "revised editions" of the past ("Fragment and Analysis of a Case of Hysteria," 116), and Robert Stolorow's self-psychological *transference,* which he defines as "serving therapy when a developmental process . . . is set in motion wherein the formerly sequestered painful reactive states, the heritage of a patient's traumatic history, gradually become integrated and transformed" ("The Nature and Therapeutic Action of Psychoanalytic Interpretation," 123).

12 Mann et al., "Demonstration in Vivo," 174.

13 Kaasinen et al., "Sex Differences in Extrastriatal Dopamine D2-Like Receptors."

14 Stotland, "Gender-Based Biology"; Meyer et al., "The Effect of Paroxetine."

15 Money and Erhardt, *Man and Woman, Boy and Girl,* 74. In "How to Build a Man" and *Myths of Gender,* Anne Fausto-Sterling offers an important critique of Money and Erhardt's research.

16 Friedman and Downey, "Biology and the Oedipus Complex," 234. I also wish to allude to Friedman and Downey's earlier work on biology and sexual orientation (see, e.g., "Neurobiology and Sexual Orientation") in my discussions of Blackbridge's character Jam.

17 Stone, *Healing the Mind,* 321.

18 The headline of a Prozac ad that appeared, among other places, in *Health,* March 1998, 19. Also relevant is the 2002 Serafem campaign: "Bloated Feeling? Think It's PMS? Think Again . . . Serafem/fluoxitine hydrochloride" (http://www.sarafem.com [accessed 24 June 2002]).

19 The brain, suddenly functional, suddenly demystified, became just one of many body organs.

For a discussion of the psychoanalytic notion of excavation, see Freud's use of Wilhelm Jensen's *Gradiva: A Pompeiian Fantasy*—a novel about a German archaeologist who dreams of "Gradiva," a young woman he sees in an ancient Roman relief—in "Delusion and Dream in Wilhelm Jensen's *Gradiva.*" Freud found in Gradiva a metaphor for how art imitates dreams and how archaeology imitates the "excavation" of psychoanalysis. Of relevance here, Freud's "Delusion and Dream" was his first study of a work of literature apart from his comments on *Oedipus Rex* and *Hamlet* in chap. 2 of *The Interpretation of Dreams.*

20 "Alleged Gunman Took Antidepressant," C4.

21 "The Best of 1990," D1.

22 Angier, "Grumpy, Fearful Neurotics," A1. As another example of this point, see Wade, "Cow's Cells."

23 Kramer, *Listening to Prozac,* chap. 1.

24 "The air is so thin you can barely breathe. You've made it—and the world says you're a hero. But it was more fun at the bottom, when you started" (Susann, *Valley of the Dolls,* 1). The thirty-six-year-old housewife figures in "Pills for the Mind," Neely in *Valley of the Dolls.*

25 Menkes, "Fearless Heroines with Looks to Match," C1.

26 As an illustration of this point, see figure 32. Similarly, the 2000 Effexor "I Got My Mommy Back" ads go to great lengths to show "Mommy" in a business suit.

With no need for the exhausting work of backlash, men could finally begin to (or were given the cultural space to) look at their own problems, perhaps creating an opening for Viagra.

27 Kramer, *Listening to Prozac,* 16–17. Attuned to such implications, Jacqueline Zita writes of *Listening to Prozac,* "Feminism is rescripted by Kramer's Prozac industry to help produce middle-class, 'hyperthymic babes' in a rhetorical stroke that not only redefines Prozac as the drug for feminist hypernormalization but also calms the panic surrounding the newly emerging postmodern body" (*Body Talk,* 62).

28 This vocabulary also divided homosexuals from rapists (see chapter 2).

29 Freeman, *Fight against Fears,* 248.

30 Green, *I Never Promised You a Rose Garden,* 114, 122, 217. See also Gordon's description of her male psychoanalyst: "I looked at the carefully pressed suit, the white shirt, the characterless tie, the angular face, the sterile room. How old was he? I realized I had no idea" (*I'm Dancing as Fast as I Can,* 31).

31 Slater, "Black Swans," 156.

32 Kennedy, "Shrinks," 57, 58.

33 Krist, "Medicated," 245.

34 For an interesting play on the connection between Prozac and castration anxiety, see Peter Lefcort's novel *Abbreviating Ernie.*

35 Kramer, *Listening to Prozac,* 23; Wurtzel, *Prozac Nation,* 315.

36 Glenmullen, *Prozac Backlash,* 7–8. Relevant here as well is Glenmullen's patient Maura, also discussed in chapter 1.

37 Thus my selection of "Black Swans"—a narrative that speaks nothing of marriage—as opposed to the later *Prozac Diary.* The dedication of the latter reads "For You, Ben," and in the book Slater describes how treatment with Prozac helped her get married. This progression—from essay in an obscure literary journal to bestseller—might reveal a great deal about the space between alternative and mainstream tellings of Prozac.

38 Danquah's *Willow Weep for Me* is one of the very few mental-illness memoirs written by a person of color.

39 Moreover, three of the four texts were published by alternative presses or journals: Kennedy's "Shrinks" (in her collection *Stripping and Other Stories*) by High Risk Books; Blackbridge's *Prozac Highway* by Press Gang; and Slater's "Black Swans" by the *Missouri Review*). Perhaps ironically, these are the three works by women. While I deal only indirectly with the differences between my four focal texts, I believe that the fact that Krist is male and that his book was published by a major trade house (Harcourt Brace) is important to keep in mind. Perhaps, in the early stages of Prozac fiction, it was more acceptable for a man, writing in skirt, as it were, to gain public acceptance. In time, however, and with Prozac, the historical stereotype of melancholia as the source of a man's creativity underwent a chemical reassignment. Slater was subsequently published by Random House, and Wurtzel's book was a national best-seller. Now, at the beginning of the twenty-first

century, men write as doctors, but hardly ever as depressed patients. Women (with the help of Prozac) become the latter-day rendition of Dürer's *Melancholia I,* suffering in the name of literary productivity.

40 *Lambda Book Report* quoted on the back cover of *Prozac Highway.* The adjective *postmodern* is used in several reviews of the book. For example, Julie Canigula writes in the *Village Voice* that "Blackbridge handles the various facets of Jam's life like an expert player in some postmodern literary card game" (review of *Prozac Highway,* by Persimmon Blackbridge, 119).

41 Blackbridge, *Prozac Highway,* 9.

42 Ibid., 108.

43 Ibid., 107, 110.

44 Kennedy, "Shrinks," 54–55, 60.

45 Slater, "Black Swans," 149, 150.

46 Stack, "Psychoanalysis Meets Queer Theory," 75.

47 Ironically so, in part, because many feminist critiques employ a psychoanalytic methodology. The stories, however, draw a clear line between theory and praxis.

48 Gilman, "The Yellow Wallpaper," 41. Or, to use a more contemporary example, the scene connects Slater with the narrator of Susanna Kaysen's autobiographical memoir *Girl, Interrupted,* who is confined to McLean Hospital in 1967, long before Elizabeth Wurtzel would become a patient there, and long before a later generation of McLean researchers would discover that Prozac was effective against affective spectrum disorder. Kaysen is imprisoned both by the locked door of the psychiatric ward and by a diagnostic model that views her only as the result of her familial past. In an ironically named "progress note," Kaysen's psychiatrist writes that, "She expressed her fears regarding her parents and her lack of communication, the fact that she has been unable to make satisfactory decisions throughout her life to the present time" (105).

49 As Slater explains, "I don't completely discount the importance of origins. And I have always believed the mind as an entity that at once subsumes the body and radiates beyond it" ("Black Swans," 150).

50 Krist, "Medicated," 52.

51 Slater, "Black Swans," 146. Similarly, Sara in "Shrinks" describes "the prescriptions doctor": "as long as she got Prozac, it would be worth dealing with this guy" (62).

52 Krist, "Medicated," 248.

53 Ibid.

54 Slater, "Black Swans," 155.

55 I quote here the headline of a Prozac advertisement that ran for two years on the back cover of the *Psychiatric News* and the *Psychiatric Times* in 1996–97. This convention also plays out in other literary texts. For example, in Philip Roth's *Sabbath's Theater,* Mickey learns that, within the twelve-stepped horizon of the detox center, Prozac comes to symbolize psychological complexities no longer recog-

nized or discussed. "The answer to every question," he is told, "is either Prozac or incest" (47).

56 Stone, *Healing the Mind,* 360.

57 Blackbridge, *Prozac Highway,* 132.

58 Slater, "Black Swans," 156.

59 Gerald Klerman quoted in Allen, "Red, White and Truly Blue," B1 (Klerman is explaining the spread of depression nationwide). See also Benjamin Sadock and Harold I. Kaplan's discussion of depression as the phenomenon that "sets in when a person becomes aware of the discrepancy between extraordinarily high ideals and the reality of his or her situation" (*Kaplan and Sadock's Synopsis of Psychiatry,* 544).

60 See Pies, *Handbook of Essential Psychopharmacology,* 86.

61 Blackbridge, *Prozac Highway,* 218.

62 Kennedy, "Shrinks," 62.

63 Slater, "Black Swans," 157–58.

64 As opposed to an impersonal or reciprocal subjectivity or even a purely grammatical subjectivity (see Lacan, *Écrits,* 207–8).

65 Slater, "Black Swans," 158, 159.

66 Kennedy, "Shrinks," 66.

67 Blackbridge, *Prozac Highway,* 161, 266.

68 Slater, "Black Swans," 160.

69 Blackbridge, *Prozac Highway,* 263.

70 Zita, *Body Talk,* 76.

71 Gardiner, "Can Ms. Prozac Talk Back?" 515.

72 Gilman, "The Yellow Wallpaper," 42.

73 Millett, *Sexual Politics,* 197. See also the description of psychiatry in Gordon, *I'm Dancing as Fast as I Can,* 278–81.

74 See Klerman, "The Advances of *DSM-III.*" See also "An Interview with Frank Berger"; Stone, *Healing the Mind,* 321.

75 Slater, "Black Swans," 159.

76 Did this liberation extend to men? In the "meatworld," variables such as the destigmatization of mental illness, increased awareness of depression and its etiologies, the wide acceptance of SSRIs, and a pharmaceutical-company-sponsored push for the masculinization of "social phobia" combined to close the gender gap in prescription rates between women and men. In the "textworld," however, things were somewhat more complicated. Narratives such as William Styron's *Darkness Visible* and, to a lesser extent, William Coleman's *A Light in the Shadows* describe men's ability to "conquer" depression as if it is a satanic, military enemy, victory leading to a requisite return to the productive, heterosexual order.

A far more nuanced and complicated version of what it means to be a man on medication in the early years of the twenty-first century is seen in Andrew Solomon's *The Noonday Demon.* Likely the era's most high-profile depression memoir written by a man, the book vacillates powerfully between the poles of science and emotion, father and mother, active and passive, and drug ingestion and talk therapy. The ultimate effect of this vacillation is a text that both enacts Solomon's confusion about gender choice and constructs medications as the signifiers of this bisexuality. For instance, Solomon's enthusiastic opening endorsement of psychotropic drugs and of the father whom they represent (the book is dedicated to "my father, who gave me life not once, but twice," a point referenced in the contention that, "after his experience of my depression, my father extended the research of his company into the field of antidepressants" [13]), not to mention the cold precision of Solomon's descriptions of neuropsychotropic research (which mirror his father's reserved, "uncaring behavior" [47]), exists in an almost schizophrenic state of tension with the book's equally prominent feminine ("sensitive," "maternal") half. Yet, instead of embracing the language of Solomon's father's science, the book's narrative structure in chapters 1–4, leading up to Solomon's treatment with medication, flows in ways uncannily similar to the women's Prozac narratives that I describe in this chapter. Solomon's mental illness is insufficiently addressed by psychotherapy, which treats him like a woman, much as the Prozac narratives treat their protagonists like men. In turn, he visits a "pills shrink" ("the psychopharmacologist seemed to have come out of some movie about shrinks" [51]), has a strong initial response, falls from grace, discovers a new self, and so on. Perhaps as a result of this gender instability, the true self that Solomon invariably finds while "on" medication is a self ultimately *less* able to exist in the world of masculine reason. When Solomon moves in with his father and begins taking psychotropic medications, he becomes the exact opposite of hyperthymic—passive to the state of flaccidity and withdrawn from the world. "My first day on medication," he writes, "I moved into my father's apartment. . . . I was hardly able to get out of bed for the next week" (51). Solomon's identification with his father is textually undermined by the possibility that the father's medications (and the narrative baggage that they bring with them) threaten to create Solomon, not as a man with a developed superego, but as a woman without one. In other words, the treatment that Solomon gets from Prozac is exactly the opposite of that which the women protagonists discussed in this chapter get.

77 Freud, "Some Psychical Consequences of the Anatomical Distinction between the Sexes," 248.

78 See Freud, *Civilization and Its Discontents,* 97.

79 Ibid., 98.

80 Slater, "Black Swans," 156–57.

81 As John Schilb argues in "Autobiography after Prozac." Schilb's point that "Black Swans" is a class statement is important to keep in mind in the light of Costello et al.'s finding, reported in "The Great Smoky Mountains Study," that poverty was the strongest correlate of psychiatric diagnosis. However, Schilb's almost auto-

matic dismissal of gender in Slater's (and Sharon Lerner's) work results in an unfortunate misreading of the meaning of the superego.

82 Blackbridge, *Prozac Highway,* 217.

83 Stone, *Healing the Mind,* 321.

84 According to Lacan (and, of course, with deference to Mickey Smith), the "law"—the structure that governs all forms of social exchange and the set of universal principles that make social existence possible—emanates from the murder of the father. "This law then," Lacan writes in *Écrits,* "is revealed clearly enough as identical with an order of language. For without kinship nominations, no power is capable of instituting the order of preferences and taboos that bind and weave the yarn of lineage through succeeding generations" (66). Perhaps this notion of law extends to the law of the wonder drug. Here, a new order, built on the Oedipal regicide of the psychoanalytic father (in much the same way as Freud describes the death of Moses, who is killed by his followers; see also McHugh, "The Death of Freud and the Rebirth of Psychiatry"), produces a drug that regulates and normalizes in the name of kinship and civilization. Not only does this drug exert a direct, in vivo effect on the bodies of its subjects. So too, the drug works on the larger, cultural body as well, discursively maintaining a specifically gendered narrative structure in the face of pathology. All the while, resistance is at constant risk of censure, specifically because it threatens this structure, and is, thus, coded as taboo.

85 Slater, "Black Swans," 160. However, given the sharp contrast drawn between her character and the mountain women, if not Eli Lilly's current claims of Prozac's efficacy against premenstrual dysphoria, the implication is clearly that her regression is menstrual as well.

86 Interestingly, this dynamic is not seen in Krist's "Medicated."

87 Stotland, "Gender, What's the Difference?" 813. Or, as Lacan realized, the symptom is constitutive of the system.

SIX *Conclusion*

1 Freud, "The Uncanny," 237.

2 Rasanen, Hakko, Isohanni, et al., "Maternal Smoking during Pregnancy," 857. "One possible explanation for our finding that maternal smoking during pregnancy increases the rate of violent offenses in male offspring as adults may be altered central nervous system monoamine function" (ibid.).

3 Freud, "The Unconscious," 118.

Bibliography

Abstracts from the Conference on Meprobamate and Other Agents Used in Mental Disturbances. New York: New York Academy of Sciences Press, 1956.

Alexander, Frank, and Sheldon Selesnick. *The History of Psychiatry.* New York: Harper and Row, 1966.

"Alleged Gunman Took Antidepressant." *Washington Post,* 10 November 1990, C4.

Allen, Henry. "Red, White, and Truly Blue." *Washington Post,* 10 November 1990, B1.

Altschule, Mark D. *Bodily Physiology in Mental and Emotional Disorders.* New York: Grune and Stratton, 1953.

Alvarez, Walter C. "Live with Your Nerves and Like It: A Famous Doctor Tells How to Conquer the Hazards of the Frantic Fifties by Making Our Nerves Work for Us Rather Than against Us." *Cosmopolitan,* February 1957, 40–45.

"The American Male: Why Do Women Dominate Him." *Look,* March 1959, 21–25.

Angell, Marcia. "Is Academic Medicine for Sale?" *New England Journal of Medicine* 342 (2000): 1516–18.

Angier, Natalie. "Grumpy, Fearful Neurotics Appear to Be Short on a Gene." *New York Times,* 29 November 1996, A1.

Ayd, Frank. "A Preliminary Report on Marsilid." *American Journal of Psychiatry* 114 (1957): 84.

———. "The Early History of Modern Psychopharmacology." *Neuropsychopharmacology* 5, no. 2 (1991): 71–84.

Ayd, Frank, and Barry Blackwell, eds. *Discoveries in Biological Psychiatry.* Philadelphia: Lippincott, 1970.

Bailey, Percival. "The Great Psychiatric Revolution." *American Journal of Psychiatry* 113 (1956): 387–406.

Bal, Mieke. *Reading Rembrandt: Beyond the Word-Image Opposition.* Cambridge: Cambridge University Press, 1991.

Balter, M., et al. "Cross-National Study of the Extent of Anti-Anxiety/Sedative Drug Use." *New England Journal of Medicine* 290 (1974): 769–74.

Barnet, Sylvan. *A Short Guide to Writing about Art.* New York: Longman, 1997.

Barsa, Joseph, "Use of Chlorpromazine Combined with Meprobamate." *American Journal of Psychiatry* 115 (1958): 79–80.

Bateman, Anthony, and Peter Fonagy. "Treatment of Borderline Personality Disorder with Psychoanalytically Oriented Partial Hospitalization: An 18 Month Follow-Up." *American Journal of Psychiatry* 158 (2001): 36–42.

Beauvoir, Simone de. *The Second Sex.* Translated by J. M. Parshley. New York: Vintage, 1974.

Berger, Frank. "The Pharmacological Properties of Miltown, a New Interneuronal Blocking Agent." *Journal of Pharmacological and Experimental Therapies* 112 (December 1954): 413–18.

———. "The Tranquilizer Decade." *Journal of Neuropsychiatry* 5 (1964): 403–10.

———. "Anxiety and the Discovery of the Tranquilizers." In *Discoveries in Biological Psychiatry,* ed. Frank Ayd and Barry Blackwell, 115–29. Philadelphia: Lippincott, 1970.

Berkwits, Michael. "Health-Industry Advertising in Medical Journals: Conflict of Interest or Much Ado about Nothing?" *Journal of Law, Medicine, and Ethics* 27 (1999): 122–25.

"The Best of 1990." *San Francisco Chronicle,* 29 November 1990, D1.

Bieber, Irving, et al. *Homosexuality: A Psychoanalytic Study.* New York: Basic, 1962.

Blackbridge, Persimmon. *Prozac Highway.* Vancouver: Press Gang, 1997.

Bloom, Lynn Z. *Dr. Spock: Biography of a Conservative Radical.* Indianapolis: Bobbs-Merrill, 1972.

Bordo, Susan. "Braveheart, Babe, and the Contemporary Body." In *Enhancing Human Traits: Ethical and Social Implications,* ed. Erik Parens, 189–222. Washington, D.C.: Georgetown, 1998.

Bowman, Karl M., and Bernice Engle. "A Psychiatric Evaluation of Laws of Homosexuality." *American Journal of Psychiatry* 112 (1956): 577–83.

Braslow, Joel T. *Mental Ills and Bodily Cures: Psychiatric Treatments in the First Half of the Twentieth Century.* Berkeley: University of California Press, 1997.

Breggin, Peter R., and Ginger Breggin. *Talking Back to Prozac.* New York: St. Martin's, 1994.

———. *Talking Back to Ritalin.* New York: Courage, 1998.

Breuer, Josef, and Sigmund Freud. *Studies in Hysteria.* 1895. New York: Nervous and Mental Diseases Publishing Co., 1956.

Brown, Bertram S. "The Life of Psychiatry." *American Journal of Psychiatry* 133 (1976): 489–95.

Buhle, Mari Jo. *Feminism and Its Discontents: A Century of Struggle with Psychoanalysis.* Cambridge: Harvard University Press, 1998.

Burt, Vivien K., Rita Suri, Lori Altshuler, et al. "The Use of Psychotropic Medications during Breast-Feeding." *American Journal of Psychiatry* 158 (2001): 1001–9.

Butler, Judith. *Gender Trouble: Feminism and the Subversion of Identity.* New York: Routledge, 1990.

———. *Bodies That Matter: Outside the Discursive Limits of Sex.* London: Routledge, 1993.

Cade, John. "Lithium Salts in the Treatment of Manic Excitement." *Medical Journal of Austria* 36 (1949): 349–52.

Canigula, Julie. Review of *Prozac Highway,* by Persimmon Blackbridge. *Village Voice* 43, no. 6 (10 February 1998): 119.

Cant, Gilbert. "Valiumania." *New York Times Magazine,* 1 February 1976, 34–54.

Cartwright, Lisa. *Screening the Body: Tracing Medicine's Visual Culture.* Minneapolis: University of Minnesota Press, 1992.

Cartwright, Lisa, Constance Penley, and Paula Treichler, eds. *The Visible Woman: Imaging Technologies, Gender, and Science.* New York: New York University Press, 1998.

Chafe, William Henry. *The American Woman: Her Changing Social, Economic, and Political Roles, 1920–1970.* New York: Oxford University Press, 1990.

Chambers, C. "An Assessment of Drug Use in the General Population." In *Drug Use and Social Policy,* ed. J. Sussman, 50–61. New York: AMS, 1972.

Cherlin, Andrew. *Marriage, Divorce, Remarriage.* Cambridge: Harvard University Press, 1981.

Chesler, Phyllis. *Women and Madness.* New York: Doubleday, 1972.

Chodorow, Nancy J. *Reproduction of Mothering: Psychoanalysis and the Sociology of Gender.* Berkeley: University of California Press, 1999.

Ciechanowski, Paul S., Wayne J. Katon, Joan E. Russo, and Edward A. Walker. "The Patient-Provider Relationship: Attachment Theory and Adherence to Treatment in Diabetes." *American Journal of Psychiatry* 158 (2001): 29–35.

Coleman, William. *A Light in the Shadows: Emerging from the Darkness of Depression.* Grand Rapids: Servant, 2000.

Collins, Patricia Hill. *Black Feminist Thought.* Boston: Unwin Hyman, 1995.

Concar, D. "Design Your Own Personality." *New Scientist* 141 (March 1994): 22–26.

Cook, Kay K. "Medical Identity: My DNA/Myself." In *Getting a Life: Everyday Uses of Autobiography,* ed. Sidonie Smith and Julia Watson, 63–88. Minneapolis: University of Minnesota Press, 1996.

Cooley, Donald. "The New Nerve Pills and Your Health." *Cosmopolitan,* January 1956, 70–75.

Coopersmith, S. *The Antecedents of Self-Esteem.* New York: Freeman, 1967.

Cooperstock, R., and H. Lennard. "Some Social Meanings of Tranquilizer Use." *Sociology of Health and Illness* 1 (1979): 331–47.

Corrodi, H., et al. "The Effect of Some Psychoactive Drugs on Central Monoamine Neurons." *European Journal of Pharmacology* 1 (1967): 363–68.

Costello, E. J., A. Erkanli, E. Federman, et al. "The Great Smoky Mountains Study of Youth: Goals, Design, Methods, and the Prevalence of *DSM-III-R* Disorders." *Archives of General Psychiatry* 53 (1996): 1129–36.

Courtney, A., and T. Whipple. *Sex Stereotypes in Advertising.* Lexington, Mass.: Lexington, 1983.

Crews, Frederick. "Analysis Terminable." *Commentary* 70, no. 1 (July 1980): 25–34.

Cuordileone, K. A. "'Politics in an Age of Anxiety': Cold War Political Culture and the Crisis in American Masculinity, 1949–1960." *Journal of American History* 87, no. 2 (September 2000): 515–45.

Cyyle, Joseph, and Steven Hyman. "The Neuroscientific Foundations of Psychiatry." In *Essentials of Clinical Psychiatry,* 3d ed., ed. Robert Hayles and Stuart Yudofsky, 3–28. Washington, D.C.: APA Press, 1999.

Daniels, R. S. "The Crisis of Financing Residency Training in Psychiatry: A Diagnosis." *American Journal of Psychiatry* 130 (1973): 496B–497B.

Danquah, Meri Nana-Ama. *Willow Weep for Me: A Black Woman's Journey through Depression.* New York: One World, 1998.

Delay, J., P. Deniker, et al. "The Treatment of Excitement and Agitation States by a Method of Medication Derived from Hibernotherapy." *Annals of Medical Psychology* 110 (1952): 267–73.

De Titta, M., and C. B. Robinowitz. "The Future of Psychiatry: Psychiatrists of the Future." *American Journal of Psychiatry* 148 (1991): 853–58.

Diagnostic and Statistical Manual of Mental Disorders (DSM-I). 1st ed. Washington, D.C.: APA Press, 1952.

Diagnostic and Statistical Manual of Mental Disorders (DSM-II). 2d ed. Washington, D.C.: APA Press, 1967.

Diagnostic and Statistical Manual of Mental Disorders (DSM-III). 3d ed. Washington, D.C.: APA Press, 1980.

Diagnostic and Statistical Manual of Mental Disorders (DSM-III-R). 3d ed., rev. Washington, D.C.: APA Press, 1987.

Diagnostic and Statistical Manual of Mental Disorders (DSM-IV). 4th ed. Washington, D.C.: APA Press, 1995.

Dickel, H. A., et al. "Electromyographic Studies on Meprobamate and the Working Anxious Patient." *Annals of the New York Academy of Science* 67 (1957): 12–13.

Divrey, P., et al. "R 1625—New Symptomatic Treatment of Psychomotor Agitation." *Acta Neurolica Psychiatria Belgica* 10 (1958): 878–88.

Dixon, N. M. "Meprobamate, a Clinical Evaluation." *Annals of the New York Academy of Science* 67 (1957): 11–12.

Domino, E. F. "Human Pharmacology of Tranquilizing Drugs." *Clinical Pharmacological Therapy* 3 (1962): 599–664.

Douglas, Susan. *Where the Girls Are: Growing Up Female with the Mass Media.* New York: Times Books, 1994.

Dumit, Joseph. *Picturing Personhood: Brain Scans and Diagnostic Identity.* Princeton: Princeton University Press, in press.

Durkheim, Emile. *Suicide.* Translated by J. A. Spaulding. New York: Free Press, 1951.

Eaton, J. S., and L. S. Goldstein. "Psychiatry in Crisis." *American Journal of Psychiatry* 134 (1977): 432–34.

Elliott, Carl. "Pursued by Happiness and Beaten Senseless: Prozac and the American Dream." *Hastings Center Report* 30, no. 2 (2000): 7–12.

Eugene, A. M., A. Alfredo, W. Nolen, et al. "Mood Improvement from Transcranial Magnetic Stimulation." *American Journal of Psychiatry* 156 (April 1999): 669.

Evans, S. M. *Born for Liberty: A History of Women in America.* New York: Free Press, 1989.

Eysenck, Hans J. "Training in Clinical Psychology: An English Point of View." *American Psychologist* 4 (1949): 173–76.

———. "The Effects of Psychotherapy: An Evaluation." *Journal of Consulting Psychology* 16 (1957): 319–24.

Fairman, Kathleen A., Wayne C. Drevets, et al. "Course of Antidepressant Treatment, Drug Type, and Prescriber's Specialty." *Psychiatric Services* 49 (1998): 1180–86.

Farnham, Marynia, and Ferdinand Lunberg. *Modern Woman: The Lost Sex.* New York: Harper and Bros., 1947.

Fausto-Sterling, Anne. *Myths of Gender: Biological Theories about Women and Men.* New York: Basic, 1992.

———. "How to Build a Man." In *The Gender and Sexuality Reader: Culture, History, Political Economy,* ed. Roger Lancaster and Micaela di Linanardo, 244–48. New York: Routledge, 1997.

Fleischman, Martin. "Will the Real Third Revolution Please Stand Up?" *American Journal of Psychiatry* 124 (1968): 1260–62.

Flemming, Thomas J. "I Had My Husband Committed." *Cosmopolitan,* June 1961, 78–83.

Foucault, Michel. *The History of Sexuality.* Vol. 1, *An Introduction.* Translated by Robert Hurley. New York: Penguin, 1984.

Frank, Erica, Lisa Boswell, Leah Dickstein, and Daniel Chapman. "Characteristics of Female Psychiatrists." *American Journal of Psychiatry* 158 (2001): 205–12.

Franzwa, H. H. "Working Women in Fact and Fiction." *Journal of Communication* 24 (1974): 104–9.

Freeman, Lucy. *Fight against Fears.* New York: Crown, 1951.

Freud, Anna. *The Ego and Mechanisms of Defence.* New York: International Universities Press, 1946.

Freud, Sigmund. *The Interpretation of Dreams.* 1900. In Strachey, ed., *Standard Edition,* vols. 4–5.

———. "Fragment and Analysis of a Case of Hysteria." 1905. In Strachey, ed., *Standard Edition,* 7:7–122.

———. "Delusion and Dream in Wilhelm Jensen's *Gradiva.*" 1907. In Strachey, ed., *Standard Edition,* 9:7–98.

———. "Hysterical Phantasies and Their Relation to Bisexuality." 1908. In Strachey, ed., *Standard Edition,* 9:157–67.

———. "Analysis of a Phobia in a Five-Year-Old Boy." 1909. In Strachey, ed., *Standard Edition,* 10:3–152.

———. "Notes upon a Case of Obsessional Neurosis." 1909. In Strachey, ed., *Standard Edition,* 10:158–259.

———. "Case History of Schreber: Psycho-Analytic Notes on an Autobiographical Account of a Case of Paranoia (Dementia Paranoids)." 1911. In Strachey, ed., *Standard Edition,* 12:12–84.

———. "The Unconscious." 1915. In Strachey, ed., *Standard Edition,* 14:159–218. From *Papers on Metapsychology.*

———. "From the History of an Infantile Neurosis." 1917. In Strachey, ed., *Standard Edition,* 17:100–12.

———. "Mourning and Melancholia." 1917. In Strachey, ed., *Standard Edition,* 14:237–58.

———. "The Uncanny." 1919. In Strachey, ed., *Standard Edition,* 17:219–56.

———. *An Autobiographical Study.* 1925. In Strachey, ed., *Standard Edition,* vol. 20.

———. *Inhibitions, Symptoms, and Anxiety.* 1925. In Strachey, ed., *Standard Edition,* 20:77–178. Also translated as *The Problem of Anxiety.*

———. "Some Psychical Consequences of the Anatomical Distinction between the Sexes." 1925. In Strachey, ed., *Standard Edition,* 19:243–61.

———. *Civilization and Its Discontents.* 1930. In Strachey, ed., *Standard Edition,* 21:59–148.

Friedan, Betty. *The Feminine Mystique.* New York: Norton, 1963.

Friedman, R. C., and J. Downey. "Neurobiology and Sexual Orientation: Current Relationships." *Journal of Neuropsychiatry and Clinical Neurosciences* 5 (1993): 131–53.

———. "Biology and the Oedipus Complex." *Psychoanalytic Quarterly* 64 (1995): 234–64.

Fromm, Erich. *Escape from Freedom.* New York: Farrar and Rinehart, 1941.

Gabbard, Glen. "Empirical Evidence and Psychotherapy: A Growing Scientific Base." *American Journal of Psychiatry* 158 (2001): 1–3.

Gabbard, Glen, and Alice Bartlett. "Selective Serotonin Reuptake Inhibitors in the Context of an Ongoing Analysis." In *Psychoanalysis and Medication,* special issue, *Psychoanalytic Inquiry* 18, no. 5 (2000): 673–701.

Gabbard, Glen, and Krin Gabbard. *Psychiatry and the Cinema*. 2d ed. Washington, D.C.: APA Press, 1999.

Galton, Lawrence. "New Drug Brings Relief for the Tense and Anxious." *Cosmopolitan*, August 1955, 82–83.

Garb, Tamar. "Gender and Representation." In *Modernity and Modernism: French Painting in the Nineteenth Century,* ed. Francis Frascina, 219–90. New Haven: Yale University Press, 1993.

Gardiner, Judith Kegan. "Can Ms. Prozac Talk Back? Feminism, Drugs, and Social Constructionism." *Feminist Studies* 21, no. 3 (fall 1995): 501–18.

Gayle, R. Finley, Jr. "Presidential Address." *American Journal of Psychiatry* 112 (1956): 1–3.

Gerard, R. W. "The Biological Roots of Psychiatry." *American Journal of Psychiatry* 112 (August 1955): 81–98.

Gilman, Charlotte Perkins. "The Yellow Wallpaper" (1892). In *"The Yellow Wall-Paper" and the History of Its Publication and Reception,* ed. Julie Bates Dock, 27–42. University Park: Pennsylvania State University Press, 1998.

Glenmullen, Joseph. *Prozac Backlash*. New York: Simon and Schuster, 2000.

Glueck, Bernard C., ed. *Psychiatry and the Law*. New York: Grune and Stratton, 1955.

———. "Psychodynamic Patterns in the Homosexual Sex Offender." *American Journal of Psychiatry* 112 (1956): 584–89.

Goffman, Erving. *Gender Advertisements*. London: Macmillan, 1979.

Goodwin, Renee, Madelyn Gould, Carlos Blanco, and Mark Olfson. "Prescription of Psychotropic Medications to Youths in Office-Based Practice." *Psychiatric Services* 52 (2001): 1081–87.

Gordon, Barbara. *I'm Dancing as Fast as I Can*. New York: Harper and Row, 1979.

Greden, J. F., and J. I. Casariego. "Controversies in Psychiatric Education: A Survey of Residents' Attitudes." *American Journal of Psychiatry* 132 (1975): 270–74.

Green, Hannah [Joanne Greenberg]. *I Never Promised You a Rose Garden*. New York: Holt, 1964.

Greenblatt, David. "Meprobamate: A Study of Irrational Drug Use." *American Journal of Psychiatry* 127 (1971): 33–39.

Greenblatt, David, and Richard I. Shrader. "The Clinical Choice of Sedative Hypnotics." *Annals of Internal Medicine* 77 (1972): 91–100.

Grob, Gerald. "Psychiatry and Social Activism." *Bulletin of the History of Medicine* 60 (1980): 477–501.

———. "The Origins of *DSM I*." *American Journal of Psychiatry* 148 (1991): 421–31.

Guttmacher, Manfred. "The Homosexual in Court." *American Journal of Psychiatry* 112 (1956): 591–699.

Guze, S. B. "The Validity and Significance of the Clinical Diagnosis of Hysteria (Briquet's Syndrome)." *American Journal of Psychiatry* 132 (1975): 221–24.

Hackett, T. P. "The Psychiatrist: In the Mainstream, or on the Banks of Medicine?" *American Journal of Psychiatry* 134 (1977): 432–34.

Hale, Nathan, Jr. *The Rise and Crisis of Psychoanalysis in the United States.* New York: Oxford University Press, 1995.

Hamilton, J. A., M. Grant, and M. F. Jensvold. "Sex and the Treatment of Depressions: What Does It Matter." In *Psychopharmacology and Women: Sex, Gender, and Hormones,* ed. U. Jensvold and M. J. A. Halbreich, 241–60. Washington, D.C.: APA Press, 1996.

Hawkins, Joellen W., and Cynthia S. Aber. "The Content of Advertisements in Medical Journals: Distorting the Image of Woman." *Women and Health* 14, no. 2 (1988): 45–51.

Hayles, Robert, and Stuart Yudofsky, eds. *Essentials of Clinical Psychiatry.* 3d ed. Washington, D.C.: APA Press, 1999.

Healy, David. *The Antidepressant Era.* Cambridge: Harvard University Press, 1997.

———. *The Creation of Psychopharmacology.* Cambridge: Harvard University Press, 2002.

Hendley, C. D., et al. "Effect of Meprobamate on Electrical Activity of the Thalamus and Other Subcortical Areas." In *Tranquilizing Drugs,* ed. H. E. Himwich, 35–46. Washington, D.C.: American Academy for the Advancement of Science, 1957.

Hobson, J. A., and R. W. McCarley. "The Brain as a Dream State Generator: An Activation-Synthesis Hypothesis of the Dream Process." *American Journal of Psychiatry* 134 (1977): 1335–48.

Hoch, Paul H. "Progress in Psychiatric Therapies." *American Journal of Psychiatry* 112 (1955): 241–47.

Hollander, E., M. Leibowitz, et al. "Cortisol and Lactate Induced Panic." *Archives of General Psychiatry* 46 (1989): 135–39.

Horney, Karen. *The Neurotic Personality of Our Times.* New York: Norton, 1937.

———. *Feminine Psychology.* New York: Norton, 1973.

"How Tranquilizers Work." *Newsweek,* 24 December 1956, 47.

Hudson, James L., and Harrison G. Pope. "Affective Spectrum Disorder: Does Antidepressant Response Identify a Family of Disorders with a Common Pathophysiology?" *American Journal of Psychiatry* 147 (1990): 552–64.

Huebner, R. "Meprobamate in Canine Medicine: A Summary of 77 Cases." *Veterinary Medicine* 51 (October 1956): 488.

"Images in Neuroscience: Cognition, Perception." *American Journal of Psychiatry* 156 (June 1999): 815.

"An Interview with Frank Berger." *Social Pharmacology* 2 (1988): 189–204.

Irigaray, Luce. *Speculum of the Other Woman.* Translated by Gillian C. Gill. Ithaca: Cornell University Press, 1985.

Jagger, Mick, and Keith Richards. "Mother's Little Helper." On *Flowers (Aftermath),* by the Rolling Stones. London Records, PS 509, 1967.

Janicak, Philip. *Handbook of Psychopharmacotherapy.* New York: Lippincott, Williams, and Wilkins, 1999.

Jensvold, Margaret, and Uriel Halbreich, eds. *Psychopharmacology and Women: Sex, Gender, and Hormones.* Washington, D.C.: APA Press, 1996.

Johnson, Jill. *Lesbian Nation: The Feminist Solution.* New York: Simon and Schuster, 1973.

Jones, Ernest. *Sigmund Freud: Life and Work.* London: Hogarth, 1955.

Jones, Thom. "Superman, My Son." In *Cold Snap,* 18–46. Boston: Little Brown, 1995.

Josephson, Susan. *From Idolatry to Advertising: Visual Art and Contemporary Culture.* New York: Sharpe, 1996.

Kaasinen, Valtteri, et al. "Sex Differences in Extrastriatal Dopamine D2-Like Receptors in the Human Brain." *American Journal of Psychiatry* 158 (2001): 308–11.

Kalinowsky, Lothar B. "Appraisal of the 'Tranquilizers' and Their Influence on Other Somatic Treatments in Psychiatry." *American Journal of Psychiatry* 115 (1958): 294–300.

Kardiner, Abraham. *Sex and Morality.* Indianapolis: Bobbs-Merrill, 1954.

Katon, W., M. VonKorff, et al. "Adequacy and Duration of Antidepressant Treatment in Primary Care." *Medical Care* 30 (1992): 67–76.

Katzelnick, D. J., K. A. Kobak, et al. "Prescribing Patterns of Antidepressant Medications for Depression in an HMO." *Formulary* 31 (1996): 374–88.

Kaysen, Susanna. *Girl, Interrupted.* New York: Turtle Bay, 1993.

Keller, Evelyn F. *Reflections on Gender and Science.* New Haven: Yale University Press, 1986.

Kennedy, Pagan. "Shrinks." In *Stripping and Other Stories,* 49–66. New York: High Risk, 1994.

Kessler, R. C., K. A. McGonagle, et al. "Sex and Depression in the National Comorbidity Survey: 1, Lifetime Prevalence, Chronicity, and Recurrence." *Journal of Affective Disorders* 29 (1993): 85–96.

Klein, Viola. *The Feminine Character: History of an Ideology.* Urbana: University of Illinois Press, 1972.

Klerman, Gerald. "The Evolution of a Scientific Nosology." In *Schizophrenia: Science and Practice,* ed. J. C. Shershow, 99–121. Cambridge: Harvard University Press, 1978.

———. "The Advances of *DSM-III.*" *American Journal of Psychiatry* 141 (1984): 539–42.

Kletzin, M., and F. Berger. "Effect of Meprobamate on the Limbic System of the Brain." *Proceedings of the Society for Experimental Biology and Medicine* 100 (April 1959): 681–82.

Koedt, Anne. *Notes from the Third Year: Women's Liberation.* New York: Radical Feminists, 1970.

Koerner, Brendan. "Leo Sternbach: The Father of Mother's Little Helpers." *U.S. News and World Report,* 27 December 1999, 1–7.

Koran, L. "Controversy in Medicine and Psychiatry." *American Journal of Psychiatry* 132 (1975): 1064–66.

Kornstein, S. G. "Premenstrual Syndrome: An Overview." *Primary Psychiatry* 9 (1997): 56–60.

Kornstein, Susan, Alan Schatzberg, et al. "Gender Differences in Treatment Response to Sertraline versus Imipramine in Chronic Depression." *American Journal of Psychiatry* 157 (2000): 1445–52.

Kornstein, S. G., A. F. Schatzberg, M. E. Thase, et al. "Gender Differences in Chronic Major and Double Depression." *Journal of Affective Disorders* 60 (2000): 1–11.

Kornstein, S. G., A. F. Schatzberg, K. A. Yonkers, et al. "Gender Differences in Presentation of Chronic Major Depression." *Psychopharmacology Bulletin* 31 (1995): 711–18.

Kramer, Peter. *Listening to Prozac.* New York: Penguin, 1994.

———. "The Valorization of Sadness: Alienation and the Melancholic Temperament." *Hastings Center Report* 30, no. 2 (2000): 13–18.

Krist, Gary. "Medicated." In *Bone by Bone,* 239–57. New York: Harcourt Brace, 1994.

Krupka, Lawrence, and Arthur Vener. "Prescription Drug Advertising: Trends and Implications." *Social Science and Medicine* 20, no. 3 (1985): 191–97.

Kuhn, R. "The Treatment of Depressive States with an Iminodibenzyl Derivative." *Schweizer Medizinische Wochenschrift* 87 (1957): 1135–40.

Kuhn, Thomas. "The Structure of Scientific Revolutions." In *International Encyclopedia of Unified Science,* ed. Otto Neurath, 2, no. 2:1–172. Chicago: University of Chicago Press, 1962.

———. *The Structure of Scientific Revolutions.* 2d ed., enlarged. Chicago: University of Chicago Press, 1970.

Kurland, A. A., et al. "The Comparative Effectiveness of Six Phenothaiazine Compounds, Phenobarbitol and Inert Placebo, in the Treatment of Acutely Ill Patients: Global Measures of Severity of Illness." *Journal of Nervous and Mental Disorders* 133 (1961): 1–18.

Lacan, Jacques. *Écrits.* Paris: Seuil, 1966.

Lader, Malcolm. "Anxiolytic Drugs." *Practitioner* 215 (1975): 468–73.

Laing, R. D. "Transcendental Experience in Relation to Religion and Psychosis." *Psychedelic Review* 6 (1965): 7–15.

Laing, R. D., and A. Esterson. *Sanity, Madness, and the Family.* New York: Penguin, 1964.

Langer, P., et al. "The Effects of Anxiety and Induced Stress on the Structured-Objective Rorschach Test." *Perceptual and Motor Skills* 16 (1963): 919–21.

Lasagna, L. "The Role of Benzodiazepines in Nonpsychiatric Medical Practice." *American Journal of Psychiatry* 134 (1977): 565–68.

Lears, T. J. Jackson. *Fables of Abundance: A Cultural History of Advertising in America.* New York: Basic, 1994.

Leary, F., et al. "Tranquilizing Drugs and Stress Tolerance." *WADC Technical Report,* October 1958, 58–64.

Lefcort, Peter. *Abbreviating Ernie.* New York: Villard, 1997.

Leibenluft, Ellen, ed. *Gender Differences in Mood and Anxiety Disorders.* Washington, D.C.: APA Press, 1999.

———. Foreword to *Gender Differences in Mood and Anxiety Disorders,* xiii–xxii. Washington, D.C.: APA Press, 1999.

Leigh, H. "Comment: The Role of Psychiatry in Medicine." *American Journal of Psychiatry* 139 (1982): 1581–87.

Levy, Richard. "The Role and Value of Pharmaceutical Marketing." *Archives of Family Medicine* 3 (1994): 327–32.

Lewine, Richard, and Jane Caudle. "Racial Effects on Neuropsychological Functioning in Schizophrenia." *American Journal of Psychiatry* 157 (2000): 2038–40.

Lewis, Bradley. "Psychiatry and Postmodern Theory." *Journal of Medical Humanities* 21, no. 2 (2000): 71–84.

Lincheiznich, H. "Meprobamate in Children." *Medizinische Klinik* 53 (9 May 1958): 840–44.

Linn, L., and M. Davis. "Physicians' Orientation toward the Legitimacy of Drug Use." *Social Science and Medicine* 6 (1972): 199–203.

Lipscomb, W. R. "Drug Use in a Black Ghetto." *American Journal of Psychiatry* 127 (1971): 1166–69.

"Listening to Eli Lilly." *Wall Street Journal,* 31 March 1994, B1.

Ludwig, A. M., and K. Othmer. "The Medical Basis of Psychiatry." *American Journal of Psychiatry* 134 (1977): 1087–92.

Luhrman, T. M. *Of Two Minds: The Growing Disorder in American Psychiatry.* New York: Knopf, 2000.

Maciver, John, and Fredrick Redlick. "Patterns of Psychiatric Practice." *American Journal of Psychiatry* 115 (1958): 692–97.

Mamdani, Muhammad M., Sagar V. Parikh, Peter C. Austin, and Ross E. G. Upshur. "Use of Antidepressants among Elderly Subjects: Trends and Contributing Factors." *American Journal of Psychiatry* 157 (2000): 360–67.

"Man and Wife." *Time,* 7 March 1955, 60.

Manheimer, D., et al. "Psychotherapeutic Drugs." *California Medicine* 109 (1968): 445–51.

Manheimer, D. I., S. T. Davidson, M. B. Balter, et al. "Popular Attitudes and Beliefs about Tranquilizers." *American Journal of Psychiatry* 130 (1973): 1246–53.

Mann, J. John, et al. "Demonstration in Vivo of Reduced Serotonin Responsivity in the Brain of Untreated Patients." *American Journal of Psychiatry* 153, no. 2 (1996): 174–82.

"Marital Status and Living Arrangements." U.S. Bureau of the Census, Current Population Reports, ser. P-20, no. 349. Washington, D.C.: U.S. Government Printing Office, 1975.

Marks, John. "The Benzodiazepines—Use and Abuse: Current Status." *Pharmacy International* 2 (1981): 84–87.

———. *The Benzodiazepines—Use, Overuse, Misuse, and Abuse.* Boston: MTP, 1985.

Marquis, D. G., et al. "Experimental Studies on Behavioral Effects of Meprobamate on Normal Subjects." *Annals of the New York Academy of Science* 67 (1957): 701–11.

McCarley, T. "The Psychotherapist's Search for Self-Renewal." *American Journal of Psychiatry* 132 (1975): 221–24.

McHugh, Paul R. "The Death of Freud and the Rebirth of Psychiatry." *Weekly Standard,* 17 July 2000, 31–36.

McHugh, Paul R., and Phillip Slavney. *The Perspectives of Psychiatry.* Baltimore: John Hopkins University Press, 1998.

Menkes, Suzy. "Fearless Heroines with Looks to Match." *New York Times,* 4 June 1995, C1.

Merriam, Eve. "The Matriarchal Myth; or, The Case of the Vanishing Male." *The Nation,* 8 November 1958, 331–35.

Meyer, Jeffrey, et al. "The Effect of Paroxetine on 5-HT2A Receptors in Depression: An [18F]Setoperone PET Imaging Study." *American Journal of Psychiatry* 158 (2001): 78–85.

Meyers, Greg. *Writing Biology: Texts in the Social Construction of Scientific Knowledge.* Madison: University of Wisconsin Press, 1990.

Millett, Kate. *Sexual Politics.* New York: Doubleday, 1970.

———. *The Loony-Bin Trip.* New York: Simon and Schuster, 1990.

"The Mind: Science's Search for a Guide to Sanity: A Medicine Special Section." *Newsweek,* 24 October 1955, 59–65.

Minsky, Rosalind. *Psychoanalysis and Gender.* London: Routledge, 1996.

Mintz, S., and S. Kellogg. *Domestic Revolutions: A Social History of American Family Life.* New York: Free Press, 1988.

"Mirror in the Brain." *Science Digest,* May 1957, back cover.

Money, John, and Anke A. Erhardt. *Man and Woman, Boy and Girl: The Differentiation and Dimorphism of Gender Identity from Conception to Maturity.* Baltimore: Johns Hopkins University Press, 1972.

Moore, Burness. "Frigidity in Women." *Journal of the American Psychoanalytic Association* 9 (1961): 571–84.

Morris, Bob. "Divine Reinvention." *New York Times,* 2 March 1995, current events ed., C1.

Mulvey, Laura. "Afterthoughts . . . Inspired by *Duel in the Sun.*" *Framework* 15–17 (summer 1981): 12–15.

———. *Visual and Other Pleasures.* London: Macmillan, 1989.

Nathanson, C. "Social Roles and Health Status among Women: The Significance of Employment." *Social Science and Medicine* 16 (1980): 1781–89.

"New Clues about Mental Illness." *Science Digest,* July 1957, 3.

"New Drug for Mental Patients." *Science Digest,* July 1957, 28–29.

"The New Feminists: Revolt against Sexism." *Time,* 21 November 1969, 53–56.

Newmark, S. R., L. I. Rose, R. Todd, L. Birk, and F. Naftolin. "Gonadotropin, Estradiol, and Testosterone Profiles in Homosexual Men." *American Journal of Psychiatry* 136 (1979): 767–71.

Nopoulos, Peg C., and Nancy C. Andreasen. "Gender Differences in Neuroimaging." In *Gender Differences in Mood and Anxiety Disorders,* ed. Ellen Leibenluft, 1–30. Washington, D.C.: APA Press, 1999.

O'Connell, Vanessa, and Rachel Zimmerman. "Drug Pitches Resonate with Edgy Public." *Wall Street Journal,* 14 January 2002, A3.

Ohmann, Richard. *Selling Culture: Magazines, Markets, and Class at the Turn of the Century.* New York: Verso, 1996.

Olfson, Mark, Steven C. Marcus, and Harold Alan Pincus. "Trends in Office-Based Psychiatric Practice." *American Journal of Psychiatry* 156 (1999): 451–57.

Olin, Margaret. "Gaze." In *Critical Terms for Art History,* ed. Robert S. Nelson and Richard Schiff, 208–19. Chicago: University of Chicago Press, 1996.

Omunuwa, Shakoora. "Health Disparities in Black Women: Lack of Pharmaceutical Advertising in Black vs. White Oriented Magazines." *Journal of the National Medical Association* 93, nos. 7–8 (2001): 263–66.

Pappenheim, Fritz. *The Alienation of Modern Man.* New York: Monthly Review Press, 1959.

Parens, Eric. "Is Better Always Good? The Enhancement Project." *Hastings Center Report* 28, no. 1 (January/February 1998): 24B–S15.

Parry, H. "Use of Psychotropic Drugs by U.S. Adults." *Public Health Reports* 83 (1968): 799–810.

Parry, H., et al. "National Patterns of Psychotherapeutic Drug Use." *Archives of General Psychiatry* 28 (1973): 769–83.

Penfold, P. Susan, and Gillian Walker. *Women and the Psychiatric Paradox.* Montreal: Eden, 1983.

Pennington, V. M. "Meprobamate." *JAMA* 164 (8 June 1957): 638.

Perelman, S. J. *The Road to Miltown; or, Under the Spreading Atrophy.* New York: Simon and Schuster, 1957.

Phillips, Katherine, and John Gunderson. "Personality Disorders." In *Essentials of Clinical Psychiatry,* 3d ed., ed. Robert Hayles and Stuart Yudofsky, 515–38. Washington, D.C.: APA Press, 1999.

"Phobias about Marriage." *Science Digest,* March 1957, 22.

The Physicians' Reference Manual. 5th ed. New Brunswick: Wallace Laboratories, 1960.

Piderhughes, C. A. "Understanding Black Power: Processes and Proposals." *American Journal of Psychiatry* 125 (1969): 1552–57.

Pies, Ronald. *Handbook of Essential Psychopharmacology.* Washington, D.C.: APA Press, 1998.

"Pills for the Mind: New Era in Psychiatry." *Time,* 7 March 1955, 63.

"Pills vs. Worry—How Goes the Frantic Quest for Calm in Frantic Lives." *Newsweek,* 21 May 1956, 68–70.

Pollock, Griselda. *Differencing the Canon: Feminist Desire and the Writing of Art's Histories.* New York: Routledge, 1999.

Prather, Jane, and Linda Fidell. "Sex Differences in the Content and Style of Medical Advertisements." *Social Science and Medicine* 23 (1975): 23–26.

Prioleau, Leslie, et al. "An Analysis of Psychotherapy versus Placebo Studies." *Behavioral and Brain Studies* 6 (1973): 275–310.

"The Promise of Prozac." *Newsweek,* 26 March 1990, 38–41.

Propp, Vladimir. *Morphology of the Folktale.* Austin: University of Texas Press, 1968.

Pulver, Sydney E. "Survey of Psychoanalytic Practice, 1976: Some Trends and Implications." *Journal of the American Psychoanalytic Association* 26 (1978): 615–31.

Rasanen, H. Hakko, P. M. Isohanni, et al. "Maternal Smoking during Pregnancy and Risk of Criminal Behavior among Adult Male Offspring in the Northern Finland 1966 Birth Cohort." *American Journal of Psychiatry* 156 (1999): 857–62.

Regier, D. A., J. H. Boyd, et al. "One-Month Prevalence of Mental Disorders in the United States: Based on Five Epidemiologic Catchment Area Sites." *Archives of General Psychiatry* 45 (1988): 977–86.

Reik, Theodore. *Of Love and Lust: On the Psychoanalysis of Romantic and Sexual Emotions.* New York: Farrar, Strauss, 1957.

Rice, J. K., and D. G. Rice. "Implications of the Women's Liberation Movement for Psychotherapy." *American Journal of Psychiatry* 130 (1973): 191–96.

Rickels, K., et al. "An Evaluation of Tranquilizing Drugs in Medical Outpatients." *Journal of Pharmacological and Experimental Therapies* 112 (1954): 413.

Roeske, N. A. "Women in Psychiatry: A Review." *American Journal of Psychiatry* 133 (1976): 365–72.

Rogler, Loyd. "Making Sense of Historical Changes in the *Diagnostic and Statistical Manual of Mental Disorders.*" *Journal of Health and Social Behavior* 38 (1997): 9–20.

Rose, Jacqueline. *Sexuality in the Field of Vision.* London: Verso, 1986.

Rose, Luis. *The Freudian Calling: Early Viennese Psychoanalysis and the Pursuit of Cultural Science.* Detroit: Wayne State University Press, 1998.

Rosenbaum, J. F. "Behavioral Inhibition in Children of Parents with Panic Disorder and Agoraphobia: A Controlled Study." *Archives of General Psychiatry* 45 (1988): 463–70.

Rosenberg, Rosalind. *Divided Lives: American Women in the Twentieth Century.* New York: Hill and Wang, 1992.

Rossi, A. S. "Equality between the Sexes: An Immodest Proposal." *Daedalus* 93 (1964): 607–52.

Roth, Philip. *Sabbath's Theater.* New York: Houghton Mifflin, 1994.

Rothman, William. *Hitchcock: The Murderous Gaze.* Cambridge: Harvard University Press, 1982.

Russell, A. T., R. O. Pasnau, and Z. C. Taintor. "Emotional Problems of Residents in Psychiatry." *American Journal of Psychiatry* 132 (1975): 263–67.

Sadock, Benjamin, and Harold I. Kaplan, eds. *Kaplan and Sadock's Synopsis of Psychiatry: Behavioral Sciences, Clinical Psychiatry.* New York: Lippincott Williams and Wilkins, 1997.

Safford, Henry B. *Tell me Doctor: Frank Advice on the Intimate Problems of Women.* New York: Pyramid, 1955.

———. "Tell me Doctor." *Lady's Home Journal,* September 1956, 50, 55, 125.

"Sanity from Chemistry?" *Newsweek,* 23 June 1958, 13.

Satel, Sally. *How Political Correctness Is Corrupting Medicine.* New York: Basic, 2000.

Scheinfeld, Aram. "Bigger Mamas, Bigger Babies." *Cosmopolitan,* November 1955, 6–7.

———. "Marriage Crises," *Cosmopolitan,* November 1955, 6–7.

———. "Motherhood Breakdowns, Single or Double Beds, and Office Collections." *Cosmopolitan,* December 1955, 16.

Schenk, Jerome. "Anxiety-Depression and Pharmacotherapy." *American Journal of Psychiatry* 115 (1958): 78–79.

Schilb, John. "Autobiography after Prozac." In *Rhetorical Bodies,* ed. Jack Selzer and Sharon Crowley, 202–21. Madison: University of Wisconsin Press, 1999.

"Schizophrenia Linked to Racism." *BBC News Online,* 7 December 2001. http://news.bbc.co.uk. Accessed 1 May 2002.

Schlesinger, Arthur, Jr. "The Crisis in American Masculinity." *Esquire,* November 1958, 12–18.

Schreber, Daniel P. *Journal of My Nervous Illness.* 1902. Edited by Ida MacAlpine. New York: New York Review of Books, 2000.

Schudson, Michael. *Advertising, the Uneasy Persuasion.* New York: Basic, 1984.

Schultheiss, John, and Mark Schaulbert, eds. *To Illuminate Our Time: The Blacklisted Teleplays of Abraham Polonsky.* Los Angeles: Sadanlaur, 1994.

Schutzman, Mattie. *The Real Thing: Performance, Hysteria, and Advertising.* Middletown: Wesleyan University Press, 1999.

Schwalb, Harry. "Search for New 'Mental Chemicals,'" *Science Digest,* July 1956, 83–86.

Seeman, Mary. "Psychopathology in Women and Men: Focus on Female Hormones." *American Journal of Psychiatry* 154 (1997): 1641–47.

Seward, Georgine. "Sex Roles in Postwar Planning." *Journal of Social Psychology* 19 (1944): 163–85.

Sharfstein, S. S., and W. Clark. "Why Is Psychiatry a Low-Paid Medical Specialty?" *American Journal of Psychiatry* 137 (1980): 831–33.

Sharfstein, S. S., and H. L. Magnas. "Insuring Intensive Psychotherapy." *American Journal of Psychiatry* 132 (1975): 1252–56.

Shorter, Edward. "From Freud to Prozac." In *A History of Psychiatry: From the Era of the Asylum to the Age of Prozac*, 288–327. New York: Wiley, 1997.

———. *A History of Psychiatry: From the Era of the Asylum to the Age of Prozac*. New York: Wiley, 1997.

Siever, Larry J. *The New View of Self: How Genes and Neurotransmitters Shape Your Mind, Your Personality, and Your Mental Health*. New York: Macmillan, 1997.

Silverman, Kaja. *The Acoustic Mirror: The Female Voice in Psychoanalysis and Cinema*. Bloomington: Indiana University Press, 1988.

Slater, Lauren. "Black Swans." *Missouri Review* 19 (spring 1996): 144–61.

———. *Prozac Diary*. New York: Random House, 1998.

———. "Prozac Mother and Child." *New York Times Magazine*, 17 October 1999, 114–18.

Smith, Mickey C. *Small Comfort: A History of the Minor Tranquilizers*. New York: Praeger, 1985.

Solomon, Andrew. *The Noonday Demon: An Atlas of Depression*. New York: Simon and Schuster, 2001.

"Special Report: Women in Revolt." *Newsweek*, 23 March 1970, 70–75.

Spitzer, R. L., J. Endicott, and E. Robins. "Clinical Criteria for Psychiatric Diagnosis and *DSM-III*." *American Journal of Psychiatry* 132 (1975): 1187–92.

Stack, Carolyn. "Psychoanalysis Meets Queer Theory: An Encounter with the Terrifying Other." *Gender and Psychoanalysis* 4, no. 1 (1999): 71–87.

Stallybrass, Peter, and Allon White. *The Politics and Poetics of Transgression*. Ithaca: Cornell University Press, 1986.

Statistical Abstract of the United States. Washington, D.C.: U.S. Government Printing Office, 1990.

Statistical Abstract of the United States. Washington, D.C.: U.S. Government Printing Office, 1992.

Steckel, M. "Financial Insecurity as a Factor in Maladjustment of College Freshmen." *Journal of Social Psychology* 25 (1947): 247–51.

Steiner, M., D. E. Wheadon, and M. S. Kreider. "Antidepressant Response to Paroxetine by Gender." In *1993 Annual Meeting New Research Program and Abstracts*. Washington, D.C.: American Psychiatric Association, 1993.

Stolberg, Sheryl. "Study Says Clinical Guides Often Hide Ties of Doctors." *New York Times*, 6 February 2002, A17.

Stolorow, Robert. "Thoughts on the Nature and Therapeutic Action of Psychoanalytic Interpretation." In *The Widening Scope of Self Psychology*, ed. Arnold Goldberg, 121–41. Hillsdale: Analytic, 1993.

Stone, Allucquere Rosanne. *The War of Desire and Technology at the Close of the Mechanical Age*. Cambridge: MIT Press, 1993.

Stone, Michael. *Healing the Mind: A History of Psychiatry from Antiquity to the Present.* New York: Norton, 1997.

Stotland, Nada. "Gender, What's the Difference?" *American Journal of Psychiatry* 156 (1999): 813–14.

———. "Gender-Based Biology." *American Journal of Psychiatry* 158 (2001): 161–62.

Strachey, James, ed. and trans. *Standard Edition of the Complete Psychological Works of Sigmund Freud.* 24 vols. London: Hogarth, 1953–74.

Strecker, Edward R., and Vincent T. Lathbury. *Their Mothers' Daughters.* Philadelphia: Lippincott, 1954.

Sturm, Roland, and Ruth Klap. "Use of Psychiatrists, Psychologists, and Master's-Level Therapists in Managed Behavioral Health Care Carve-Out Plans." *Psychiatric Services* 50 (1999): 504–8.

Styron, William. *Darkness Visible: A Memoir of Madness.* New York: Vintage, 1991.

Sullivan, H. S. *The Interpersonal Theory of Psychiatry.* New York: Norton, 1953.

Susann, Jacqueline. *Valley of the Dolls.* New York: Random House, 1966.

Sussman, Warren. *The Transformation of American Society in the Twentieth Century.* New York: Pantheon, 1973.

Szasz, Thomas. "Blackness and Madness: Images of Evil and Tactics of Exclusion." In *Black America,* ed. John F. Szwed, 67–77. New York: Basic, 1970.

———. *Ideology and Insanity: Essays on the Psychiatric Dehumanization of Man.* New York: Doubleday, 1970.

———. *The Myth of Psychotherapy: Mental Healing as Religion, Rhetoric, and Repression.* New York: Doubleday Anchor, 1978.

———. "The Case against Psychiatric Power." In *The Construction of Power and Authority in Psychiatry,* ed. Phil Barker and Chris Stevenson, 43–56. Oxford: Butterworth, 2000.

Tasman, Alan, Michelle Riba, and Ken Silk. *The Doctor-Patient Relationship in Pharmacotherapy Improving Treatment Effectiveness.* New York: Guilford, 2000.

"Techno-Prosthetics and Exterior Presence: A Conversation with Sandy Stone." *SPEED.* http://proxy.arts.uci.edu/. Accessed 1 April 2002.

Thompson, Eva. "Sexual Bias in Drug Advertisements." *Social Science and Medicine* 13A (1979): 187–91.

Thornam, Sue. *Passionate Detachments.* London: Arnold, 1997.

Toch, Hans H., and Richard E. Farson. "How to Be a Good Listener." *Science Digest,* June 1957, 1–4.

Toland, John. "My Husband Came Home." *Cosmopolitan,* March 1956, 38–43.

Toufexis, Anastasia. "The Personality Pill." *Time,* 1 October 1993, 53.

Tourney, G., A. J. Petrilli, and L. M. Hatfield. "Hormonal Relationships in Homosexual Men." *American Journal of Psychiatry* 132 (1975): 288–90.

"The Tranquilizer." *Scientific American,* January 1957, 68–69.

"Tranquilizers Shield Brain." *Science News Letter,* 5 September 1959, 153.

"Truth about the Tranquilizers." *Science Digest,* October 1956, 3.

"Unsettling Facts about the Tranquilizers." *Consumer Reports,* January 1958, 4.

"U.S. Women Now Mothers at Younger Age." *Science Digest,* July 1956, 86.

Valenstein, Eliot. *Blaming the Brain: The Truth about Drugs and Mental Illness.* New York: Free Press, 1998.

Verhoff, J., R. A. Kulka, and E. Douvan. *Mental Health in America: Patterns of Help Seeking from 1957 to 1976.* New York: Basic, 1981.

Wade, Nicholas. "Cow's Cells, in Experiment, Offer Hope for Cloning." *New York Times,* 28 April 2000, A15.

Walker, Janet. *Couching Resistance: Women, Film, and Psychoanalytic Psychiatry.* Minneapolis: University of Minnesota Press, 1993.

Wallerstein, Robert S. "The Future of Psychotherapy." *Bulletin of the Menninger Clinic* 55 (1991): 421–43.

Wallis, Claudia. "Onward Women!" *Time,* 4 December 1989, 81–89.

"Want a Long Life? Get Married." *Science Digest,* July 1957, 28–29.

Watt, Douglas. "The Dialogue between Psychoanalysis and Neuroscience: Alienation and Reparation." *Neuro-Psychoanalysis: An Interdisciplinary Journal for Psychoanalysis and the Neurosciences* 2, no. 2 (2001): 23–29.

Weiner, L. Y. *From Working Girl to Working Mother: The Female Labor Force in the United States, 1820–1980.* Chapel Hill: University of North Carolina Press, 1985.

Weissman, M. M., R. Bland, et al. "Sex Differences in Rates of Depression: Cross-National Perspectives." *Journal of Affective Disorders* 29 (1993): 77–84.

Wexler, B. E. "Cerebral Laterality and Psychiatry: A Review of the Literature." *American Journal of Psychiatry* 137 (1980): 279–91.

"What's on Your Mind." *Science Digest,* May 1957, 6.

Whitman, R. M., B. B. Armao, and O. B. Dent. "Assault on the Therapist." *American Journal of Psychiatry* 133 (1976): 426–29.

"Who's Come a Long Way Baby?" *Time,* 31 August 1970, 16–21.

"Why People Don't Marry." *Newsweek,* 24 December 1956, 47.

Wikler, Abraham. "The Uses of Drugs in Psychiatric Research." *American Journal of Psychiatry* 112 (June 1956): 961–69.

Wilson, Mitchell. "*DSM III* and the Transformation of American Psychiatry: A History." *American Journal of Psychiatry* 150 (1993): 399–410.

Wong, David T., et al. "A Selective Inhibitor of Serotonin Uptake." *Life Sciences* 15 (1974): 471–79.

The World Almanac and Book of Facts. New York: Newspaper Enterprise Association, 1957.

Wurtzel, Elizabeth. *Prozac Nation: Young and Depressed in America.* New York: Riverhead, 1995.

Wylie, Philip. *Generation of Vipers.* 2d ed. New York: Pocket, 1955.

Zita, Jacqueline. *Body Talk: Philosophical Reflections on Sex and Gender.* New York: Columbia University Press, 1998.

Žižek, Slavoj. *Enjoy Your Symptom: Jacques Lacan in Hollywood and Out.* New York: Routledge, 1992.

———. *The Plague of Fantasies.* New York: Verso, 1997.

Zlotnick, C., et al. "Gender, Type of Treatment, Dysfunctional Attitudes, Social Support, Life Events, and Depressive Symptoms over Naturalistic Follow-Up." *American Journal of Psychiatry* 153 (1996): 1021–27.

Zube, M. J. "Changing Concepts of Morality: 1948–1969." *Social Forces* 50 (1972): 385–93.

McLean Hospital, 235n.48

MD Medical Newsmagazine, 226n.5

"Medicated" (Krist), 166, 169–70, 175–76, 177, 181–82, 186–87, 192, 234–35n.39, 238n.86

medications. *See* advertisements, pharmaceutical; psychopharmacology; psychotropic medication; SSRI antidepressants; *specific drugs*

men: anxieties/problems of, as caused by women, 76, 81–85, 87–88, 95–96, 114, 132, 157–58, 215n.25; as doctors, 13–14, 28; as doctors, in ads, 13–14, 27, 129; as patients, in ads, 225n.3; in Prozac narratives, 173–74, 233–34n.26; psychotropic medication as helpers of white, male psychiatrists, 37–38, 42–43, 44–45, 48–49, 209n.24; psychotropic medication as replacing male practitioners, 54–56, 57–58, 60–61, 65, 211nn.57–58; psychotropic medication prescribed for, 236–37n.76; and SSRI antidepressants, response to, 229–30n.54; tranquilizers used by, 71–72, 75, 213–14n.3

Menkes, Suzy, 174

Menninger, C. F., 88, 90, 91, 96

Menninger, Carl, 88, 90, 91, 93, 96

Menninger, William C., 88, 90, 91, 96, 201n.2

Menninger Hospital and Clinic, 88, 93

meprobamate. *See* Miltown

Meprosan, 130

Merriam, Eve: "The Matriarchal Myth," 138, 141, 227n.26

Meyers, Greg, 205n.47

Millett, Kate, 15, 23, 130, 221–22n.24; *The Loony Bin Trip,* 174; *Sexual Politics,* 144, 189

Miltown: ads for, 42; anxiety treated with, 72–73; and binding of anxiety, 122–23; and biological anxiety, 98–102; demand for/popularity of, 13, 73, 104, 214nn.9–10; and Deprol, 134, 227n.17; and doctor-patient interaction, 124; efficacy/neural effects of, 100, 112, 123–24, 222n.126, 224n.138; frigidity treated with, 74; hysteria treated with, 13; introduction of, 73, 98, 214n.9; and marriage, 122–23; and mothers, in popular print, 74, 76; neurosis treated with, 13; in the popular press, 19, 102–12, 221n.108, 221n.112, 223n.130; vs. Prozac, 173–74; psychoanalysis as facilitated/replaced by, 14–15, 101–2; in the scientific press, 98–102; selective action of, 99, 101; women in articles about, 113–14

"The Mind: Science's Search for a Guide to Sanity": on anxiety as irrational fear, 119; Freud and psychoanalysis conflated in, 88, 217n.59; and the maternal repressed, 95–96; and prosperity/national malaise, 91–95, 119, 218n.67; on psychoanalytic progress, 75, 88, 89–91, 92, 117

Minsky, Rosalind, 67–68, 80, 111, 209n.15

"Mirror in the Brain" (Penfield), 108–9, 110, 111, 221n.119

Moban, 68

modernism and postmodernism, 23, 168–69

Modern Woman: The Lost Sex (Farnham and Lunberg), 81, 96, 218n.73

momism, 196–97, 238n.2; and the crisis of psychoanalysis, 81, 87–88, 96; in pharmaceutical advertisements, 137–41, 227–28nn.26–27; popular appeal of, 227–28n.27

Money, John, 172

moral superego. *See* superego

"Motherhood Breakdowns, Single or
Double Beds, and Office Collections,"
84, 95, 97, 217n.50

mothers: anxiety about, 14, 74–75; and
civilization, 222n.24; domestic role
of, 80–81, 106–7, 216n.38, 216n.41,
218–19n.73, 219n.76; Freudian, 76,
81–85, 87–88, 95–96, 114, 215n.25; and
medications, in popular print, 72–73
(*see also* Miltown); and Miltown, in
popular print, 74, 76; neuroses caused
by, 14–15, 16, 18; in pharmaceutical
advertisements, 129, 131, 159, 162;
repression of, 95–96, 121, 222n.24;
smoking by, 196–97, 238n.2. *See also*
momism

"Mother's Little Helper" (Rolling
Stones), 71, 72

Mulvey, Laura, 137

Murphy, Michael, 184

Naftolin, F., 54

narcissism, 47, 68–69, 209n.31, 213n.84

narrative form and Prozac, 27–28, 165–
94; Blackbridge's *Prozac Highway,*
166, 169–70, 175–76, 177–81, 183,
185–88, 191–93, 234–35nn.39–40;
the Breggins' *Talking Back to Prozac,*
20, 177, 204–5n.46; crisis/relapse in,
184–87, 192–93; criticism of, 166–67,
176–77, 231n.2; discovery of Prozac
in, 175, 181–84; on the failure of the
past, 178–81; female vs. male writers
of, 234–35n.39, 236–37n.76; Glenmullen's *Prozac Backlash,* 10–11, 12,
177, 203n.25, 234n.36; hyperthymia
in, 191–92; Kennedy's "Shrinks,"
166, 169–70, 175–76, 177, 179–82,
185–88, 191–93, 234n.39, 235n.51;
Kramer's *Listening to Prozac,* 7, 15, 17,

153–54, 166, 174, 177, 184, 205n.48,
234n.27; Krist's "Medicated," 166,
169–70, 175–76, 177, 181–82, 186–87,
192, 234–35n.39, 238n.86; men as less
threatened in, 173–74, 233–34n.26;
postmodernism of, 166–67, 168–69,
170–71, 178, 235n.40; and Prozac ads,
172–73, 182, 233n.18, 235n.55; and
psychoanalytic narratives of gender
development/identity, 170, 175, 180–
81, 183, 192–93, 235n.47, 235n.49;
return of the repressed in, 191–94;
selfhood in, 167, 168–74, 183, 187–
89, 194; Slater's "Black Swans," 166,
169–70, 175, 177, 179–89, 191–93, 234–
35n.39, 234n.37, 235n.49, 237–38n.81,
238n.85; Slater's *Prozac Diary,* 175,
234n.37; on the trajectory of Prozac,
168, 168–69; and women in mental
illness narratives, 174–75, 234n.30;
Wurtzel's *Prozac Nation,* 165–66, 177,
235n.39

Nathanson, C., 127

neurogenetics, 60

neuroimaging, 60

neuroradiology, 222n.24

neuroreceptor binding, 6

neuroses, 10; classification of, 1; *DSM-I*
on, 21, 39–40; mothers as causing,
14–15, 16, 18; in pharmaceutical advertisements, 15, 16; psychotropic
medication for, 13, 14–15, 16

neurotic disorders, elimination of, 53

New England Journal of Medicine, 226n.5

Newmark, S. R., 54

Newsweek: on biological cures for
women's neuroses, 15; circulation of,
214n.8; on doctor-patient interactions
and wonder drugs, 13; on feminists,
143–44; "How Tranquilizers Work,"
105, 107, 109, 120–21; laboratory

feminists); definition of, 7; on depression, 171, 232–33n.11; excavation of, 233n.19; and feminists, 15, 16, 130–31, 141, 143, 144, 189, 228n.29; on gender difference, 7–8, 14, 21–23, 206n.63; and gender difference in popular print, 74–75; heterosexist categories/norms of, 7–10, 14; on homosexuality, 47–48, 209–10n.33, 234n.28; on hysteria, 212n.82; influence/popularity of, 14, 21–23, 74, 206n.63, 215n.22; on narcissism, 47, 209n.31; on the past, 171–72, 232–33n.11; pharmaceutical advertisements' assumptions of, 129, 158; on the pleasure principle, 207n.67; Prozac vs. psychoanalytic narratives, 170, 175, 180–81, 183, 192–93, 235n.47, 235n.49; and psychopharmacology, 21–26; and psychotropic medication, 14–15, 25, 207n.67; on repetition of the same thing, 195, 197; status of, 1–2, 201–2nn.1–3; on top vs. bottom, 212–13n.83; transference/countertransference in, 4–5, 55, 124, 132, 232–33n.11; on the unconscious, 2, 22, 40, 54, 69, 108, 206–7n.64 (see also *Inhibitions, Symptoms, and Anxiety;* unconscious); and the unseen, 195–96, 197. *See also* Oedipus complex; psychiatry, history of; psychoanalysis, crisis of; superego

psychoanalysis, crisis of, 77–98; and anxiety, Freudian conception of, 78, 82, 94, 215–16n.31, 218nn.71–72; and anxiety and the Oedipal crisis, 78, 94; and anxiety caused by economic/social instability, 92–95, 217n.63, 218n.66; and civilization, Freudian conception of, 78–79, 81–82, 216n.33; and diagnosis as iden-

tity formation, 96; discontent with psychoanalysis, 88, 89, 90–91, 92, 96–98, 111–12, 219n.74; divisions within psychoanalysis, 77; and external vs. internal stimuli, 94–95, 218nn.71–72; Freud's influence in popular culture, 77–79, 82, 88, 215n.26, 217n.59; and golden age of psychoanalysis, 77, 119, 215n.29; and male problems as caused by mothers/women, 76, 81–85, 87–88, 95–96, 114, 215n.25; and masculine identity in patriarchal culture, 80–81; and momism, 81, 87–88, 96; and repression, 108, 219n.76, 222n.24, 223n.138, 224n.139 (*see also* mothers: repression of); and social climate/prosperity of America, 91–95, 217n.61, 218n.66; and working women, 79–84, 96, 216n.41, 218–19n.73

"Psychodynamic Patterns in the Homosexual Sex Offender" (Glueck), 45–48, 97, 209–10n.33

psychogenetics, 1–2

psychoneurosis, classification of, 1. *See also* neuroses

psychopharmacology, 1–2, 14–15; gender differences in, 20, 21–23, 205–6n.52; in popular culture, 18–26, 204n.44, 205–6n.52, 205nn.47–48; and psychoanalysis, 21–26. *See also* advertisements, pharmaceutical; psychotropic medication; *specific drugs*

Psychopharmacology Research Branch (National Institute of Health), 49

psychosis, 29

psychotropic medication: biological psychiatry's use of, 2, 5, 202n.6; complexity of, as constructed in popular culture, 212n.74; and doctor-patient interactions, 13, 41–42, 64, 124–25;

Jonathan Michel Metzl is Assistant Professor of Psychiatry and
Women's Studies and Director of the Program in Culture, Health,
and Medicine at the University of Michigan. In addition he teaches
in the Robert Wood Johnson's Clinical Scholars Program and the
Bioethics Program and is an assistant research scientist in the Institute for Research on Women and Gender, all at the University
of Michigan. He has written for *The American Journal of Psychiatry, American Journal of Psychotherapy, Journal of Practical Psychiatry
and Behavioral Health,* and *SIGNS: The Journal of Women, Culture
and Society.*

Library of Congress Cataloging-in-Publication Data

Metzl, Jonathan.

Prozac on the couch : prescribing gender in the era of wonder
drugs / by Jonathan Michel Metzl.

p. cm.

Includes bibliographical references and index.

ISBN 0-8223-3061-X (cloth: alk. paper)

1. Neuropsychiatry. 2. Psychopharmacology. 3. Psychoanalysis.
4. Gender identity. I. Title.

RC341.M593 2003

616.89′18 — dc21   2002151959